Dedicated to Savy and Peanut, who make
every day an adventure. Thank you for
traveling the world with us.

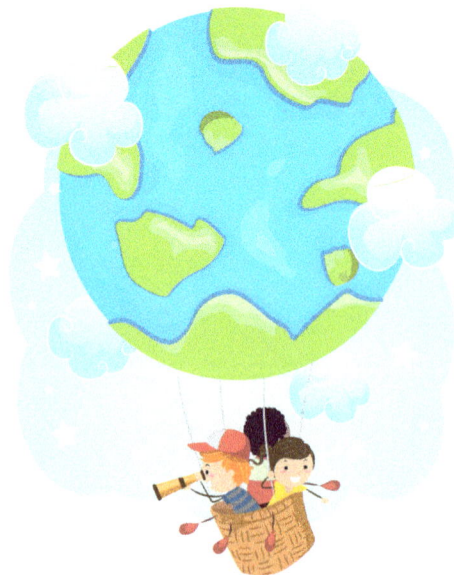

ANATOMY & HEALTH

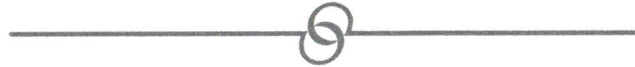

Educational Resources, Crafts & Activities for Kids

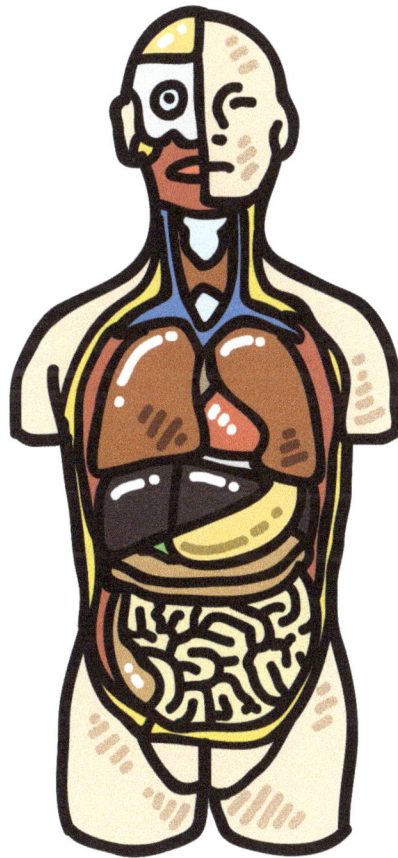

Sarah M. Prowant, MSN-Ed, RN

Savy Activities
Colorado, USA

TERMS & CONDITIONS

FOR BEST RESULTS:

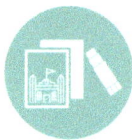

When assembling a 3D model, glue a second piece of thick paper with a craft glue stick to back of each sheet of model pieces (prior to cutting pieces) to provide additional stability when assembled.

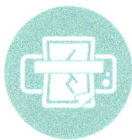

Laminate all cards & posters with at least 3 ml lamination for additional protection.

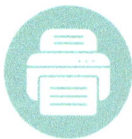

If printing from an ebook, cardstock paper (>60 lbs) provides best results for cards, models and manipulative activities, while standard printer paper is adequate for recipes, lessons, etc. Please set printer to "FIT TO PAGE" when printing for best results.

FOLLOW US ON SOCIAL MEDIA!

@savyactivities

/SavyActivities

www.SavyActivities.com

WHATS INCLUDED:

- Order of Organization & Cell Size Comparison Poster
- Parts of a Human Cell Poster & Gelatin Cell Activity
- Systems of the Human Body Flashcards
- *The Most Important Body Organ* Mini-Book
- Anatomy ABC's Poster & Word Tracing
- Timeline of Medical History
- Candy DNA Model
- Organs of the Human Body Poster & Body Tracing w/Organs
- Connectable Skeleton
- Dry Erase Teeth Brushing
- Articulating Hand Model
- Joint Types Flashcards
- Arm Muscle Model
- Mechanisms of Breathing
- Anatomy of the Heart Matching
- Blood Sensory Tray & Components of Blood Slide Flashcards
- Cardiopulmonary Circulation
- Coffee Filter Kidney
- Pom Pom Lymph Node Craft
- Immune Cells & Response Flashcards
- Better Choice Matching Cards
- Female & Male Urinary/Reproductive System Anatomy
- Development of the Human Fetus Spinner
- Stages of Digestion Matching & Making Poop Sensory Activity
- Healthy Plate Sorting
- Layers of the Skin Model
- Balloon Fingerprints
- Brain Hemisphere Hat & Lobes of the Brain Poster
- Playdough Neuron Anatomy
- Emotion Matching
- Endocrine System Matching
- The Five Major Senses Worksheet
- Sensory: Sight (Snellen Chart, Ishihara Test)
- Sensory: Taste Activity
- Sensory: Smell Activity
- Sensory: Hearing Activity
- Sensory: Touch Activity
- Anatomy Art Study Cards

Order of Organization

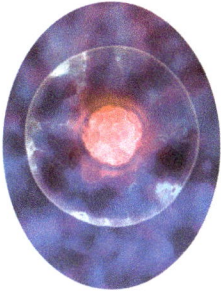

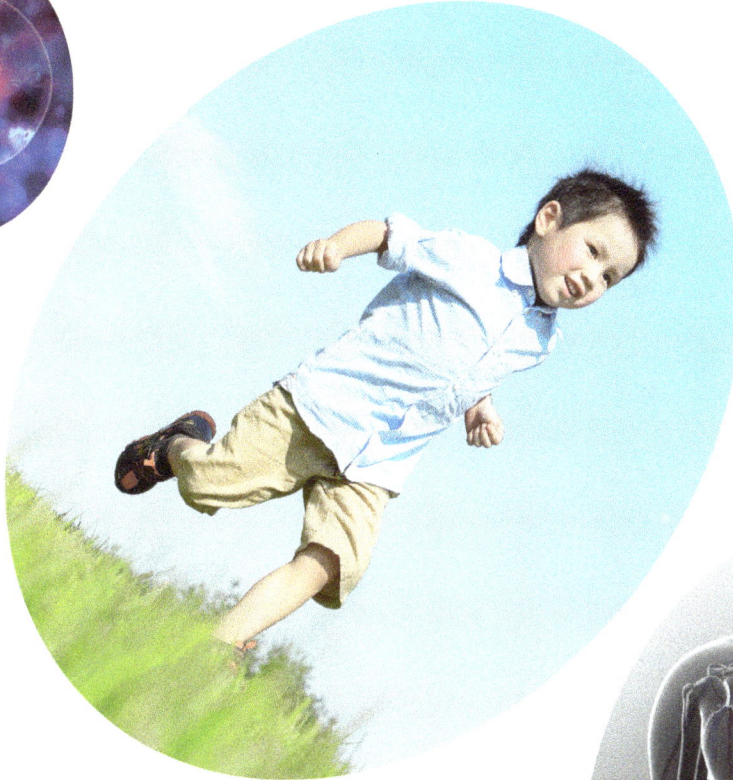

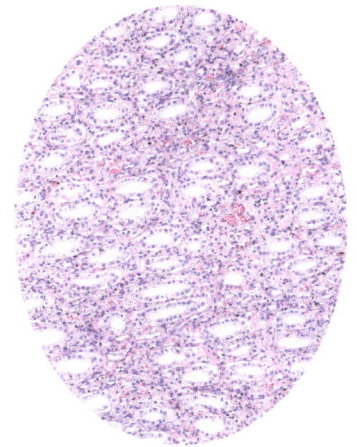

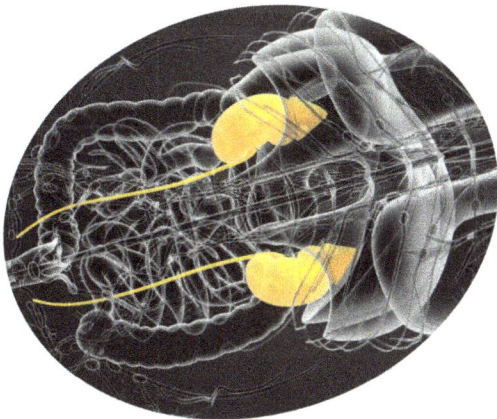

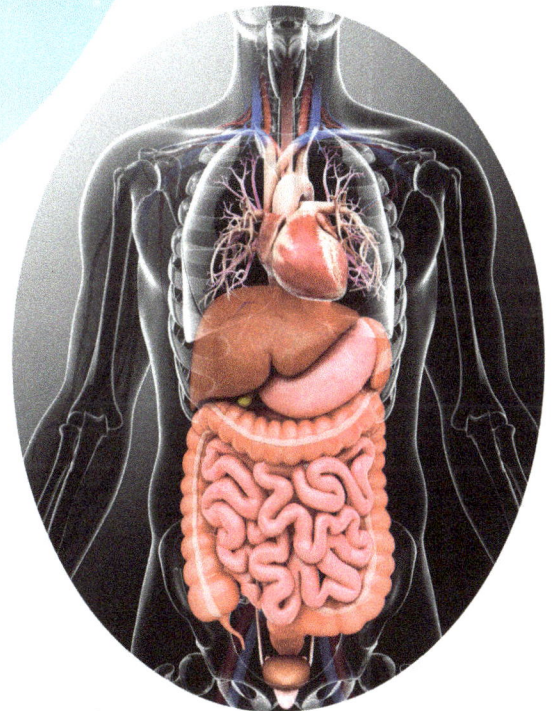

Place each photo in order of complexity. Label using labels.

Cell	Tissue	Organ

Organ System	Organism

Cell Size Comparison

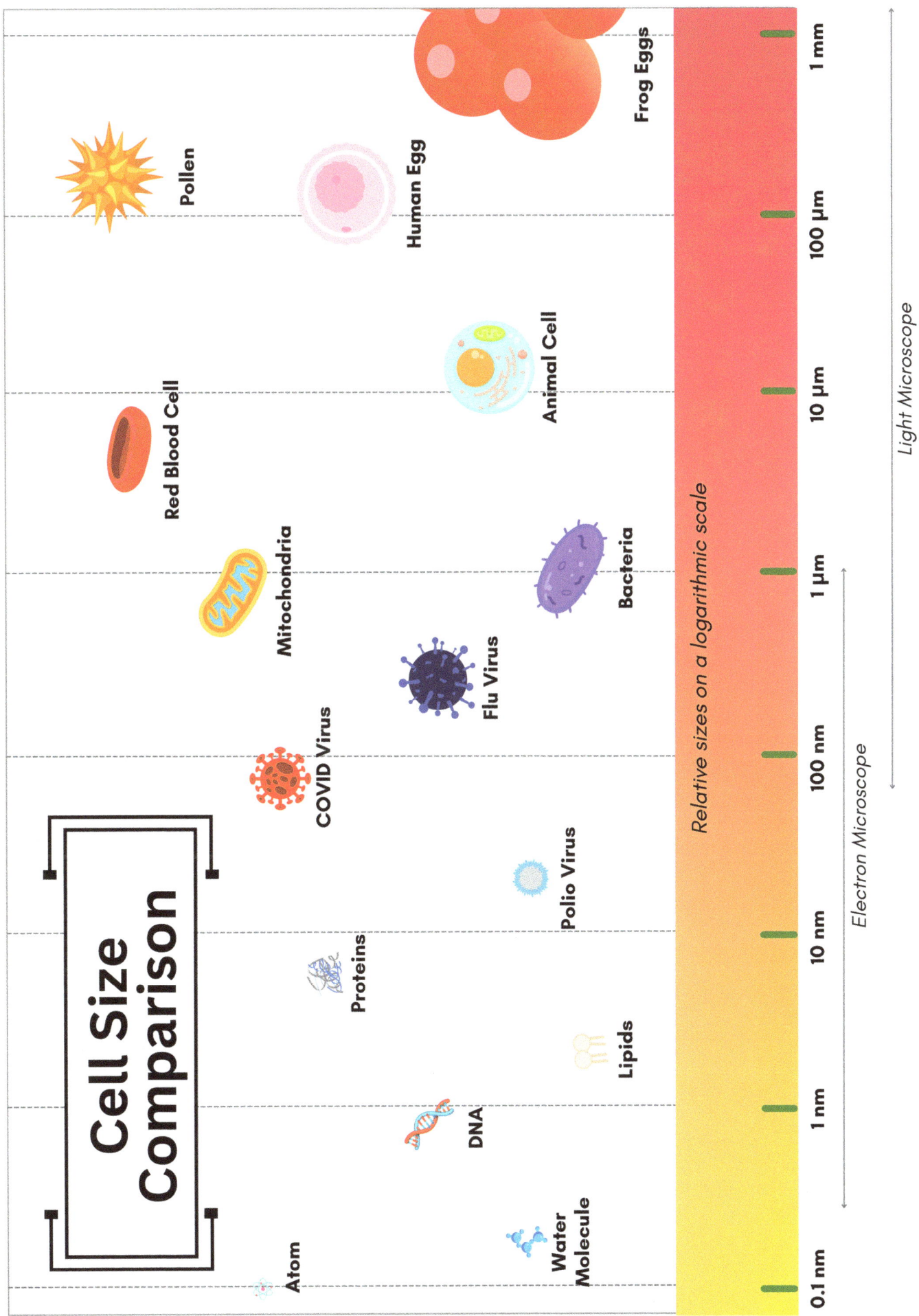

Atom

Water Molecule

DNA

Lipids

Proteins

Polio Virus

COVID Virus

Flu Virus

Mitochondria

Red Blood Cell

Bacteria

Animal Cell

Pollen

Human Egg

Frog Eggs

Relative sizes on a logarithmic scale

| 0.1 nm | 1 nm | 10 nm | 100 nm | 1 μm | 10 μm | 100 μm | 1 mm |

Electron Microscope

Light Microscope

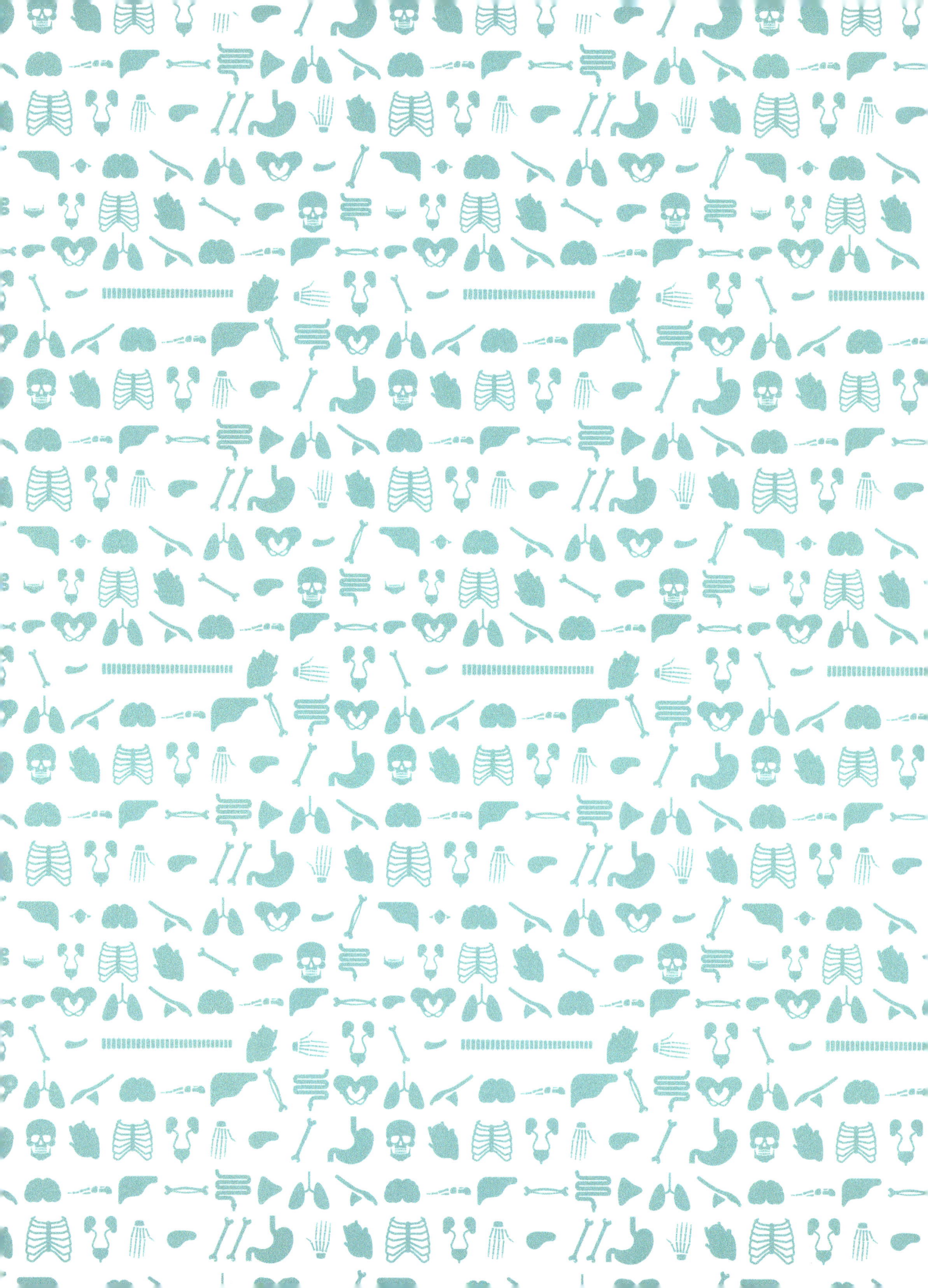

Parts of a Human Cell

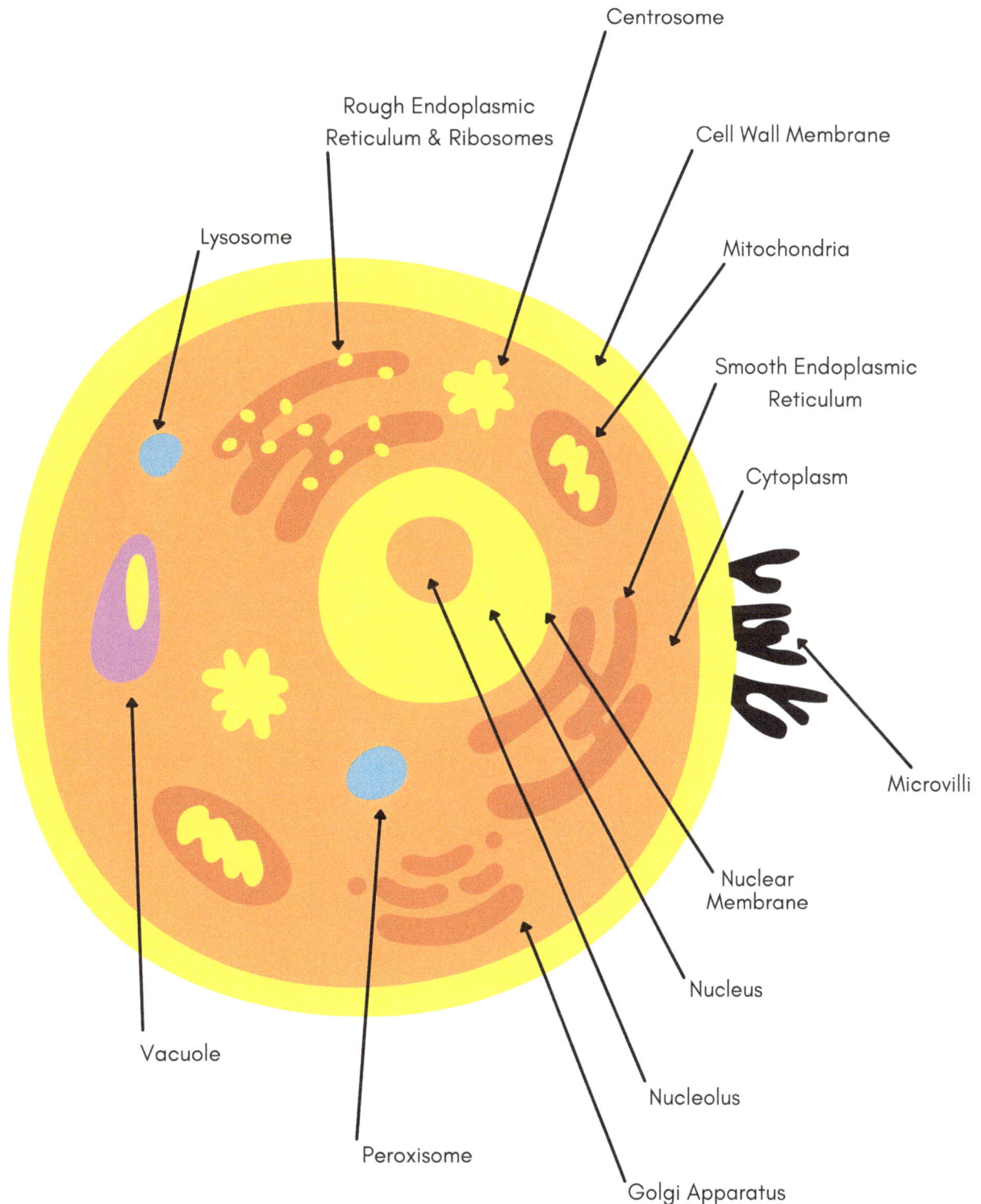

Centrosome

Rough Endoplasmic
Reticulum & Ribosomes

Cell Wall Membrane

Lysosome

Mitochondria

Smooth Endoplasmic
Reticulum

Cytoplasm

Microvilli

Nuclear
Membrane

Nucleus

Vacuole

Nucleolus

Peroxisome

Golgi Apparatus

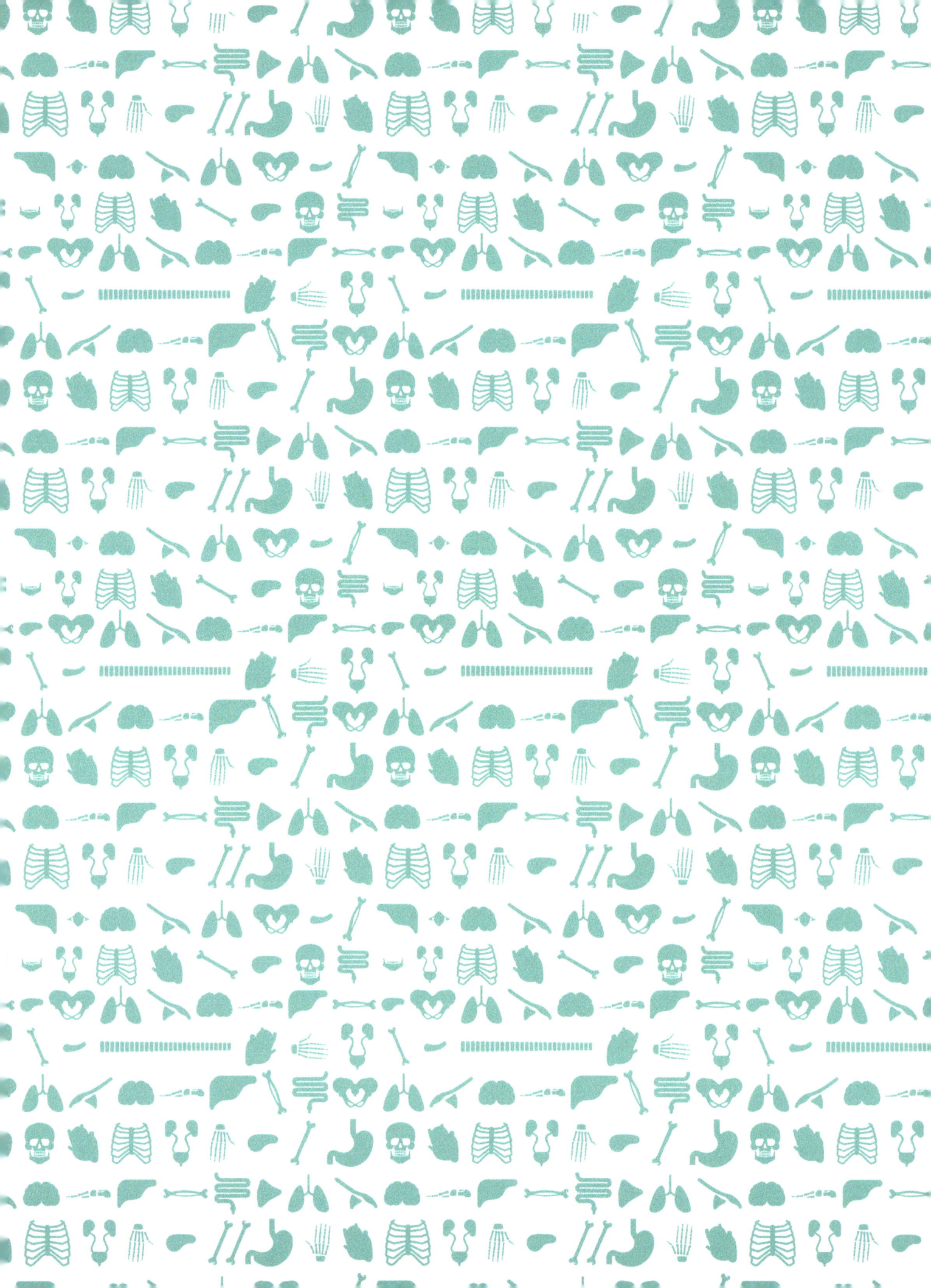

GELATIN CELL

Instructions

The average cell in the human body is approximately 10–20μm in diameter. This small size results in a large surface area-to-volume ratio that allows for efficient transport of materials in and out of cells. While each cell has readily identifiable parts, but a common optical light microscope cannot visualize them; electron microscopy is needed. Mix gelatin and add food color if desired and fill 1-2 inches of a bowl. Allow to sit until gelatin is semi-solid. Cut a hard boiled egg so that yolk is exposed. Place in center of gelatin before completely solid (This will be the nucleus). Place two pieces of ramen on either side of egg, sprinkle one with rice. (rough and smooth endoplasmic reticulum). Add 3-4 pieces of curved egg noodles (golgi apparatus), 1-2 raisins (lysosomes), 2-3 pinto beans (mitochondrion), 1-2 lentils (peroxisome) lima bean (vacuole) and two mini penne (centrosomes). Label with included labels using toothpicks or T-pins.
Discuss: How does this version compare to an illustration of a cell?

Materials

- Gelatin
- Food Coloring (Optional)
- Hard Boiled Egg
- Ramen
- Rice
- Egg Noodles
- Raisins
- Pinto Beans
- Lima Beans
- Lentils
- Mini Penne
- T-Pins/Toothpicks

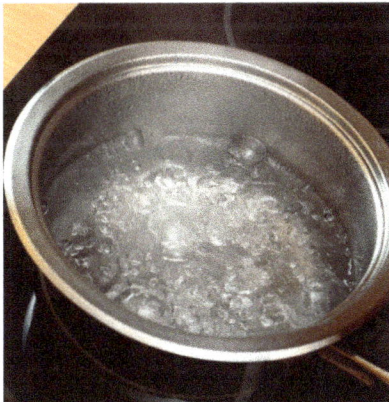

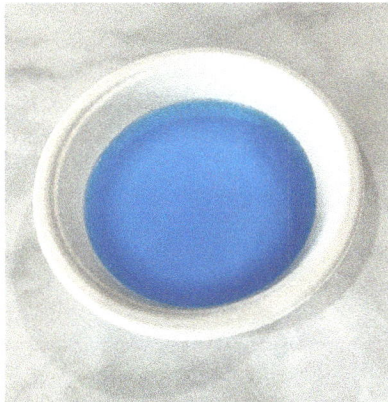

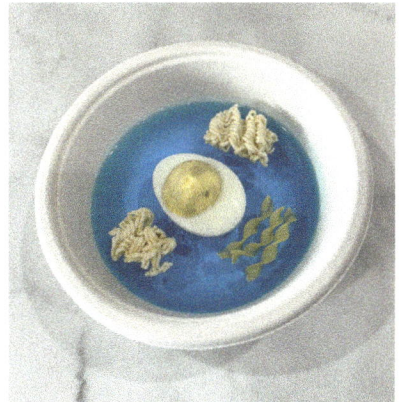

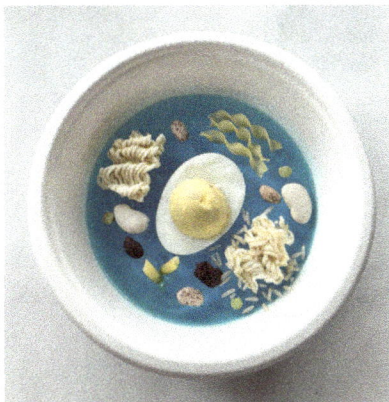

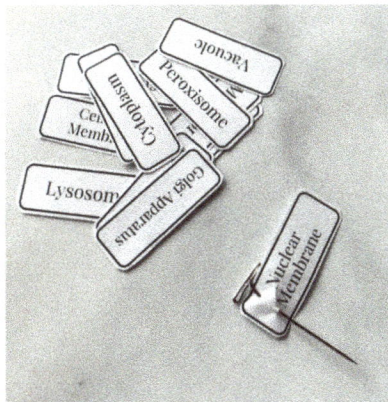

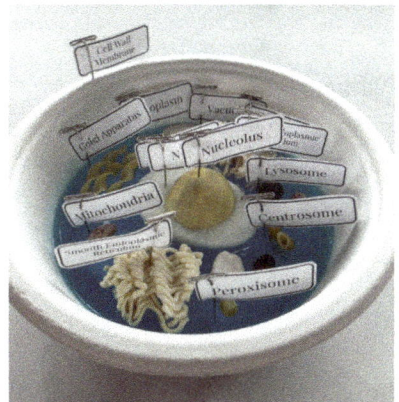

Parts of a Human Cell

Rough ER

Smooth ER

Centrosome

Cell Wall

Nuclear Membrane

Mitochondria

Lysosome

Cytoplasm

Peroxisome

Microvilli

Nucleus

Nucleolus

Vacuole

Golgi Apparatus

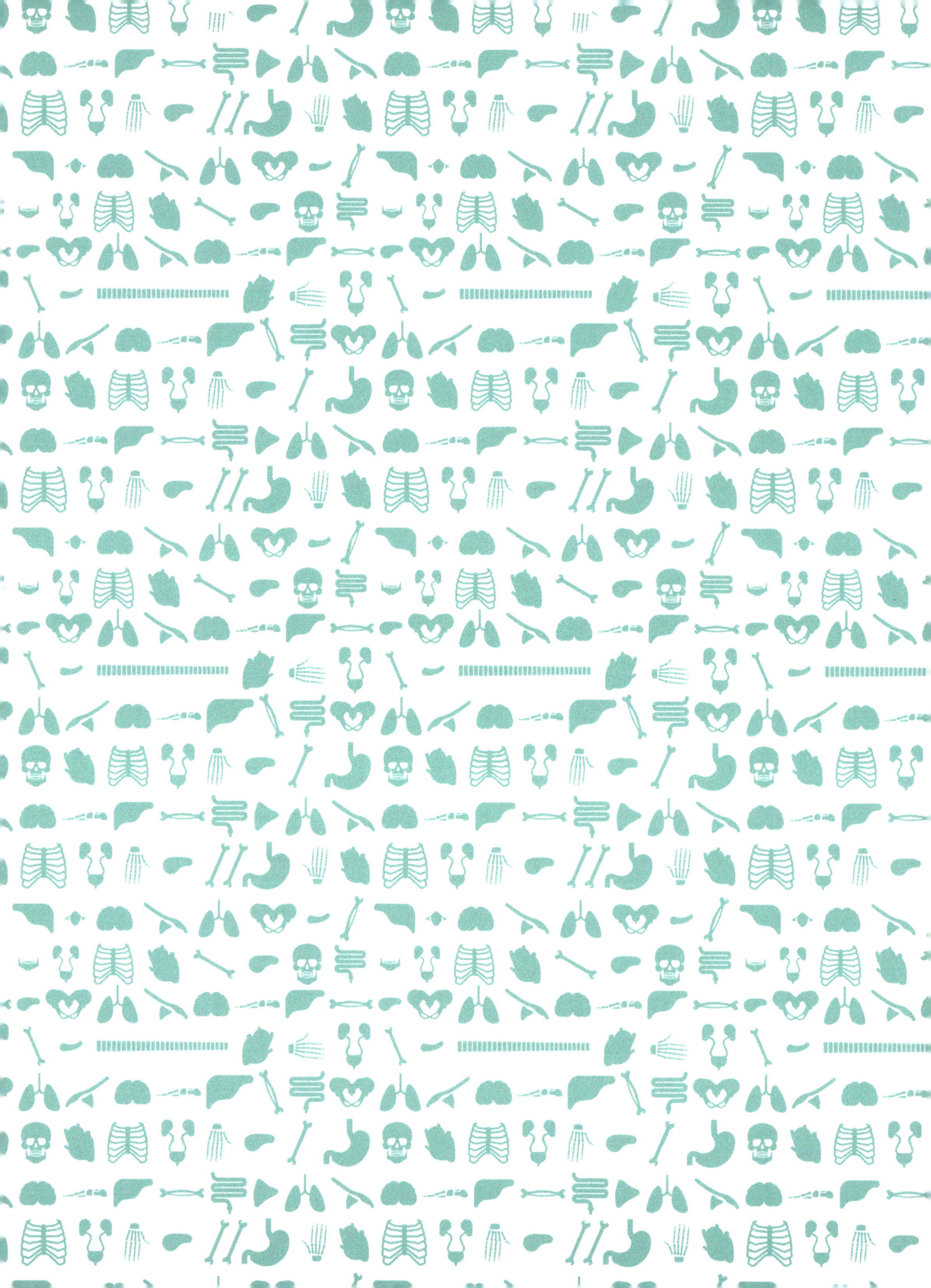

Systems of the Human Body

Use the following flashcards to compare and contrast each system, to provide structure during activities and to test knowledge.

Muscular System

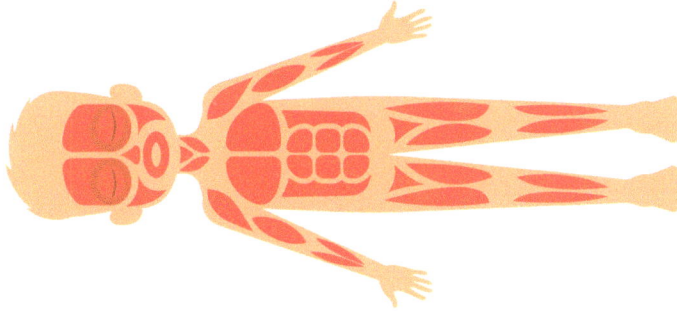

Components
Skeletal, smooth & cardiac muscles

Functions
Movement, support, protection and heat generation

Skeletal System

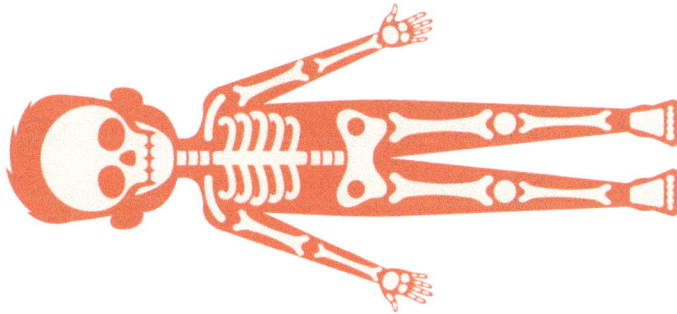

Components
Bones, ligaments, tendons, and joints

Functions
Support, protection and movement

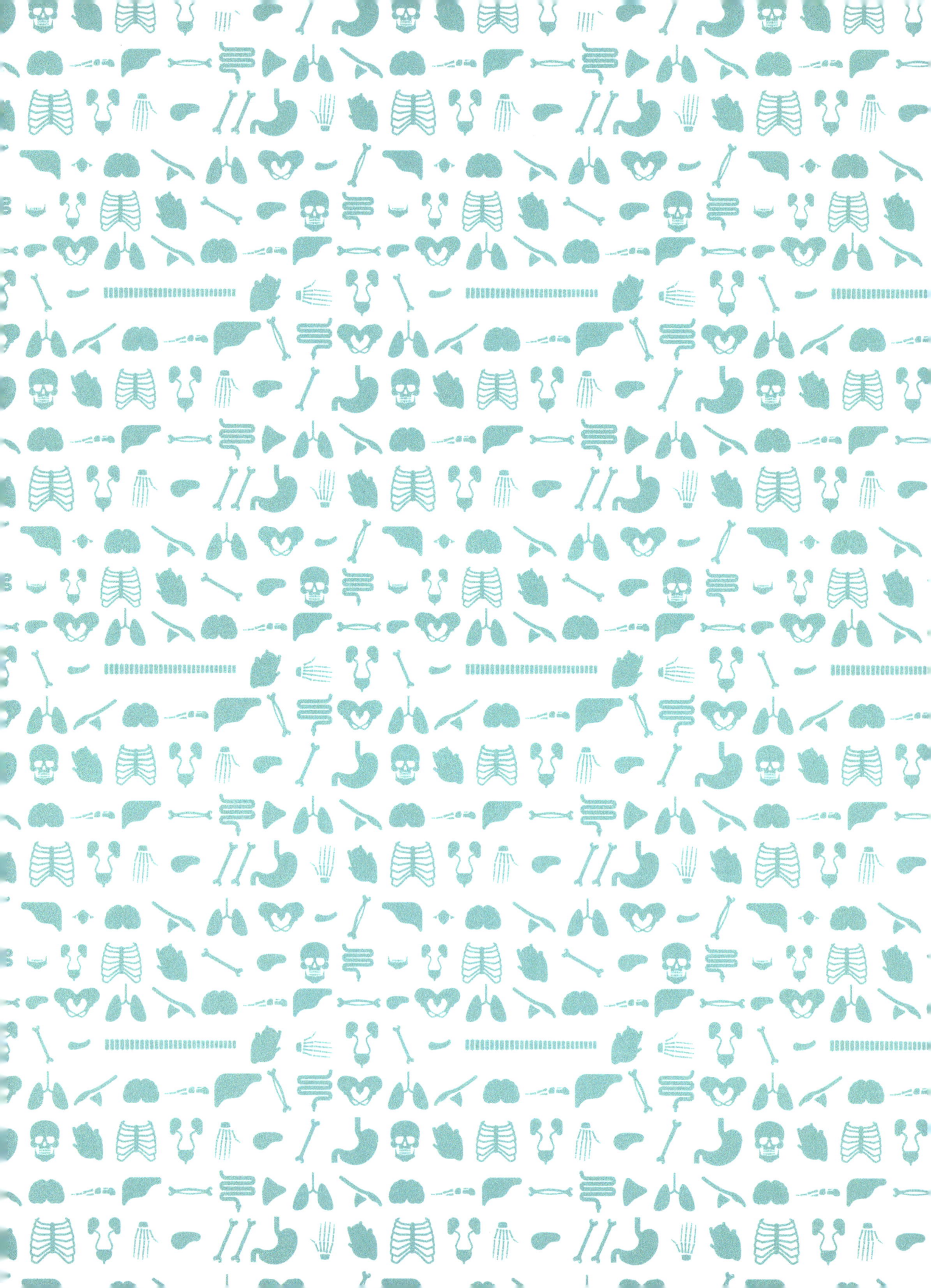

Integumentary System

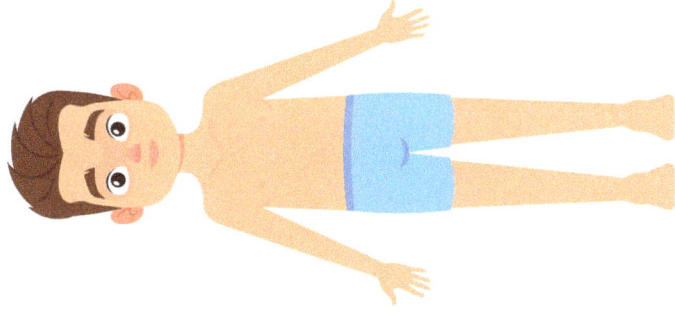

Components

Skin, hair, nails, and exocrine glands.

Functions

Protection, sensory perception and temperature regulation

Nervous System

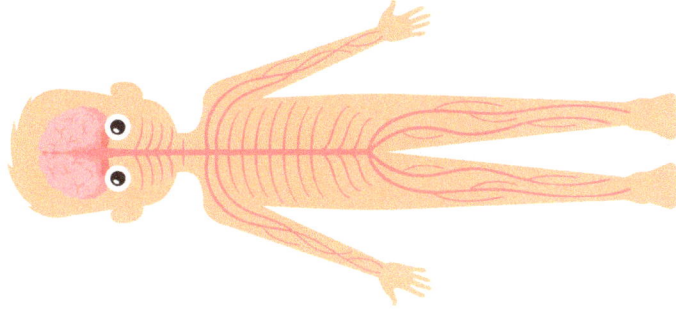

Components

Brain, spinal cord and nerves

Functions

Sensory perception, coordination and control of responses, memory, language skills and reasoning

Cardiovascular System

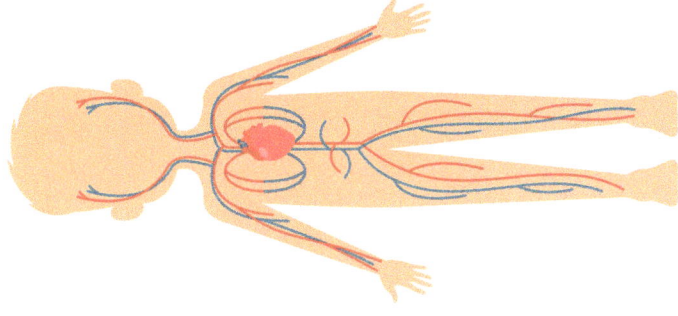

Components

Heart, veins, arteries, capillaries, and blood

Functions

Supply of oxygen and nutrients to tissues and removal of metabolic waste

Endocrine System

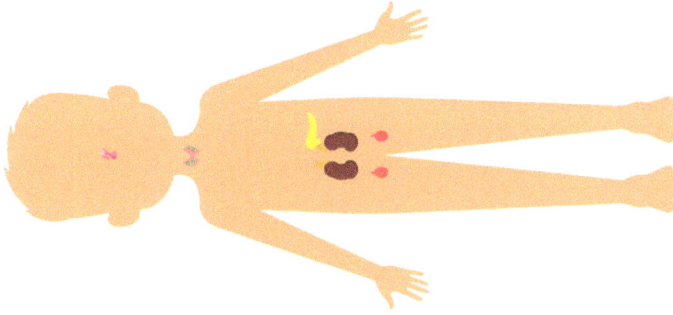

Components

Hypothalamus, pituitary, pineal, thyroid, parathyroids, adrenals, pancreas, ovaries/testes

Functions

Secretion of hormones that regulate growth, metabolism, fluid balance behavior, reproduction

Respiratory System

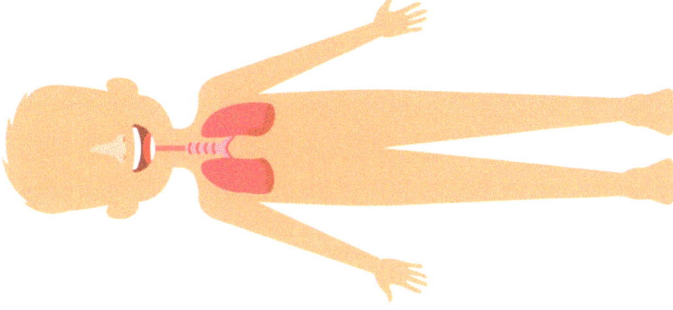

Components

Nose, mouth, throat, voice box, windpipe, and lungs

Functions

Ventilation of lungs and exchange of oxygen and carbon dioxide between the body and atmosphere

Digestive System

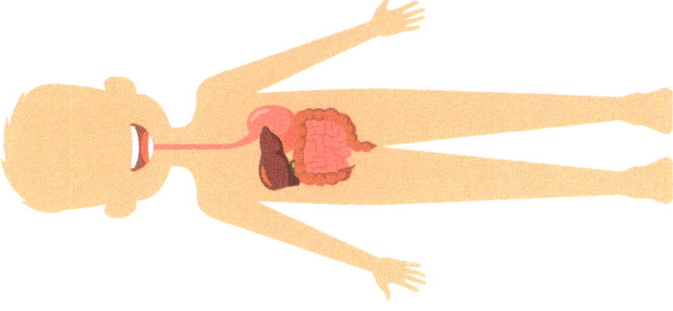

Components

Mouth, esophagus, stomach, liver, intestines, gallbladder, pancreas and anus

Functions

Breakdown of food into usable nutrients, absorption of nutrients into the circulation, elimination of waste

Urinary System

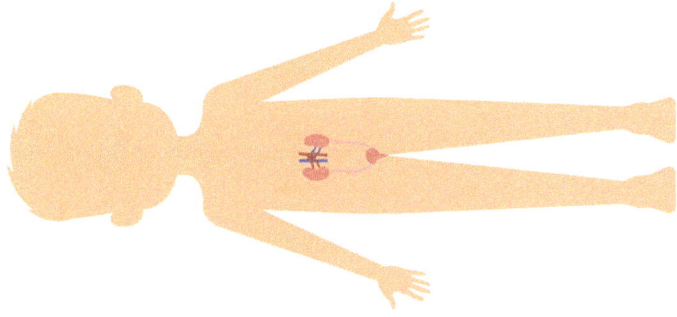

Components

Kidneys, ureters, bladder & urethra

Functions

Elimination of waste materials and water

Reproductive System

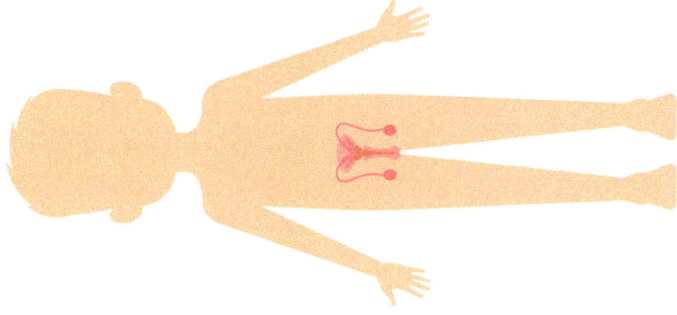

Components

Sex glands: ovaries/testes, eggs/sperm and uterus (female)

Functions

Production of offspring

Lymphatic System

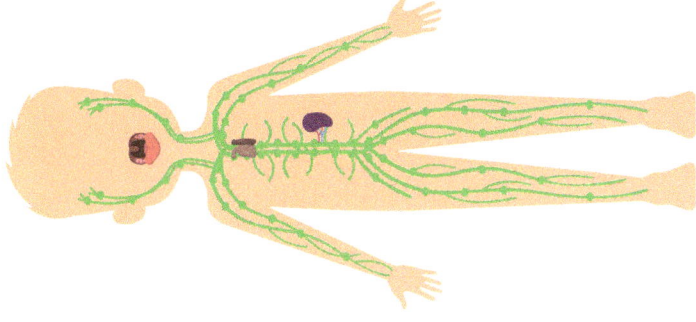

Components

Lymphatic vessels, nodes, lymph spleen, thymus and tonsils

Functions

Helps with circulation, immunity and transport of digested fats

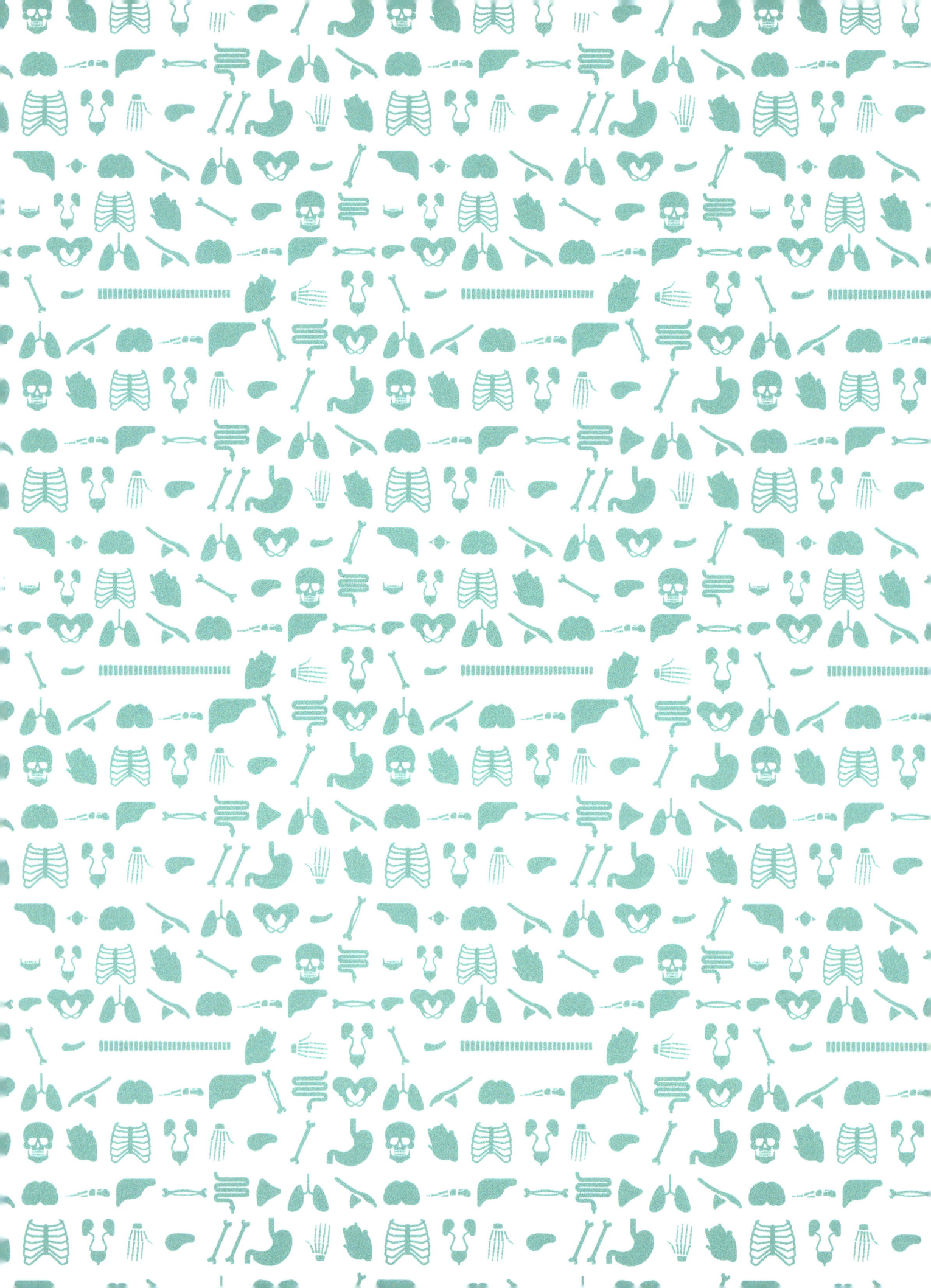

THE MOST IMPORTANT BODY ORGAN

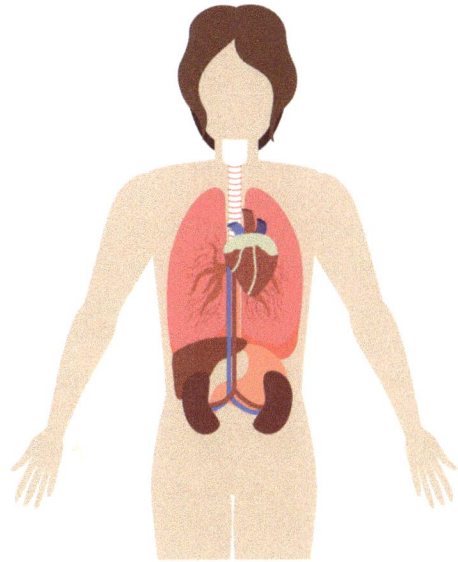

The pancreas finally spoke, "I am pretty important too, I help put nutrients into the body's cells using insulin. Without me, the nutrients would be useless!"

So the intestines stopped absorbing and the brain stopped telling the pancreas to make insulin and the body stopped working.

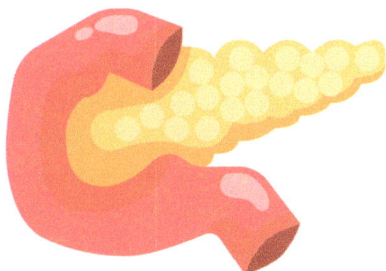

9

Then the heart said, "I am truly the most important, without me blood wouldn't go to each organ, bringing lifegiving oxygen and nutrients!"

And so the lungs stopped breathing and the kidneys stopped filtering, and the body stopped working.

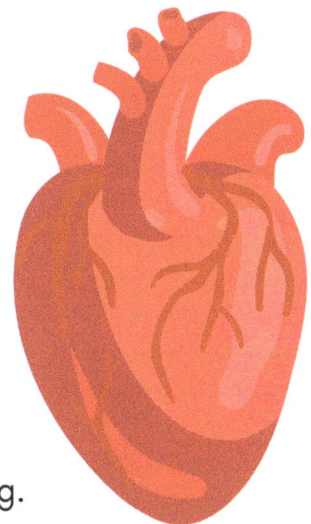

2

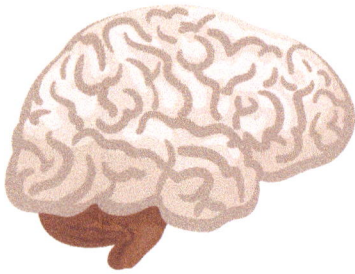

Once upon a time, the brain said to the rest of the body, "I am the most important! Without me you cannot do anything! I control every function in the body!"

And so the stomach stopped digesting and the heart stopped pumping, and the body stopped working.

1

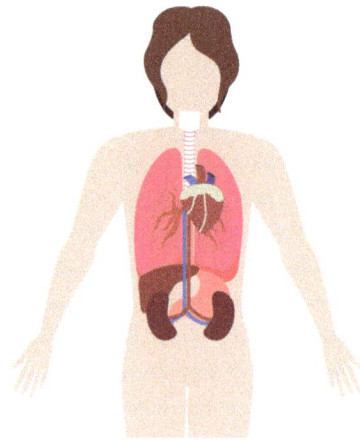

Finally all the organs agreed that each of them played an important part, and that they worked best when they all worked together.

THE END.

10

Then the lungs said, "I truly am the most important in the body, without me nobody would have life-giving oxygen!"

So brain stopped reminding the body to breath and the heart stopped pumping blood to the lungs and the body stopped working.

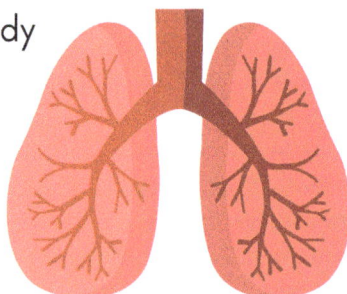

3

The intestines finally spoke up, "I have stayed quiet long enough! I am the most important because I absorb important fluids and nutrients into the body. Without me, the body would be nothing!"

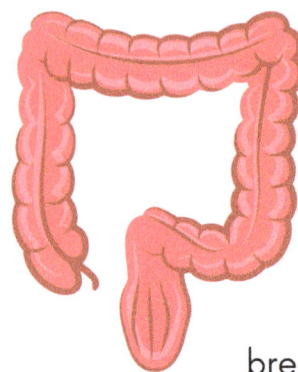

So the spleen stopped filtering and the lungs stopped breathing and the body stopped working.

8

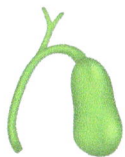

Then the gallbladder said I'm the most important, although little, I serve an important role in digestion!" The spleen retorted, "Actually people live all the time without you, I am more important because I filter damaged blood from the body!"

And the stomach stopped digesting and kidneys stopped filtering and the body stopped working.

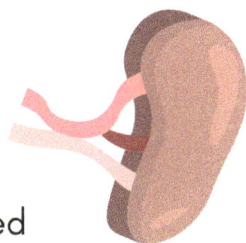

7

Then the kidneys and bladder got together and exclaimed, "We truly are the most important, without us waste products wouldn't get eliminated!"

So the intestines stopped absorbing fluids and the heart stopped pumping, and the body stopped working.

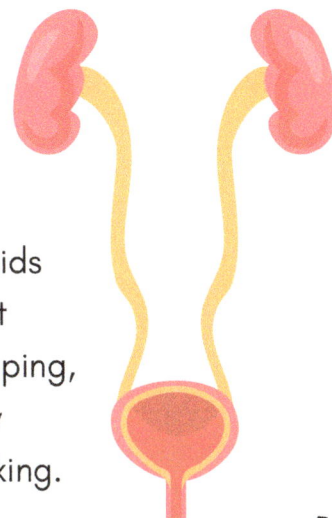

4

Assembly Instructions

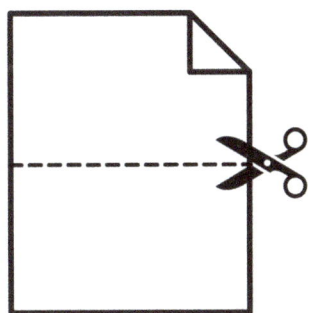

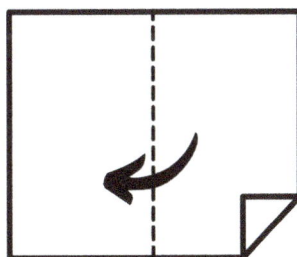

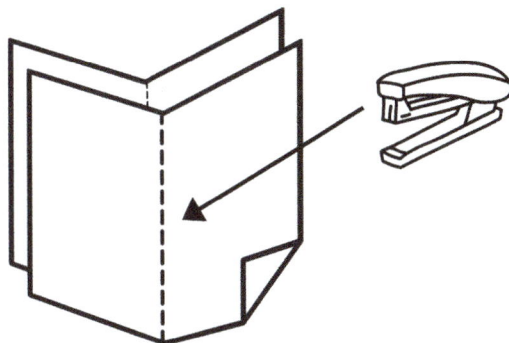

Cut paper in half on lines. Fold each page of book as indicated. Collate together so pages match up appropriately. Staple spine to hold together.

The stomach finally spoke up, "I am really the most important, without me, the body would have no nutrients to power its metabolism. I am the most important after all!"

So the pancreas stopped producing insulin and the liver stopped regulating chemicals and the body stopped working.

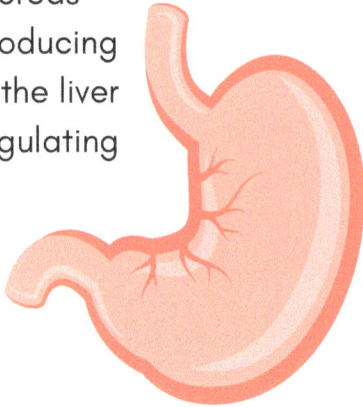

5

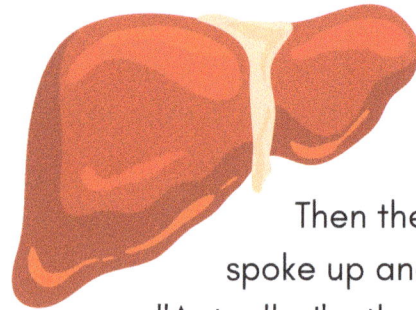

Then the liver spoke up and said "Actually, I'm the most important part, without me the chemicals in the body would be all out of whack!

So the spleen stopped removing damaged blood and the lungs stopped oxygenating it, and the body stopped working.

6

Anatomy ABC's

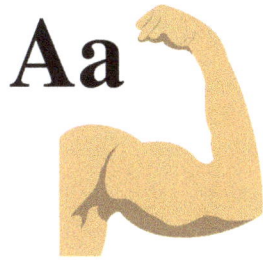 Aa

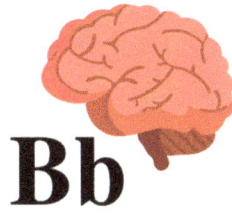 Bb

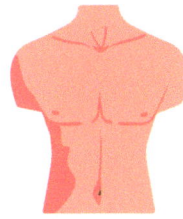 Cc

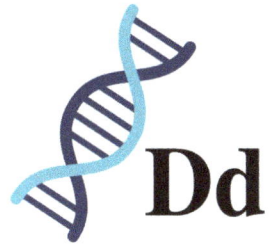 Dd

Ee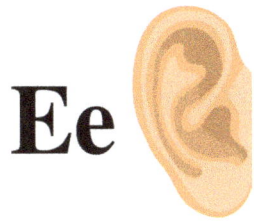

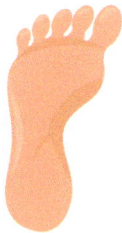 Ff

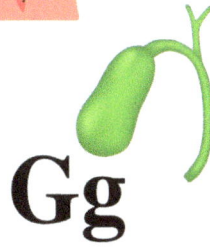 Gg

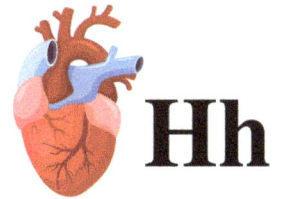 Hh

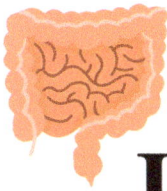 Ii

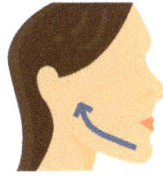 Jj

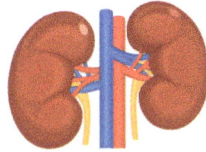 Kk

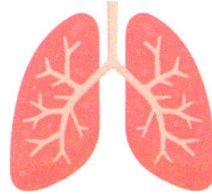 Ll

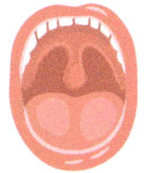 Mm

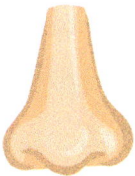 Nn

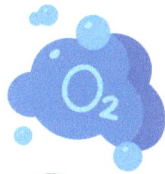 Oo

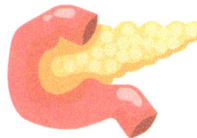 Pp

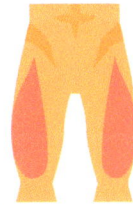 Qq

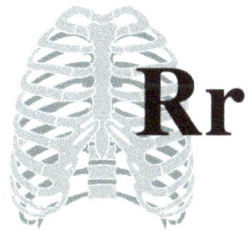 Rr

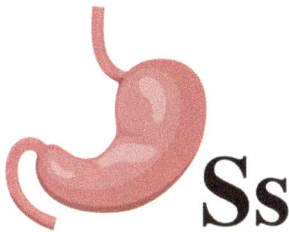 Ss

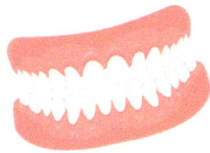 Tt

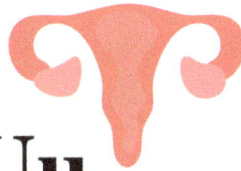 Uu

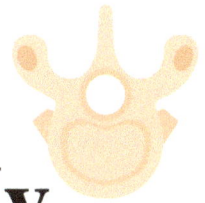 Vv

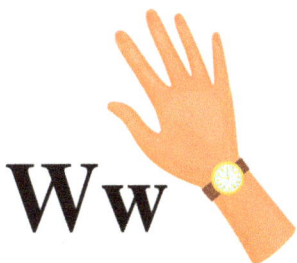 Ww

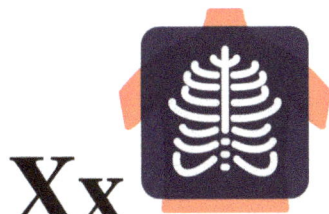 Xx

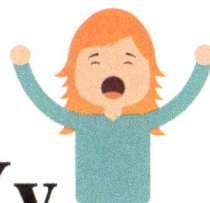 Yy

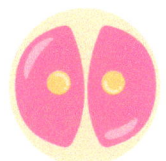 Zz

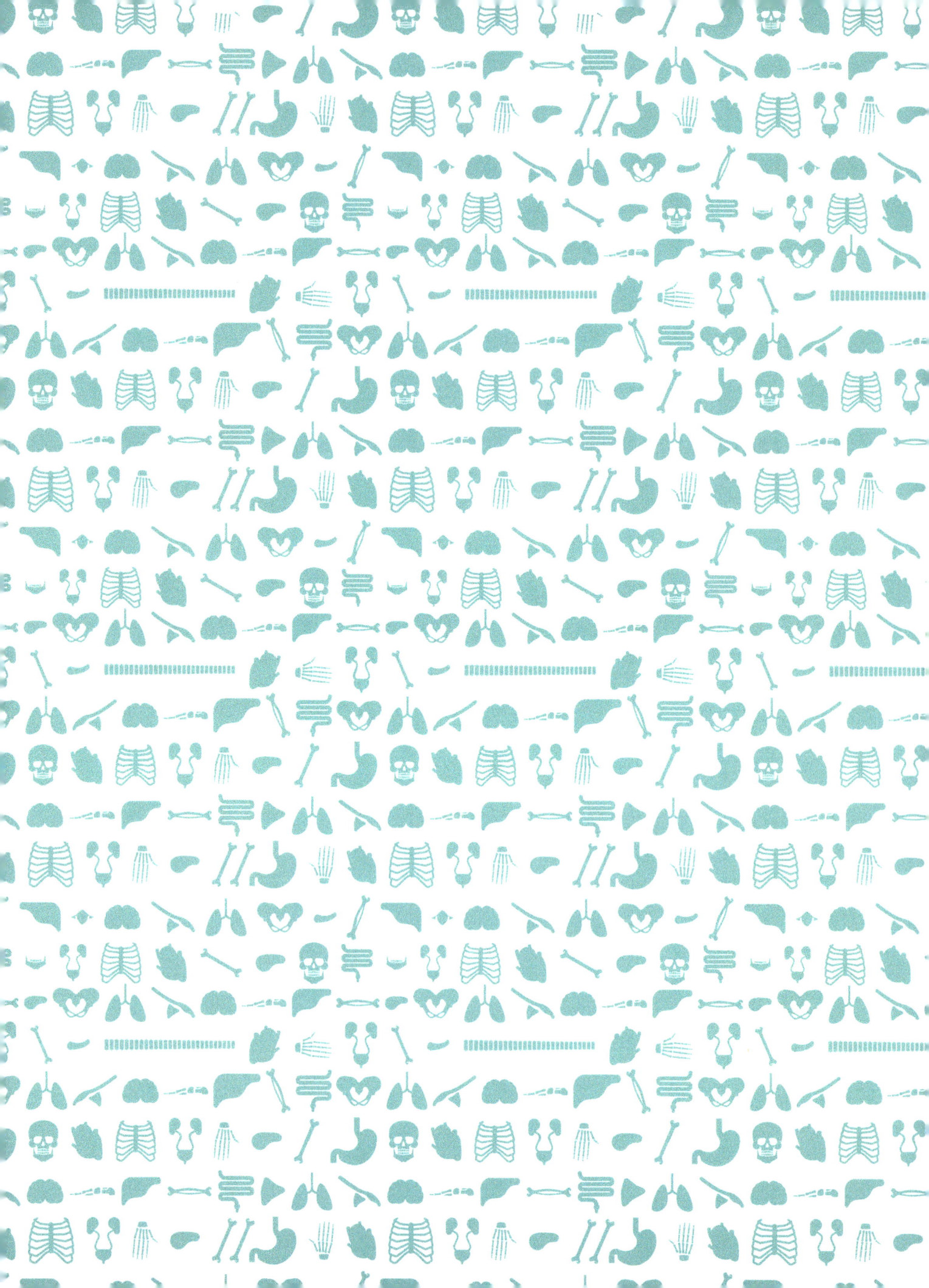

Anatomy Word Tracing

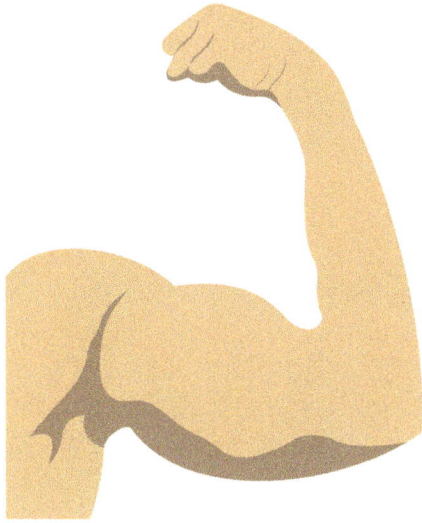

Arm

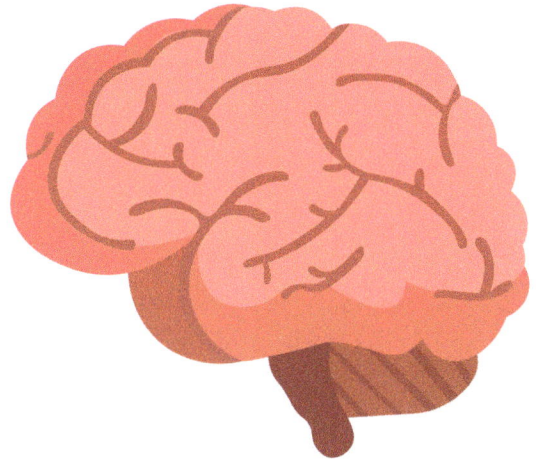

Brain

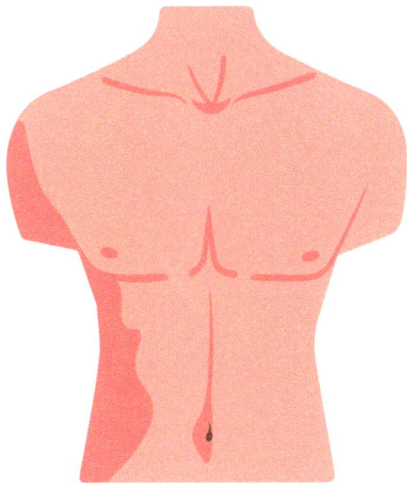

Chest

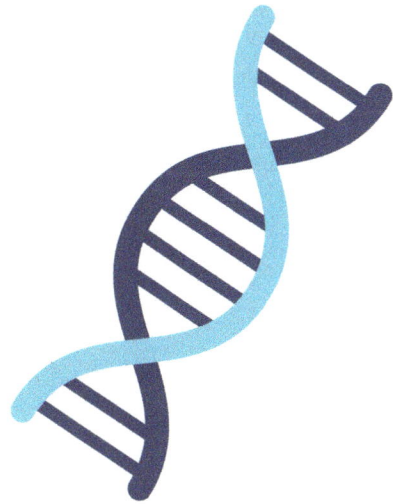

DNA

Anatomy Word Tracing

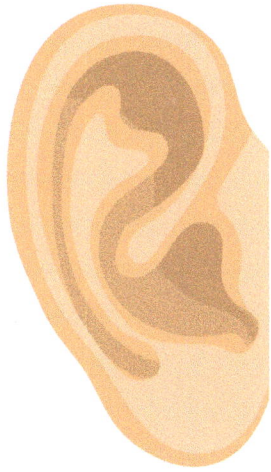

Ear

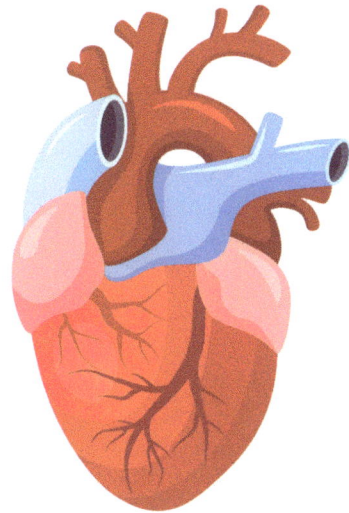

Heart

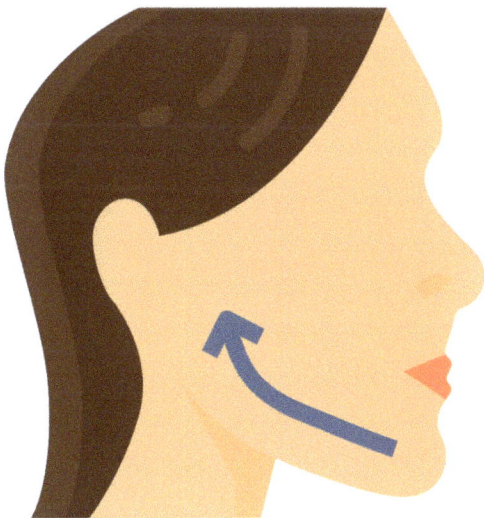

Jaw

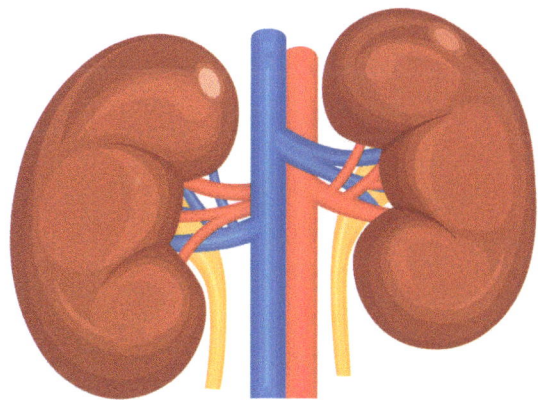

Kidney

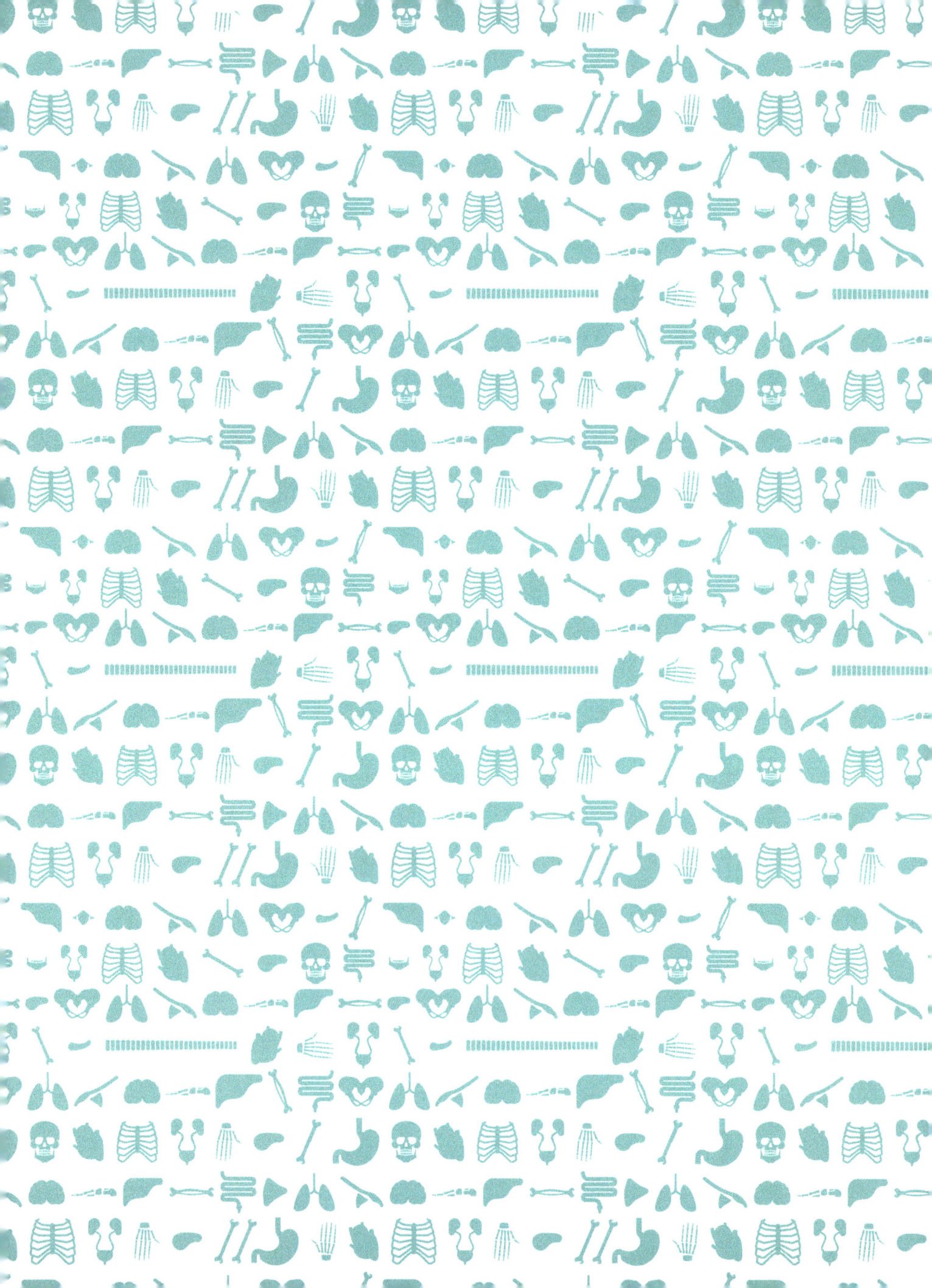

Anatomy Word Tracing

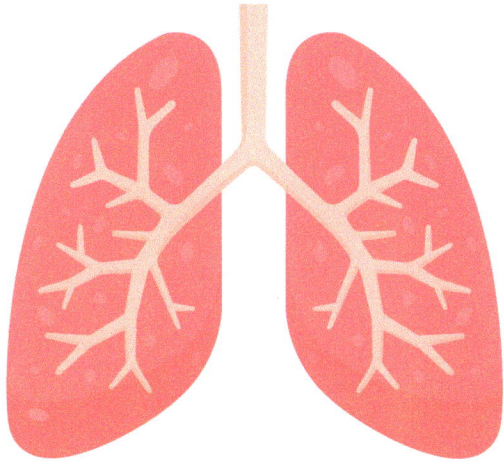

Lungs

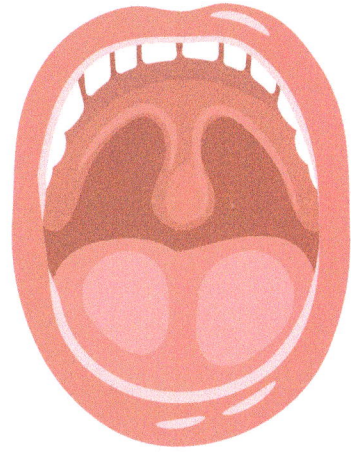

Mouth

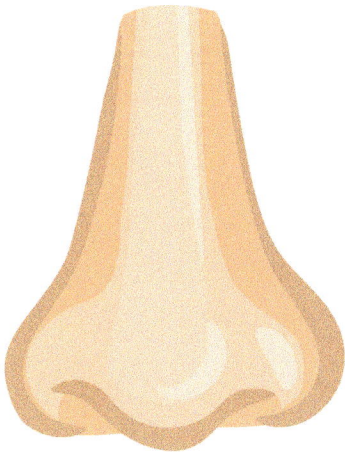

Nose

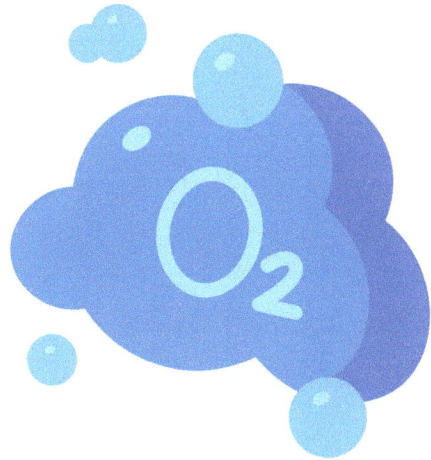

Oxygen

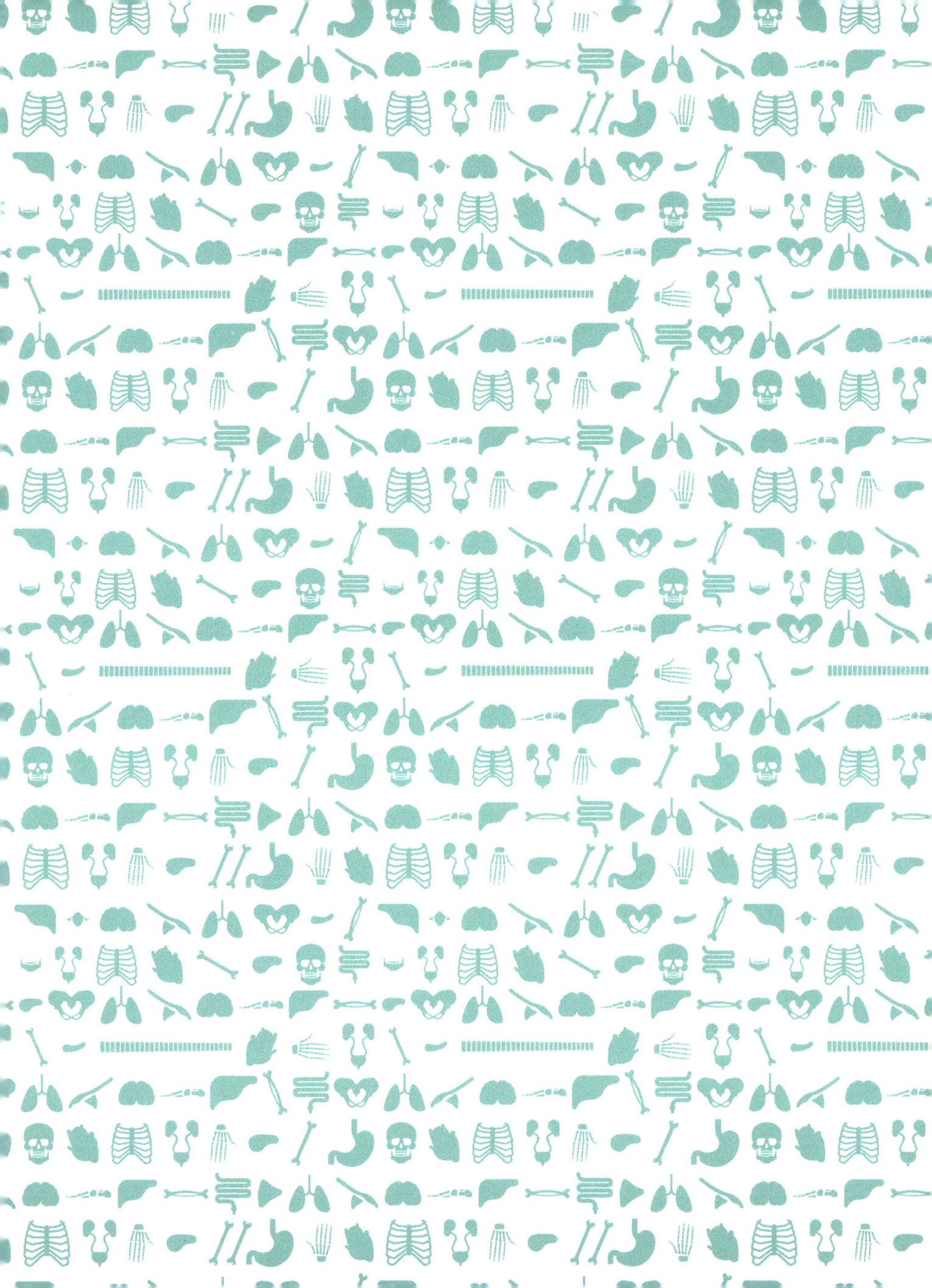

Anatomy Word Tracing

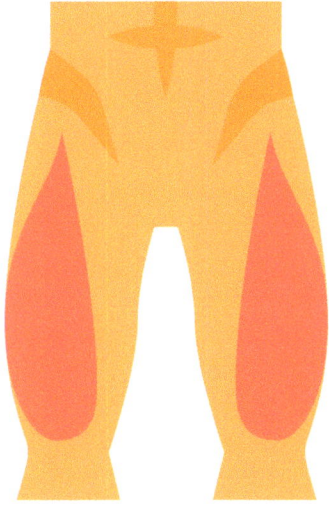

Quads

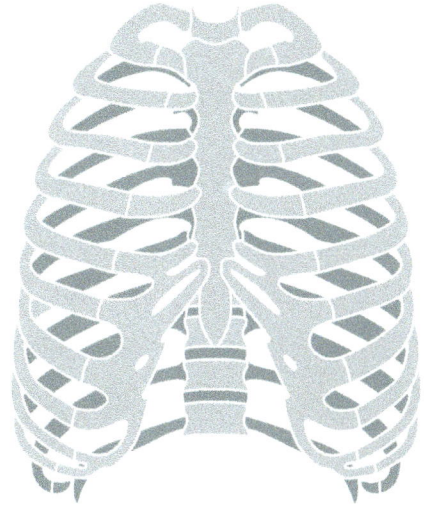

Ribs

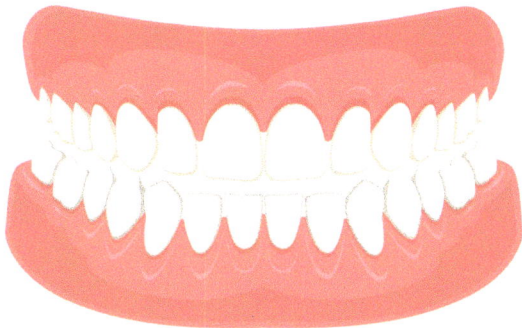

Teeth

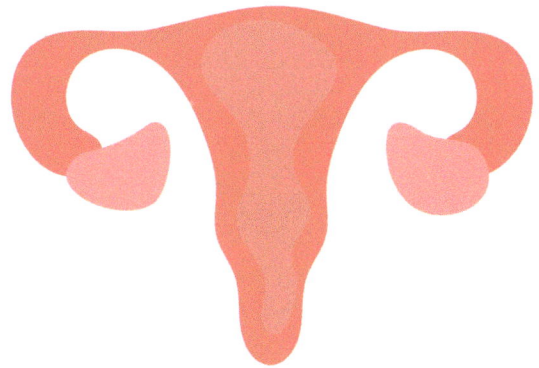

Uterus

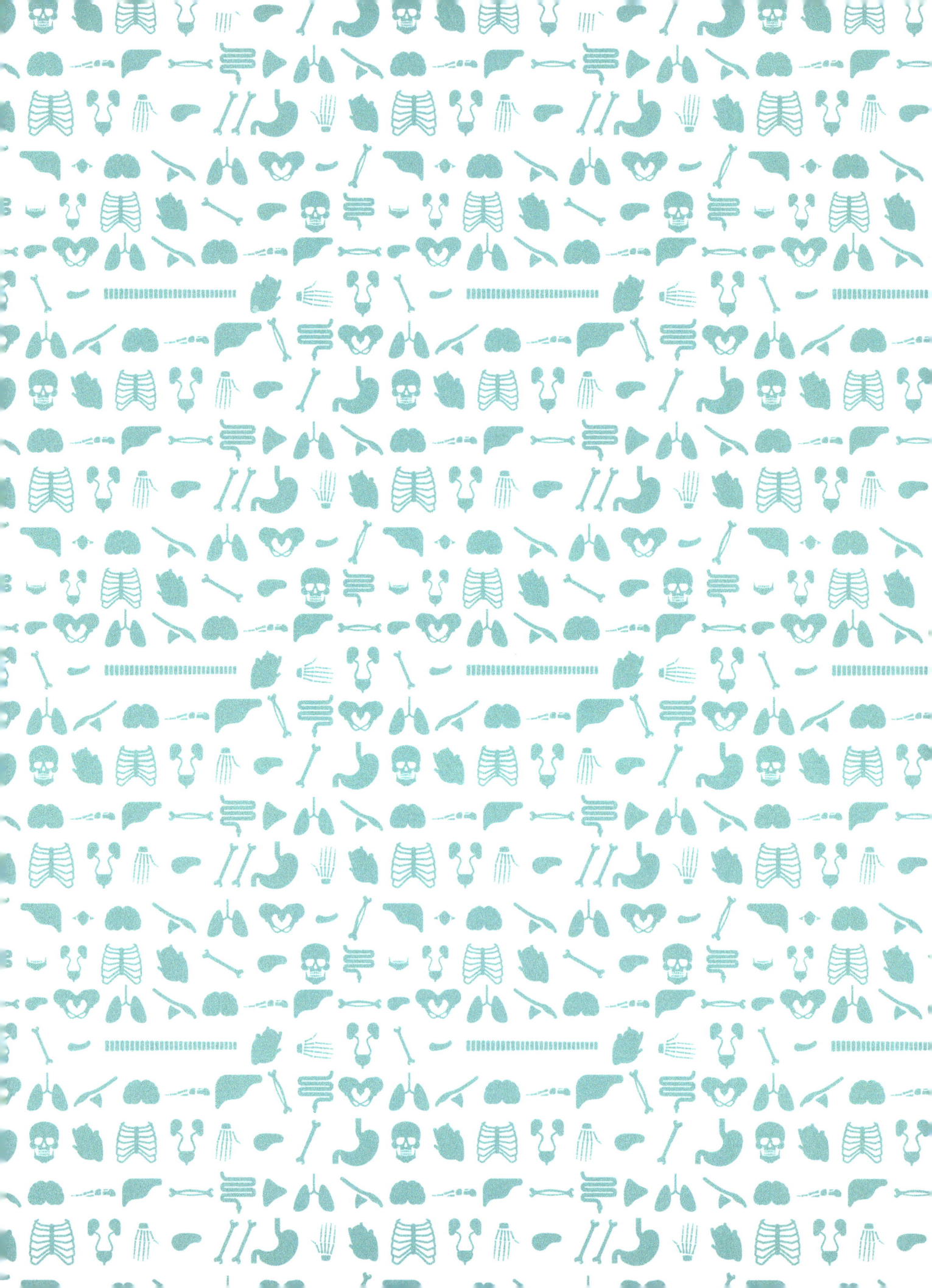

Anatomy Word Tracing

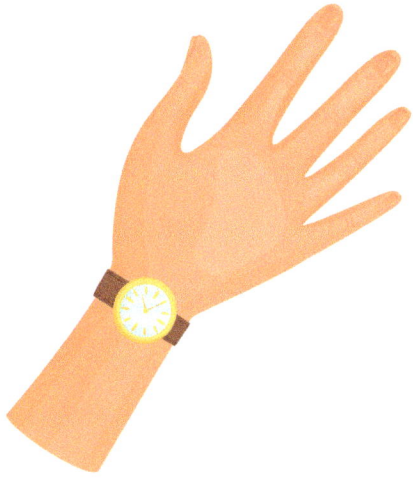

Wrist

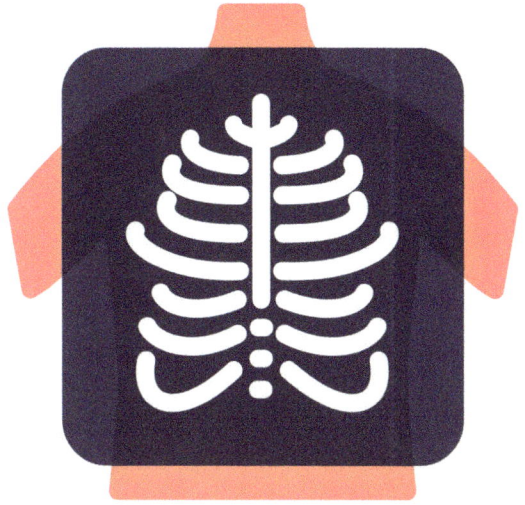

Xray

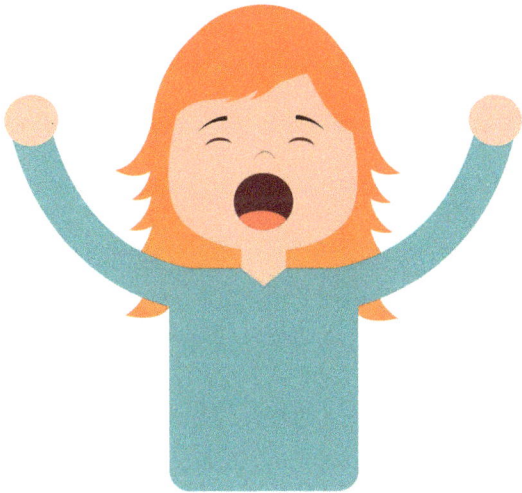

Yawn

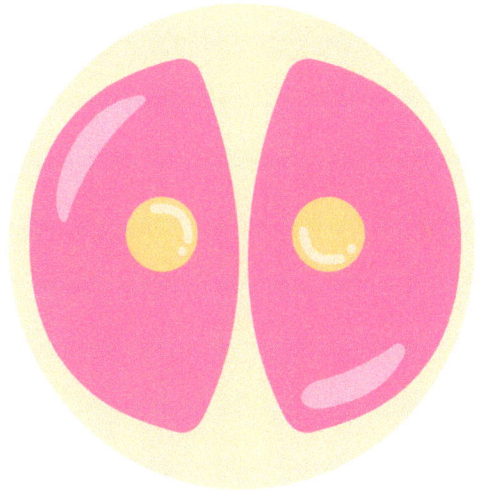

Zygote

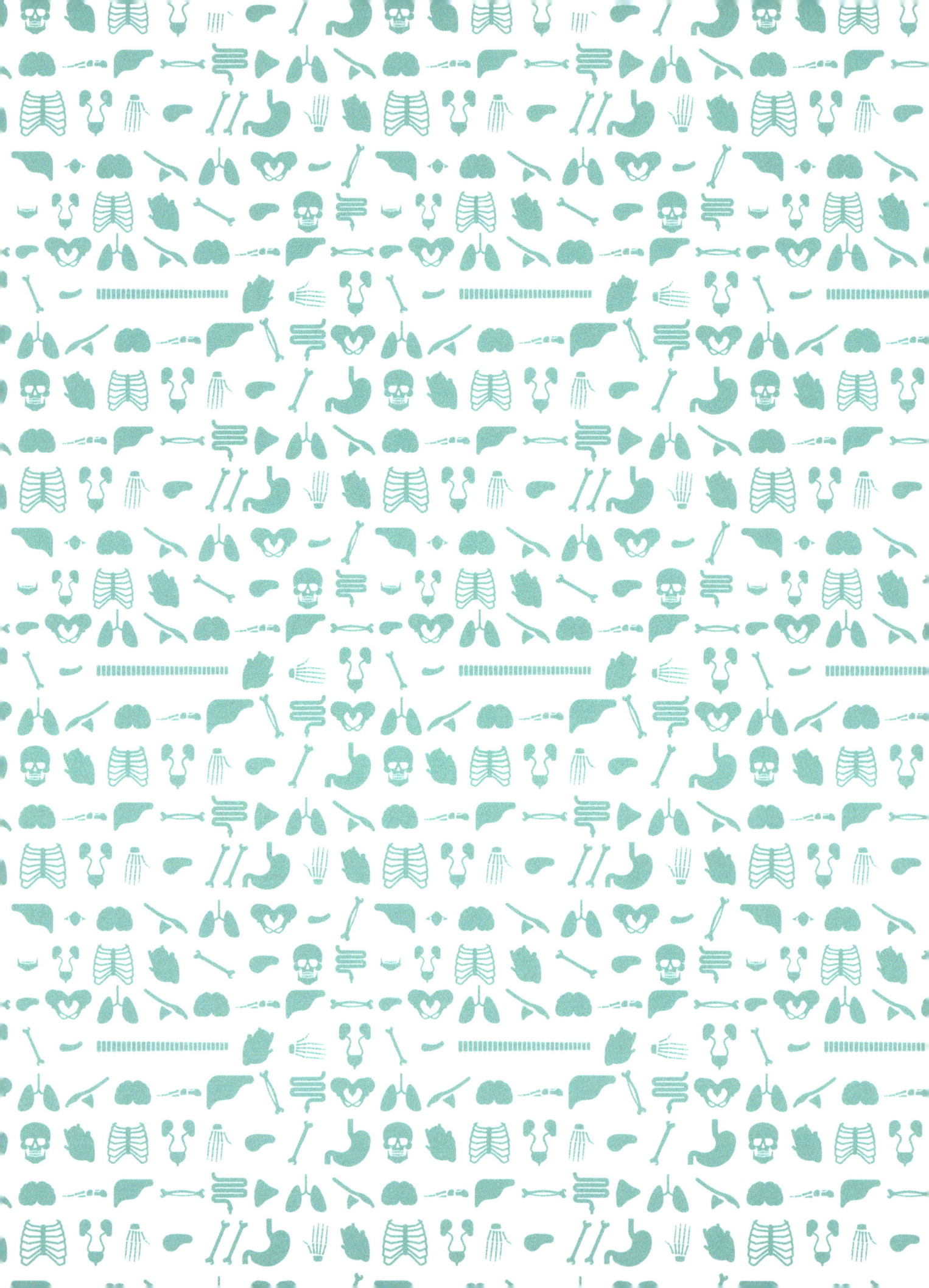

Timeline of Medical History

2600 BC
Egypt: First
Medical Book

460
Greece:
Hippocrates
is born

300
Greece:
First
Anatomy Book

200
Italy: First
Prosthetic
Limb

AD ......>

910
Persia:
Smallpox
identified

1249
England:
Eyeglasses
Invented

1489
Italy:
Cadavers are
Studied

1580
Switzerland:
First
Successful
C-Section

1590
Netherlands:
Microscope
invented

1763
France:
First
Successful
Appendectomy

1774
England:
First
Dentures

1795
USA: First
Blood
Transfusion

1796
Europe: First
Vaccine:
Smallpox

1816
France:
Stethoscope
Invented

1846
Anesthesia
Invented

1849
USA: First
Woman Doctor
(Medical
Degree)

1857
France:
Germ
Theory
Discovered

1888
USA: First
Brain Tumor
Removed

1895
Germany:
X-Rays
Invented

1921
Canada:
Insulin
Invented

1928
England:
Penicillin
Discovered

1930
USA:
Ventilator
Invented

1954
USA: First
Human Organ
Transplant:
Kidney

1978
England:
First IVF
Baby Born

1985
Netherlands:
Dialysis
Machine
Invented

2022
USA: First
Successful
Animal to
Human Organ
Transplant:
Heart

Photos used for illustration purposes and may not be of exact event or item.

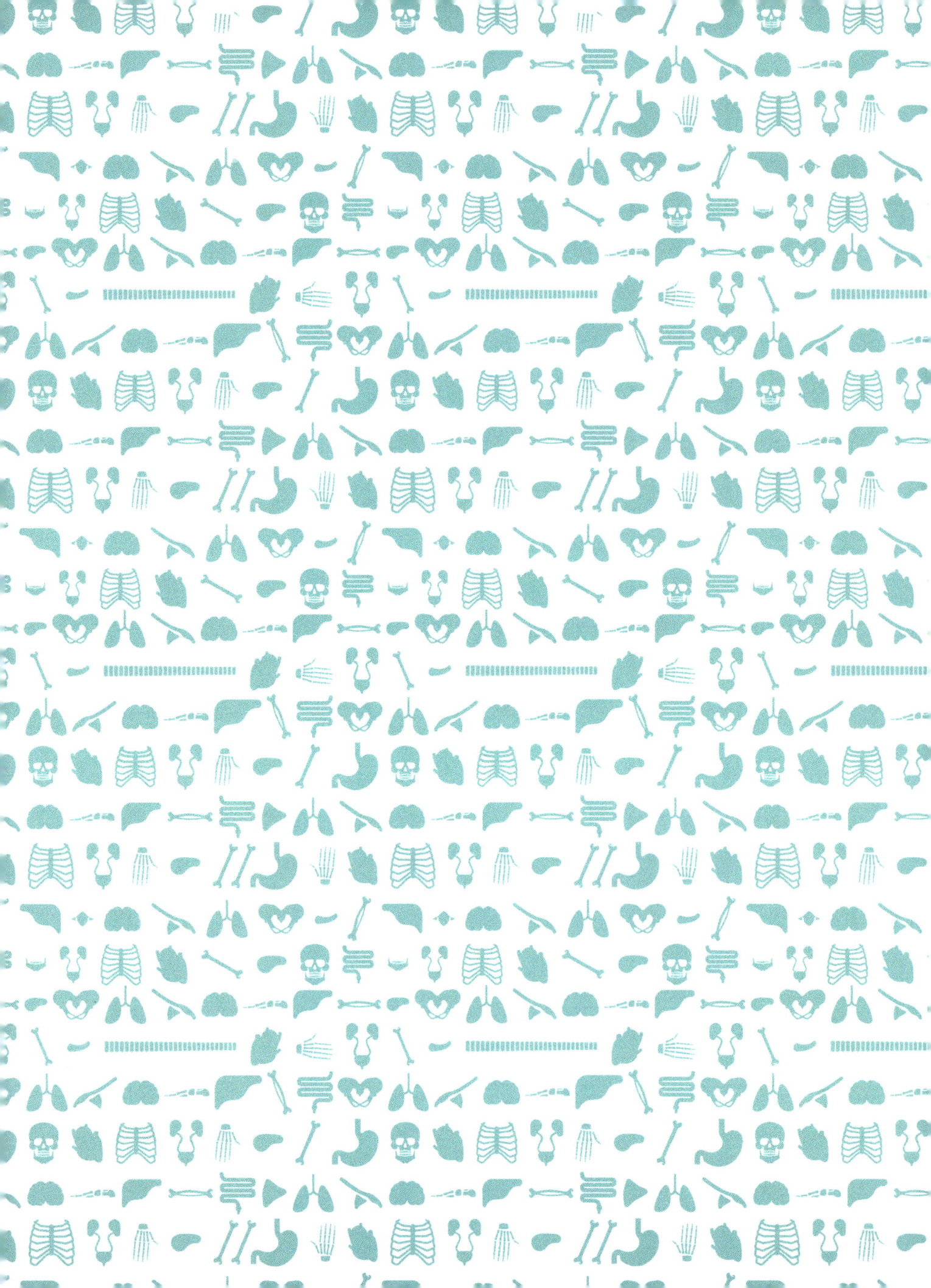

CANDY DNA MODEL

Instructions

Deoxyribonucleic acid (DNA) is the molecule that carries genetic information for the development and functioning of an organism. DNA is made of two linked strands that wind around each other to resemble a twisted ladder — a shape known as a double helix. The information in DNA is stored as a code made up of four chemical bases: adenine (A), guanine (G), cytosine (C), and thymine (T).

A deoxyribose-phosphate backbone is the portion of the DNA double helix that provides structural support to the molecule. Use multi-colored candy pieces to form the chemical bases - one for each base. Alternate the pairs on toothpicks. Insert each side onto candy rope, which illustrate the deoxyribose-phosphate backbone of DNA. Continue until rope length is filled with alternating chemical bases. Twist model to form the double helix shape.

Discuss: which colors represent which bases?

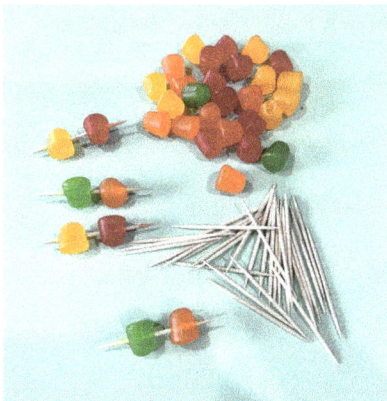

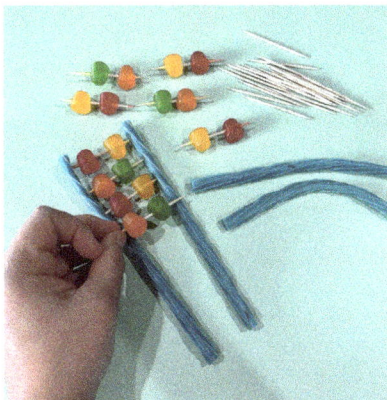

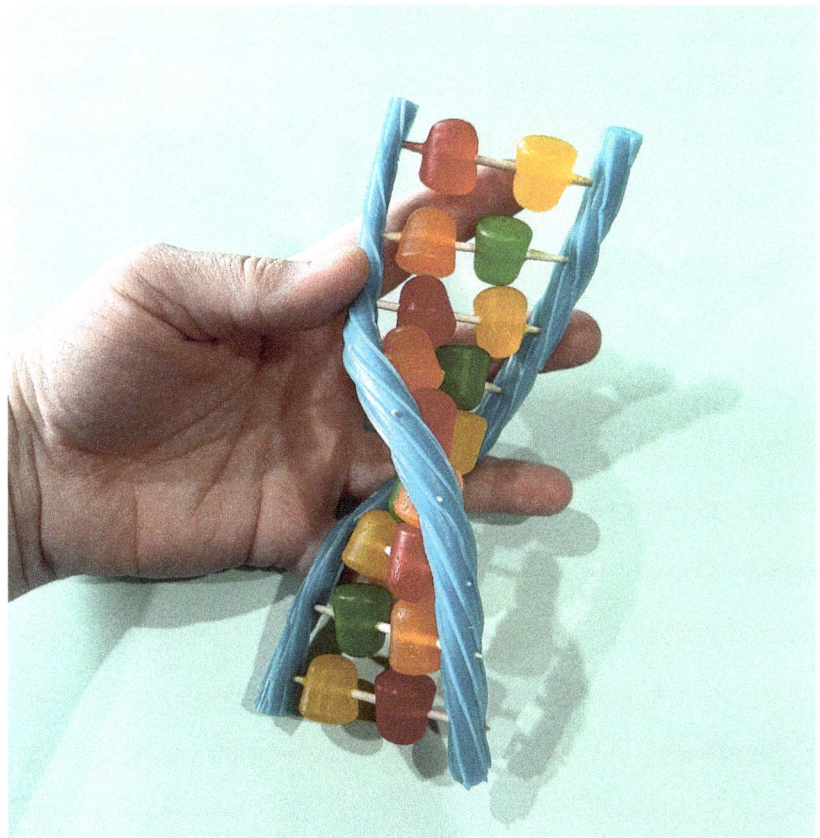

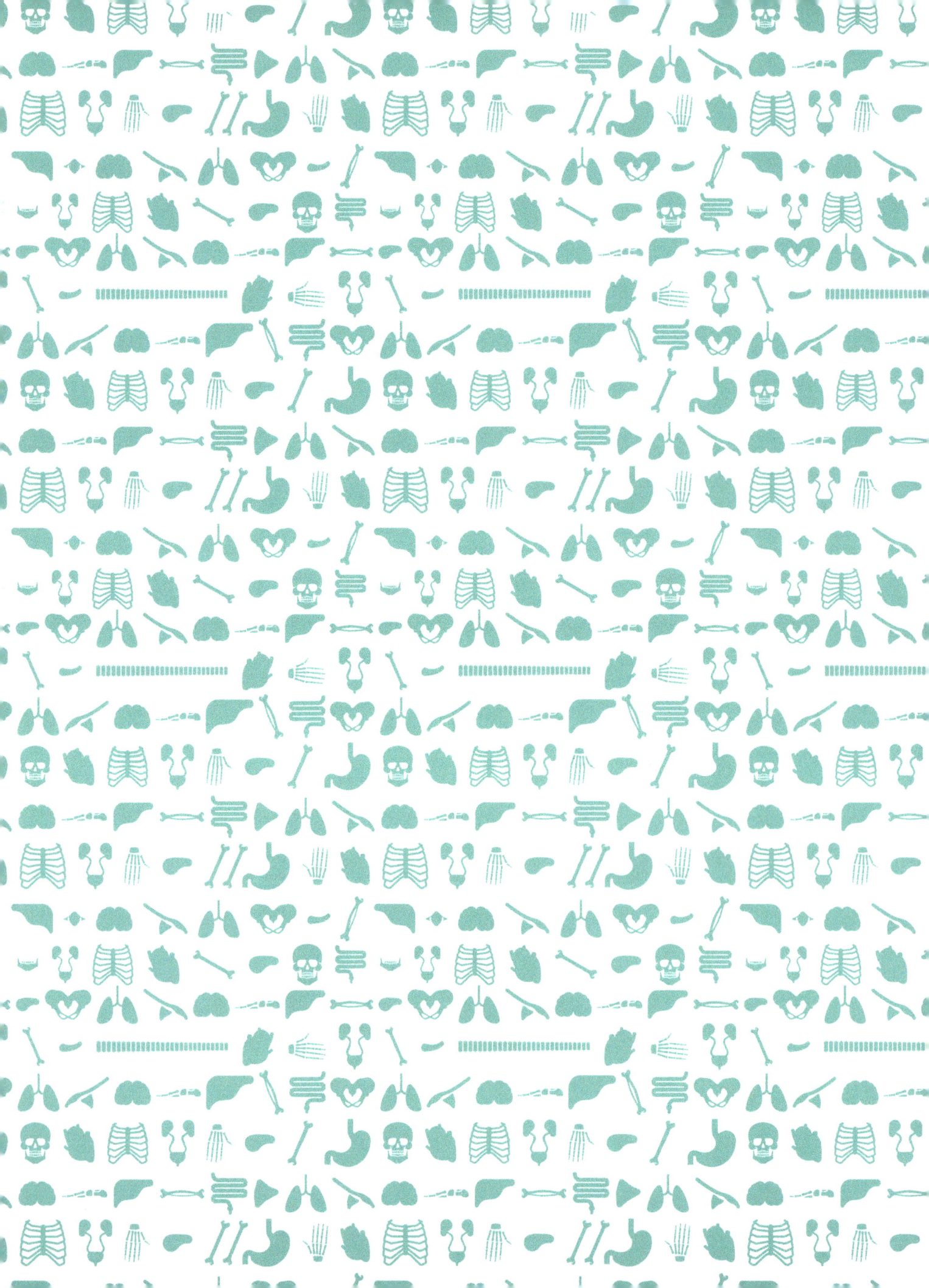

Components of DNA

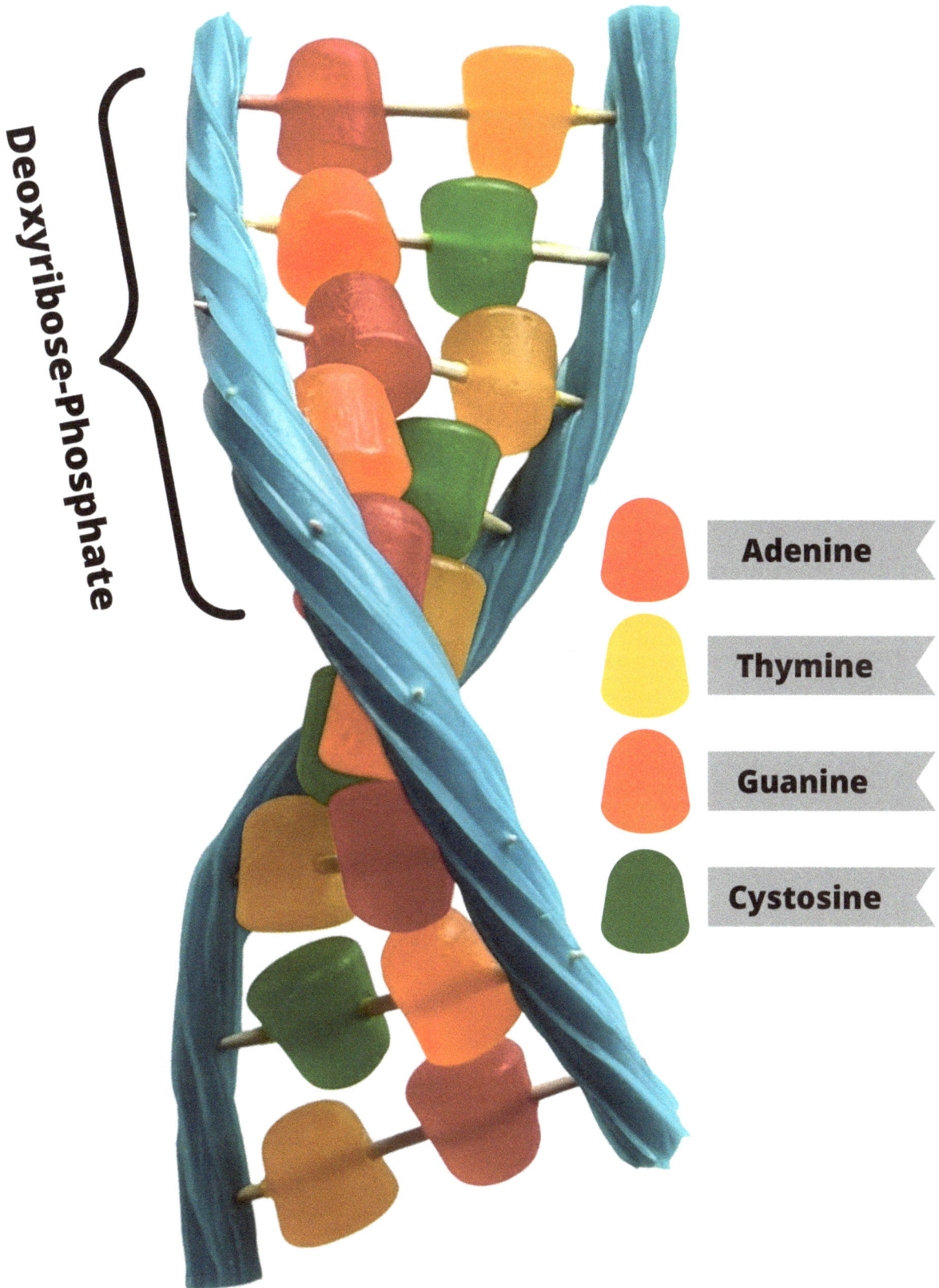

Deoxyribose-Phosphate

Adenine

Thymine

Guanine

Cystosine

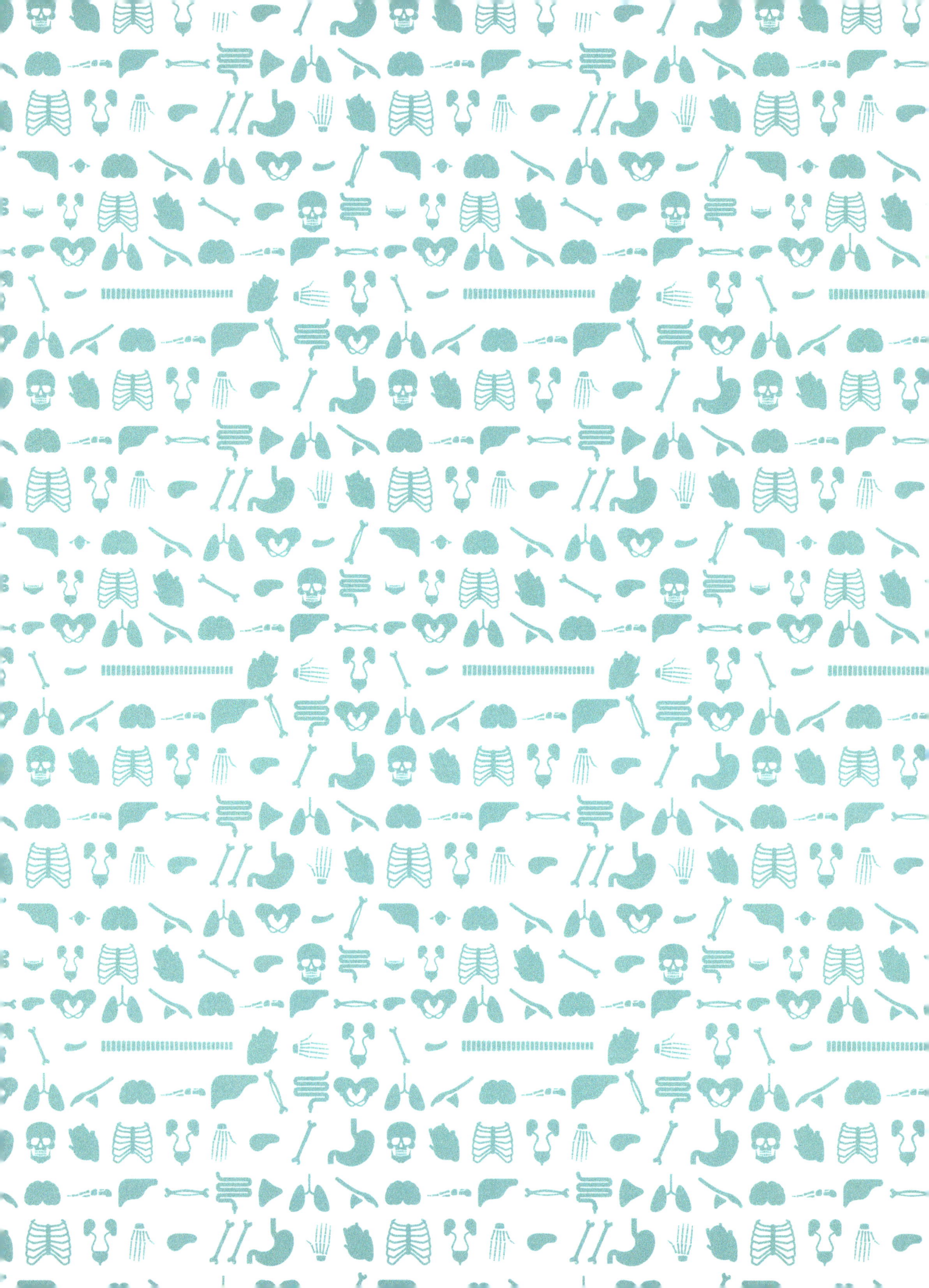

Organs of the Human Body

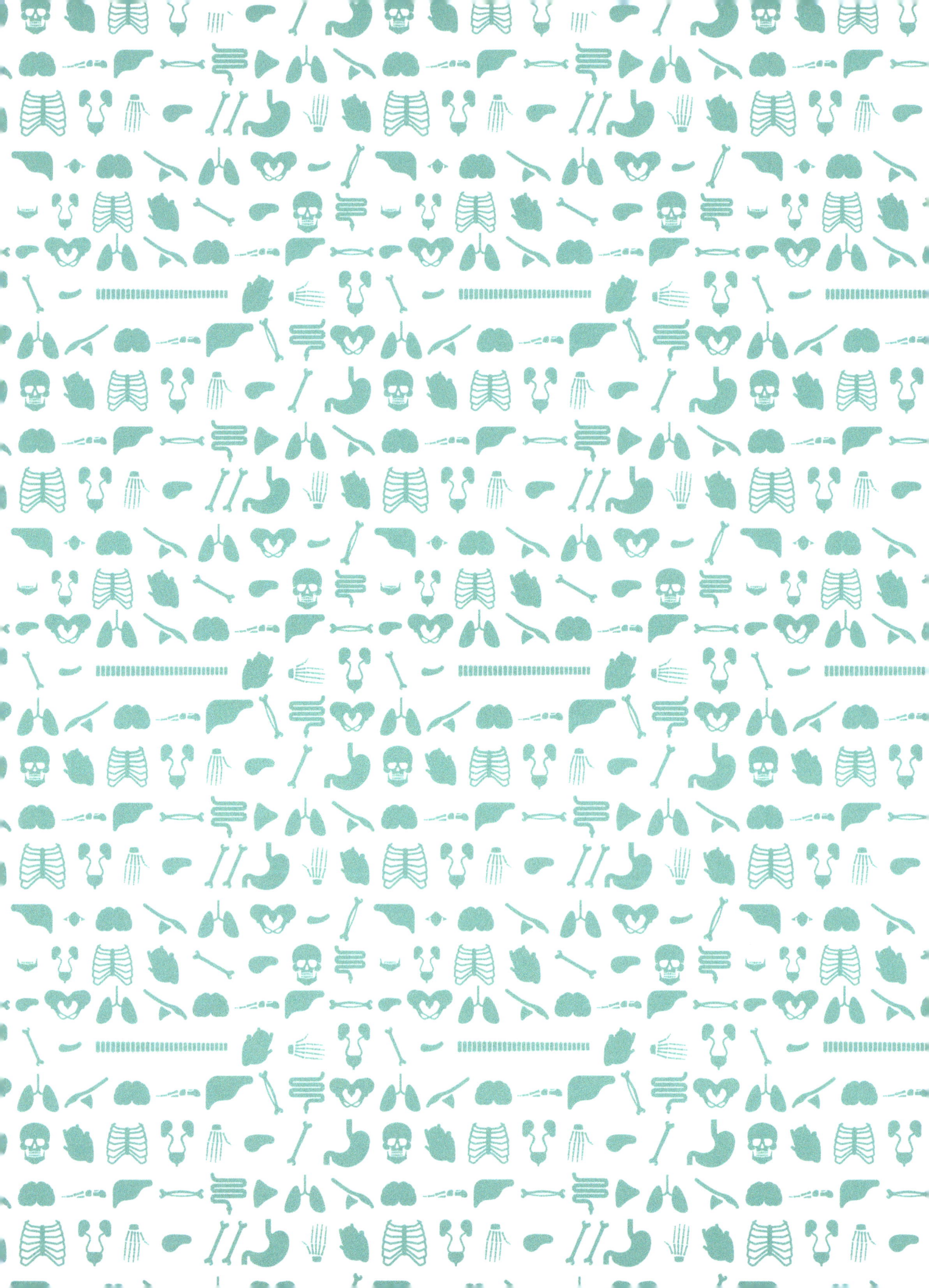

HUMAN BODY TRACING W/ORGANS

Instructions

This activity helps the child learn the different parts of the body and where they are located as related to their own body outline. Lay a large roll of craft paper on the floor. You will need paper at least as tall as the child and as wide (with their hands positioned at sides) - you can also upcycle a large shipping box.

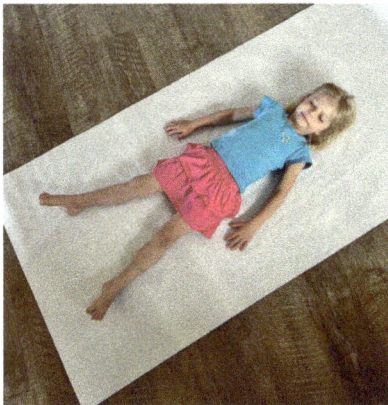

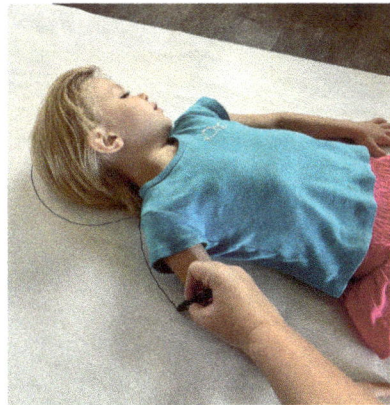

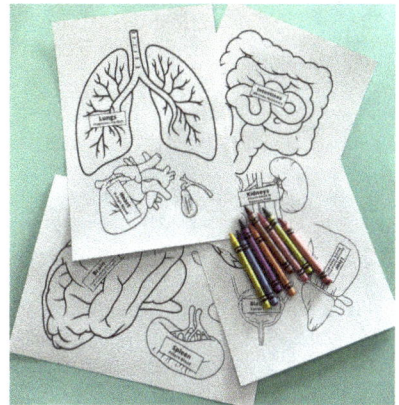

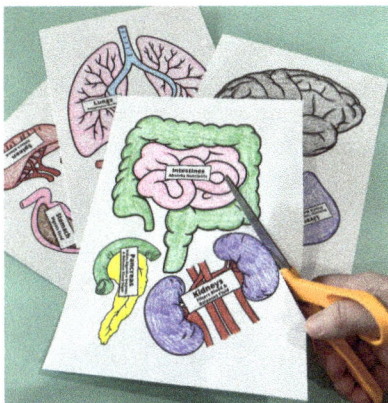

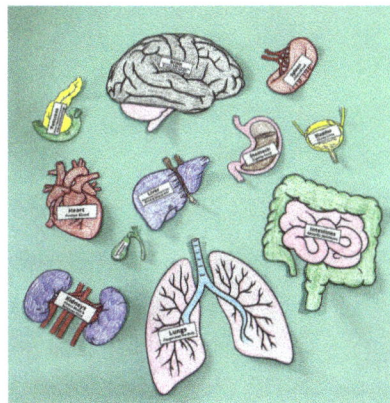

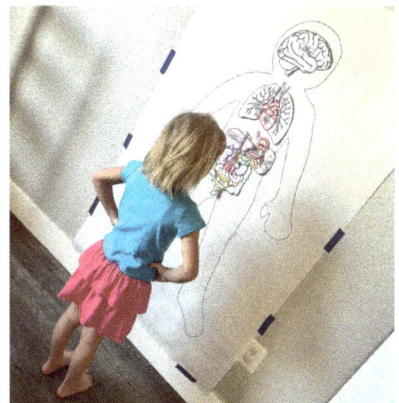

Have the child lay down on paper and trace entire body. Use painter's tape to place outline on wall. Using the included body organs template, have the child color each organ with crayons or markers. What colors are associated with each organ? Cut out the organs; younger children may need a bit of assistance. Use tape to adhere organs to appropriate location on outline. Read the function of each organ on the printouts. **Discuss:** what is the actual color of the organ in a functioning human body? How does each organ help the body work?

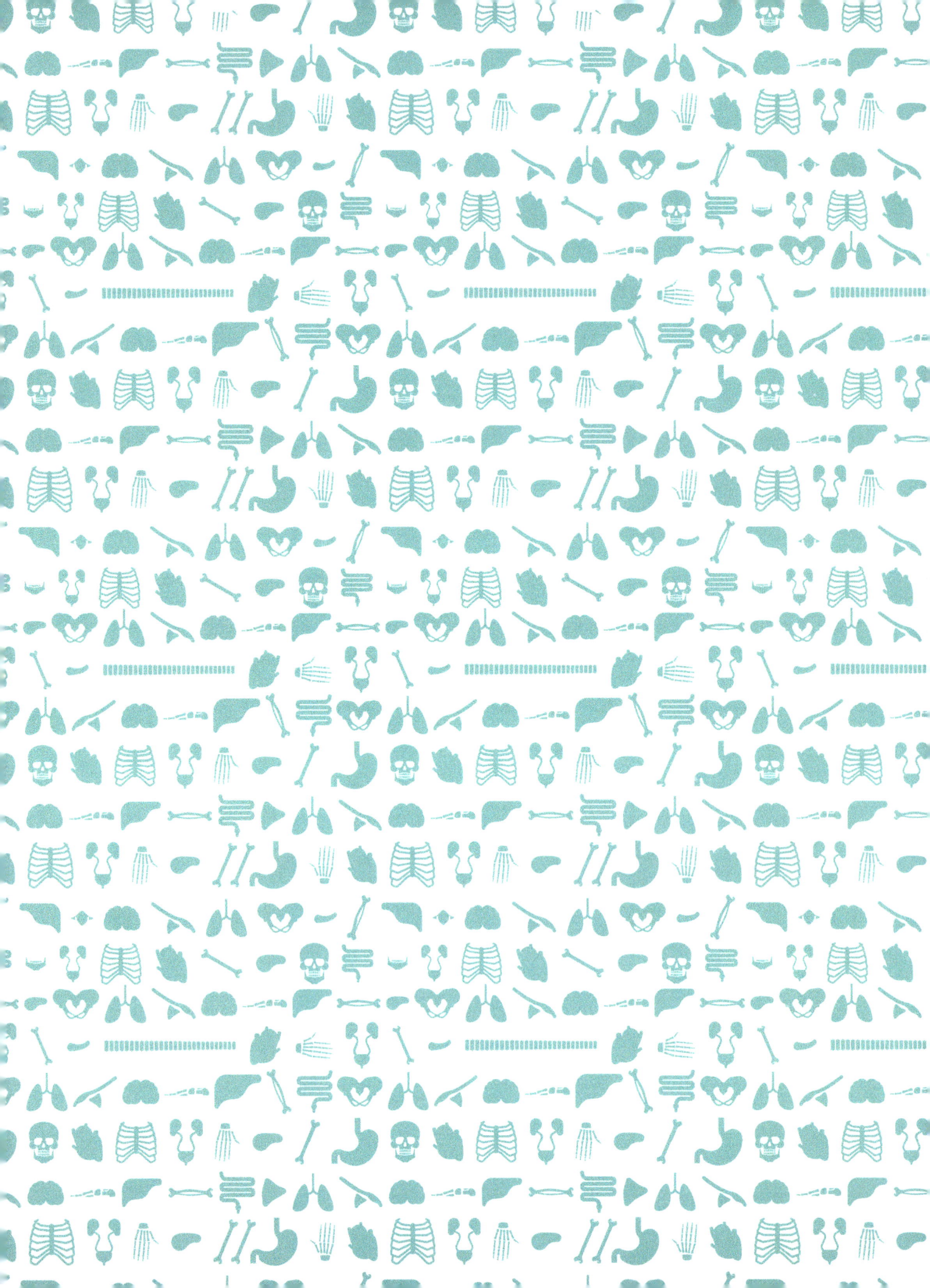

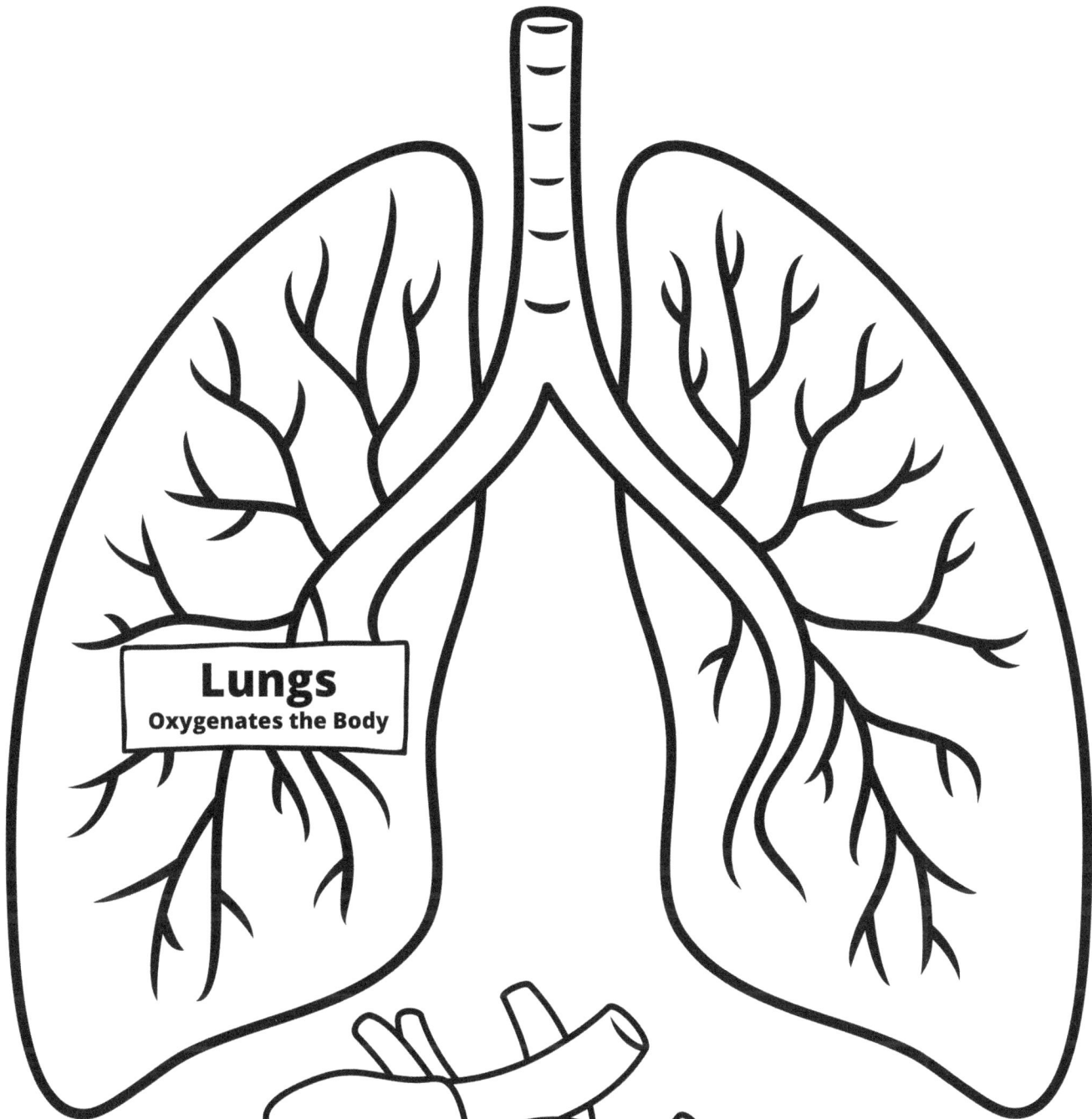

Lungs
Oxygenates the Body

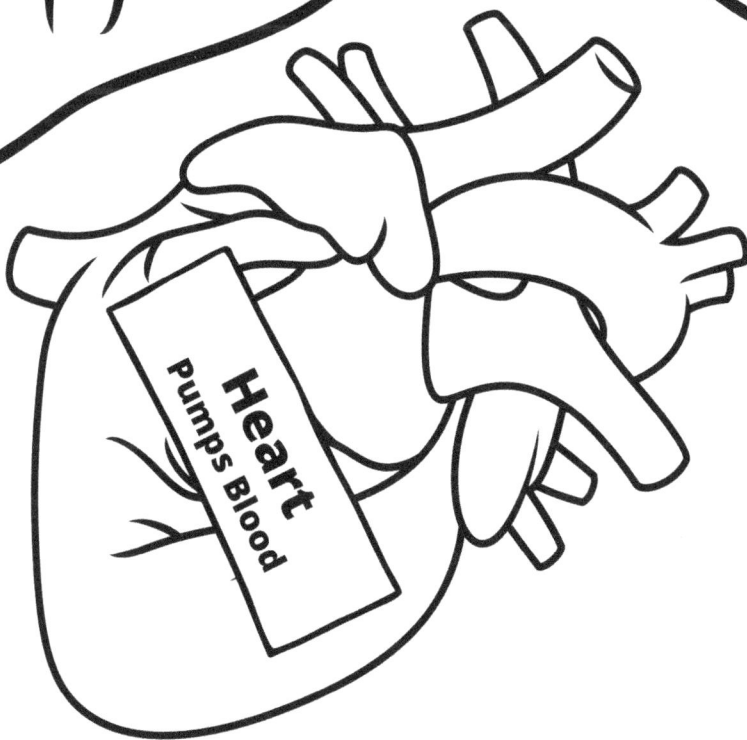

Heart
Pumps Blood

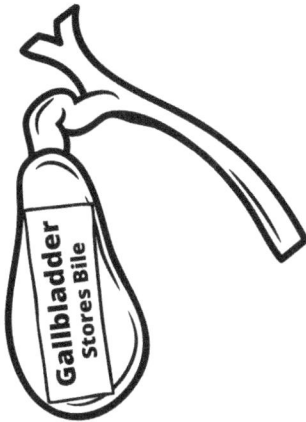

Gallbladder
Stores Bile

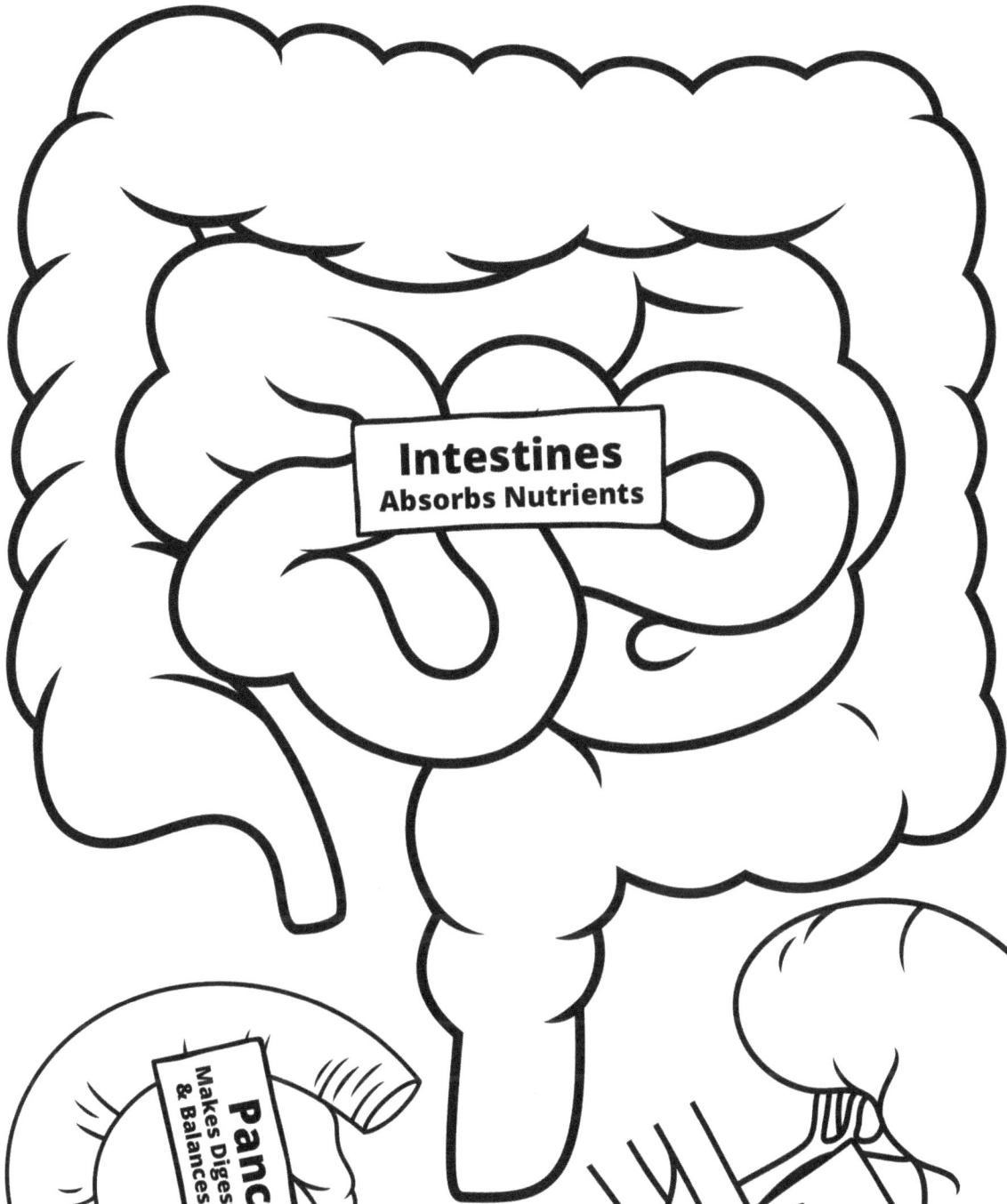

Intestines
Absorbs Nutrients

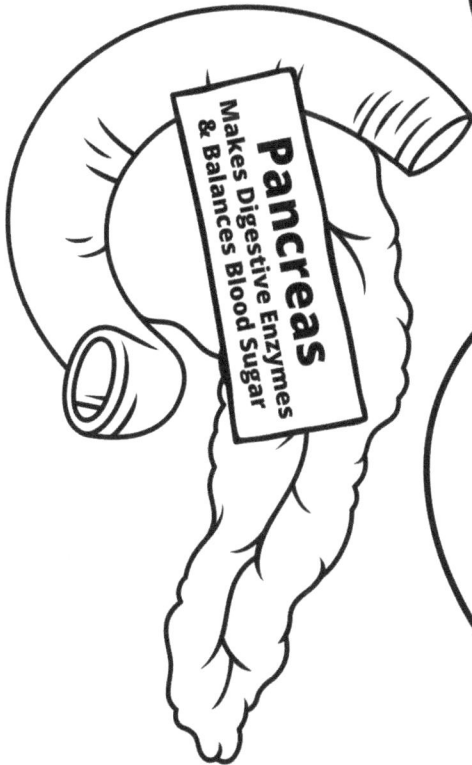

Pancreas
Makes Digestive Enzymes
& Balances Blood Sugar

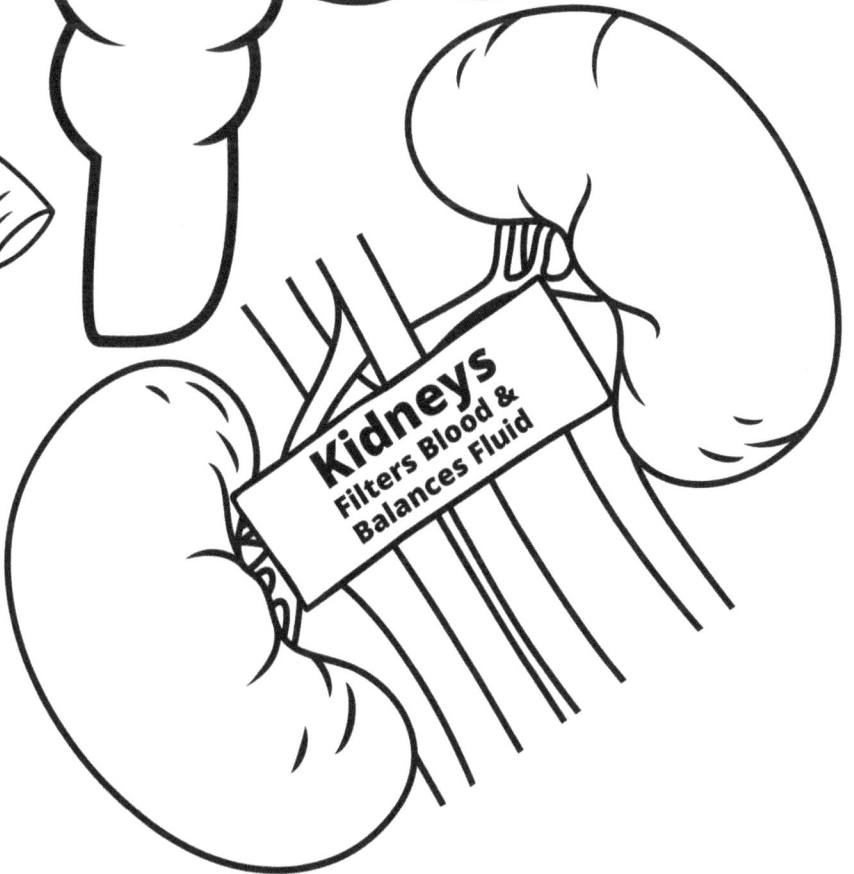

Kidneys
Filters Blood &
Balances Fluid

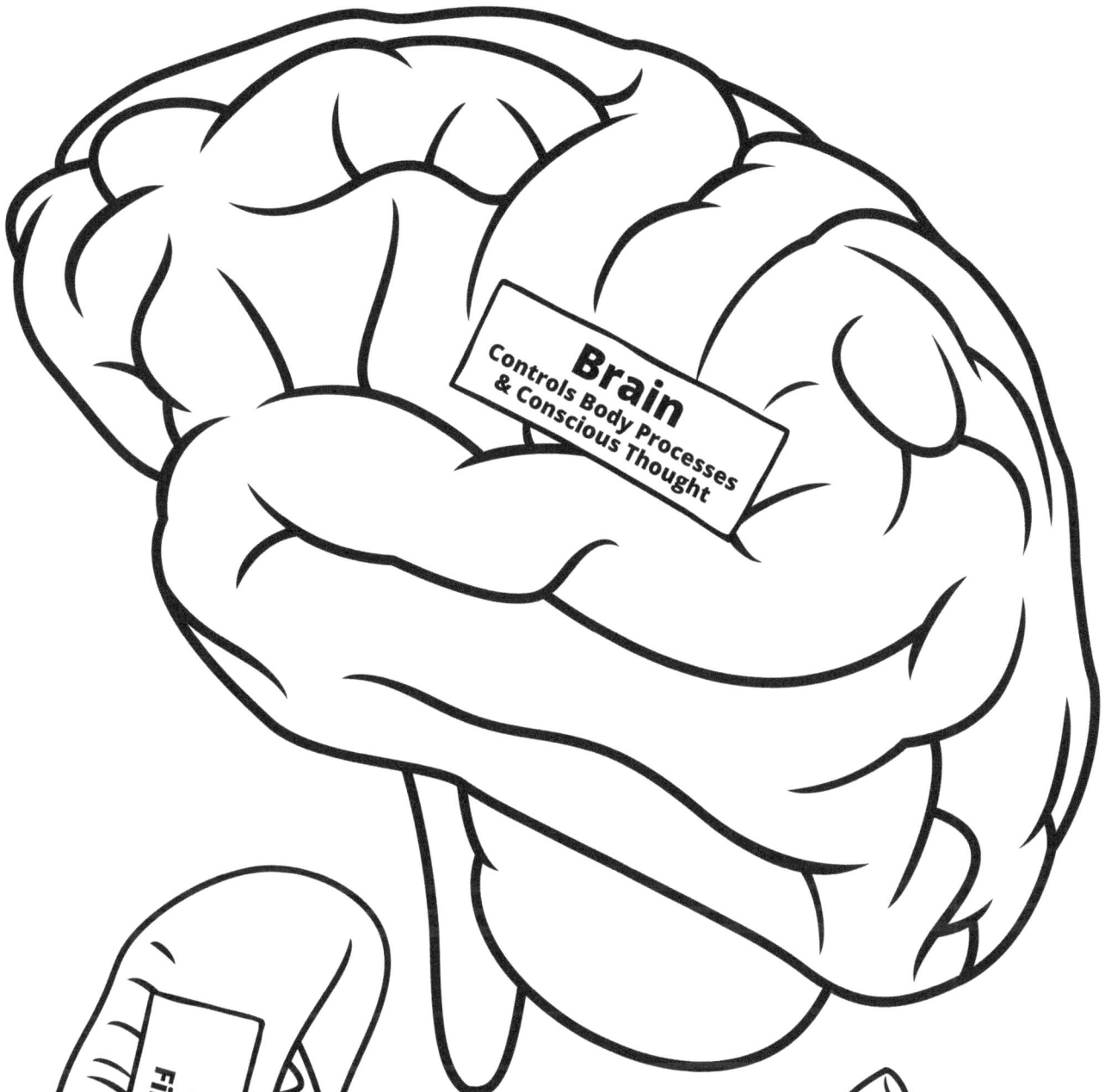

Brain
Controls Body Processes
& Conscious Thought

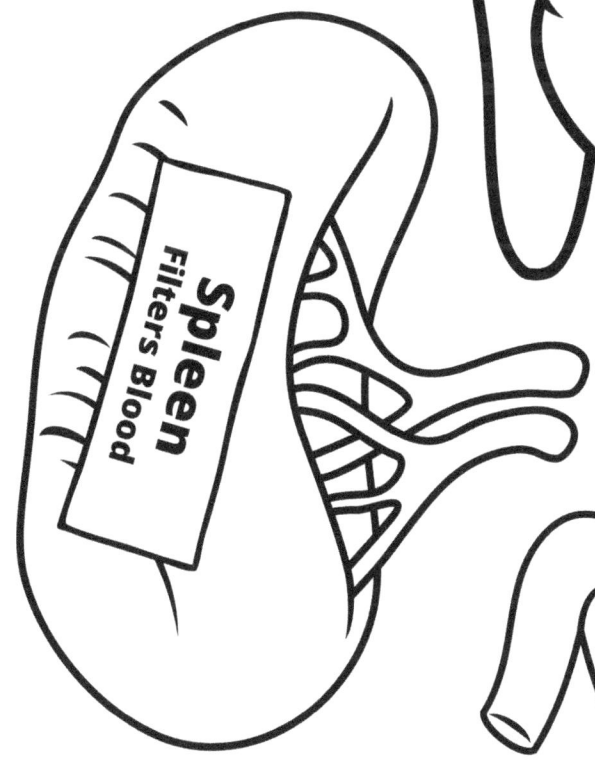

Spleen
Filters Blood

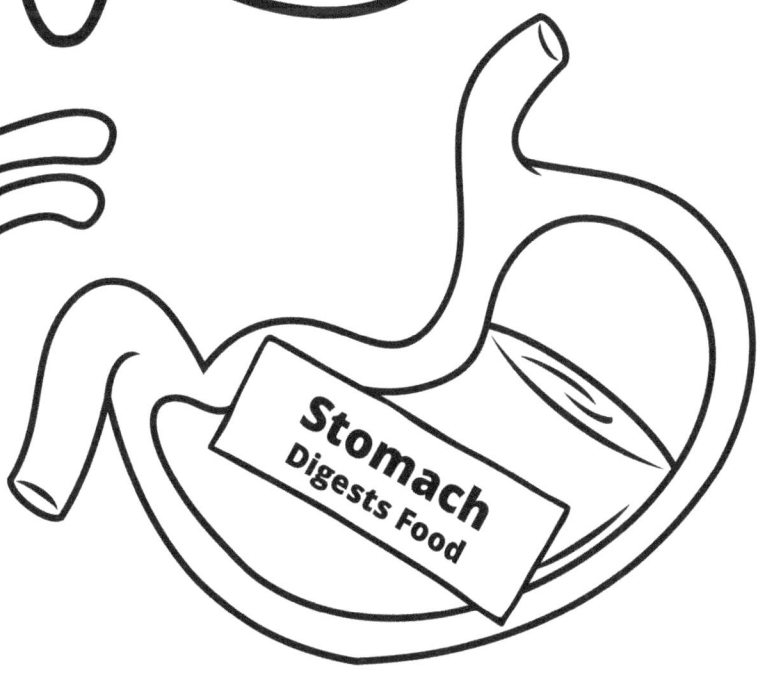

Stomach
Digests Food

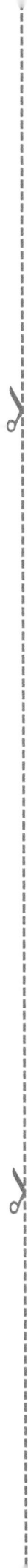

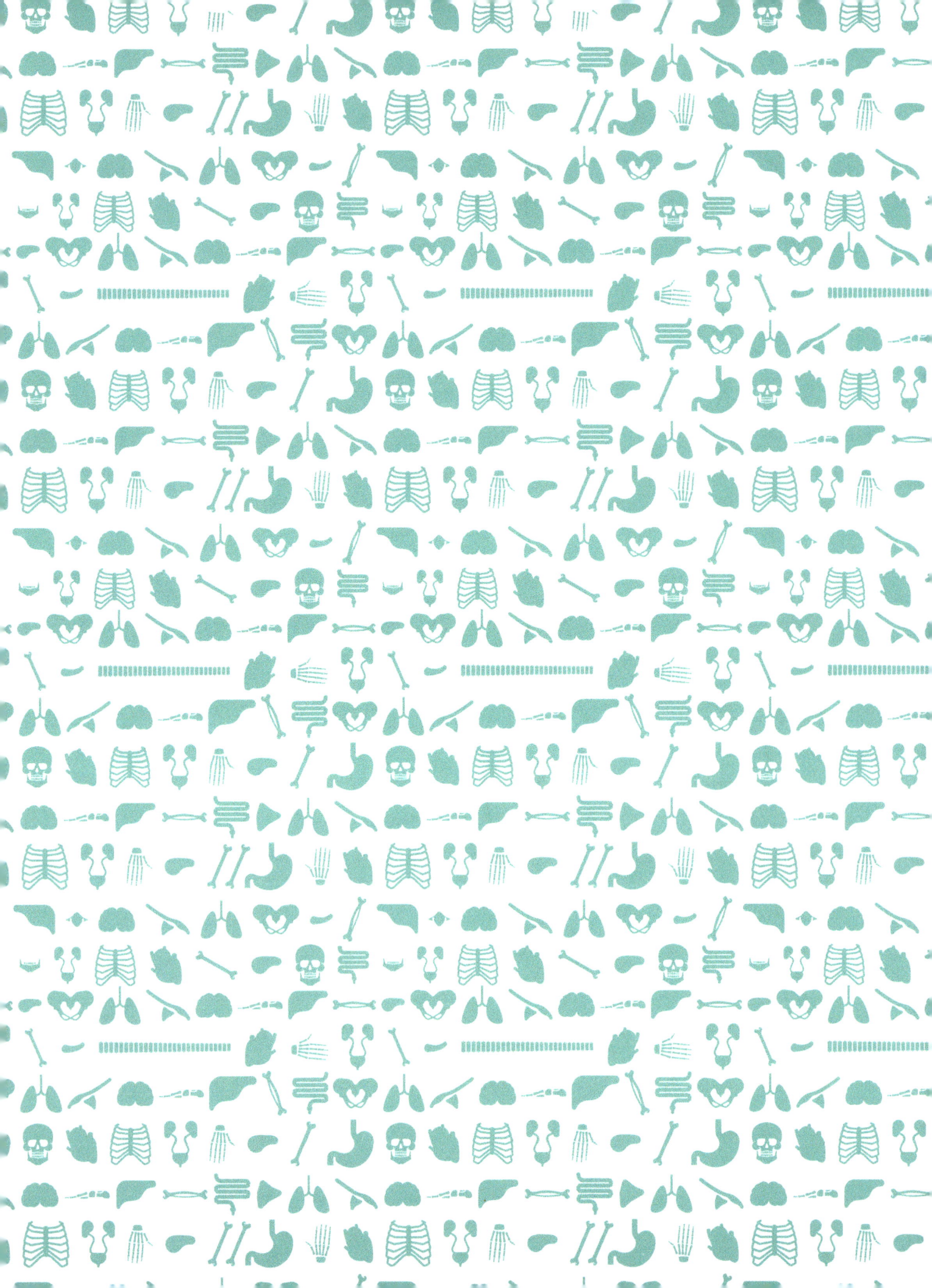

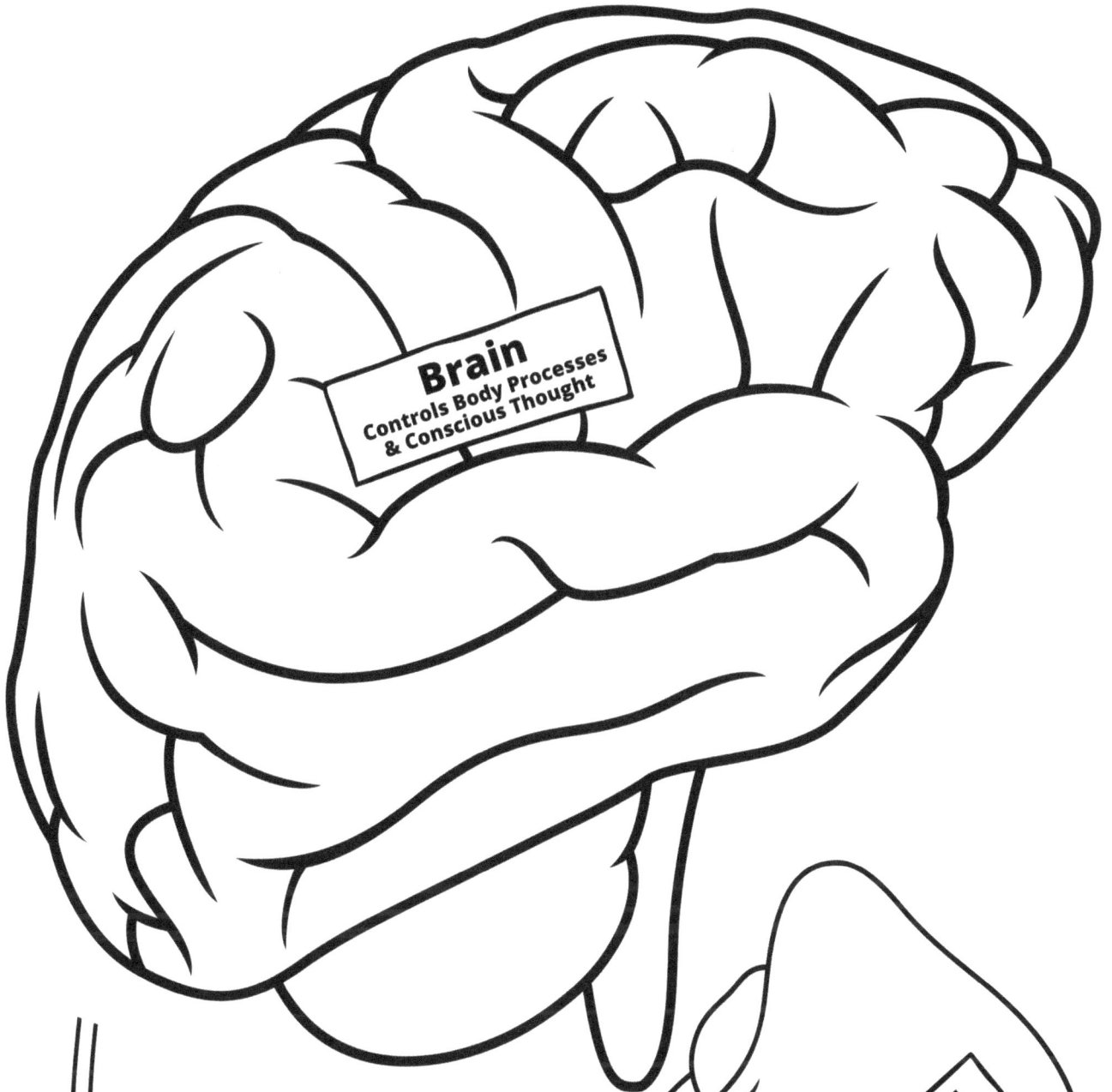

Brain
Controls Body Processes
& Conscious Thought

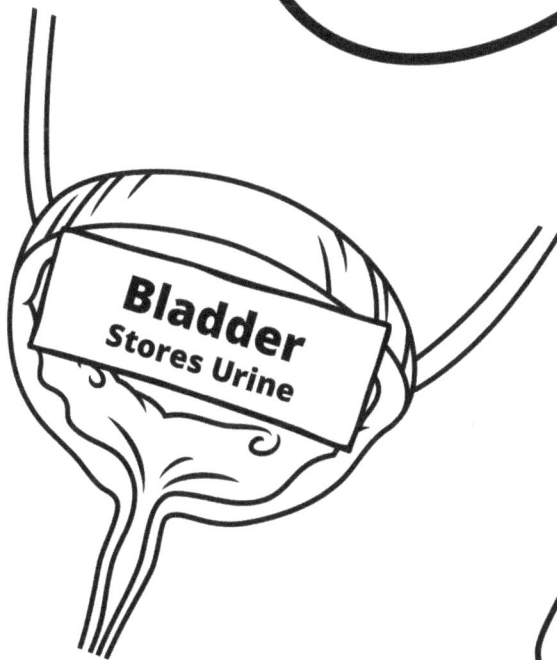

Bladder
Stores Urine

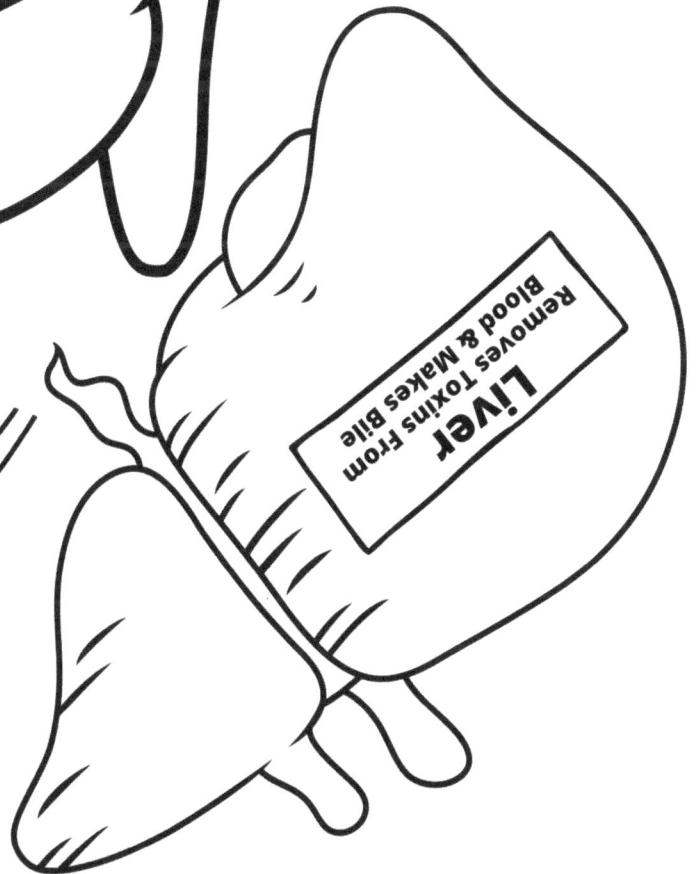

Liver
Removes Toxins From
Blood & Makes Bile

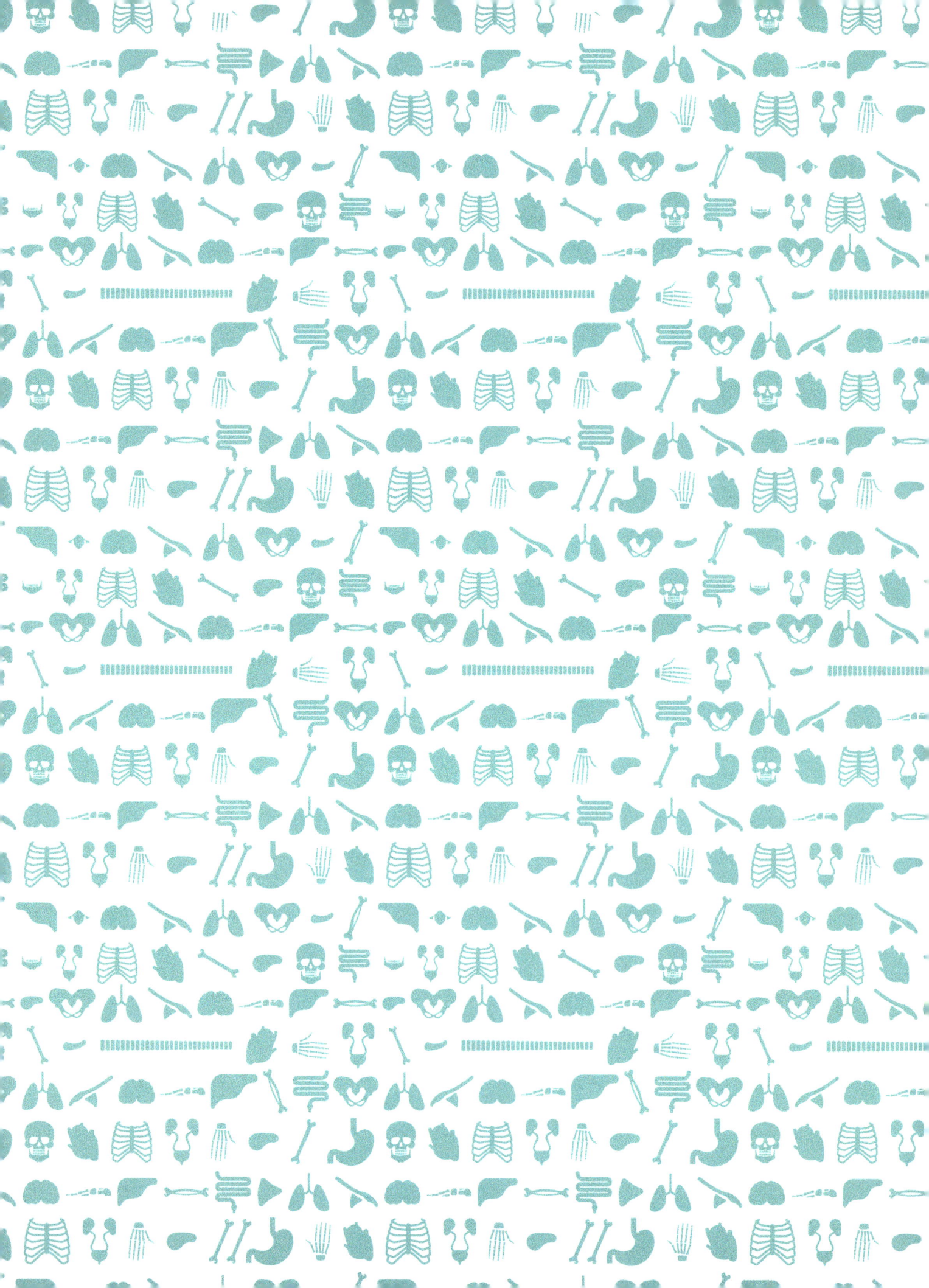

CONNECTABLE SKELETON

Instructions

The human skeletal system consists of bones, cartilage, ligaments and tendons and accounts for about 20 percent of the body weight. Bones provide a rigid framework, known as the skeleton, that support and protect the soft organs of the body. This activity helps the child visually learn what a human skeleton looks like and where the major bone(s) are located. Use the included bone templates. Laminate for protection (optional). Cut out each bone or bone groups. Assemble the cutout bones. Use a hole punch to punch holes in the indicated areas; this is where the bones will attach together. Use brads to connect the bones together - for younger children, assist them with a picture of a completed template. During the assembly process, discuss the bones of the human body. Have the child point to their skull or femur for instance. What happens if a bone breaks? For pre-school sized children, compare the completed skeleton to their body.

Materials

- Bone Templates
- Laminator (optional)
- Scissors
- Hole Punch
- Brads

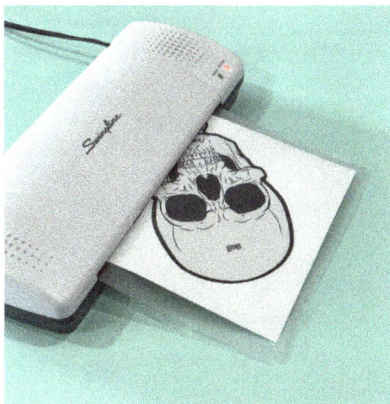

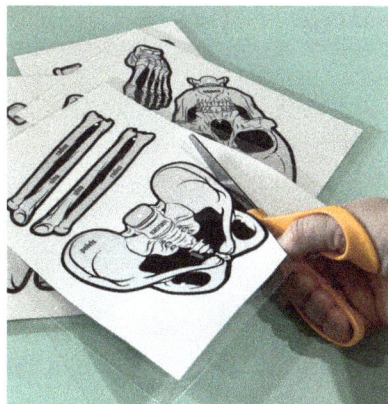

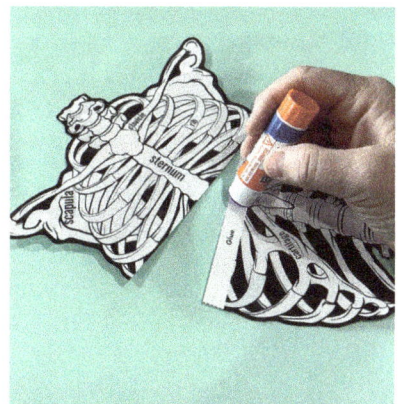

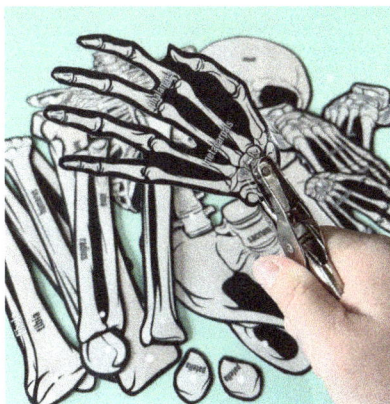

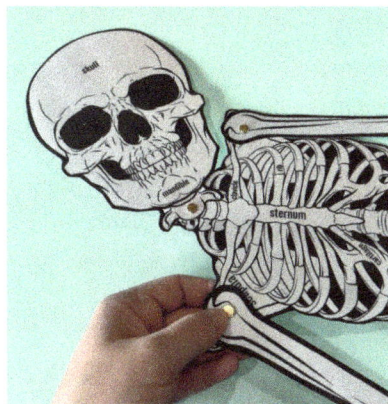

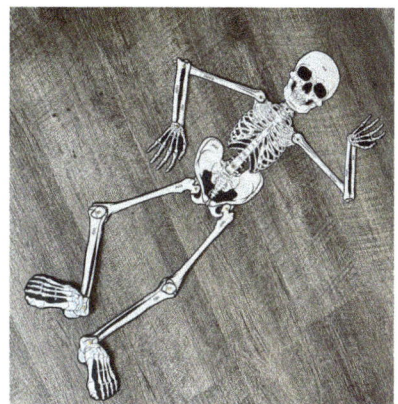

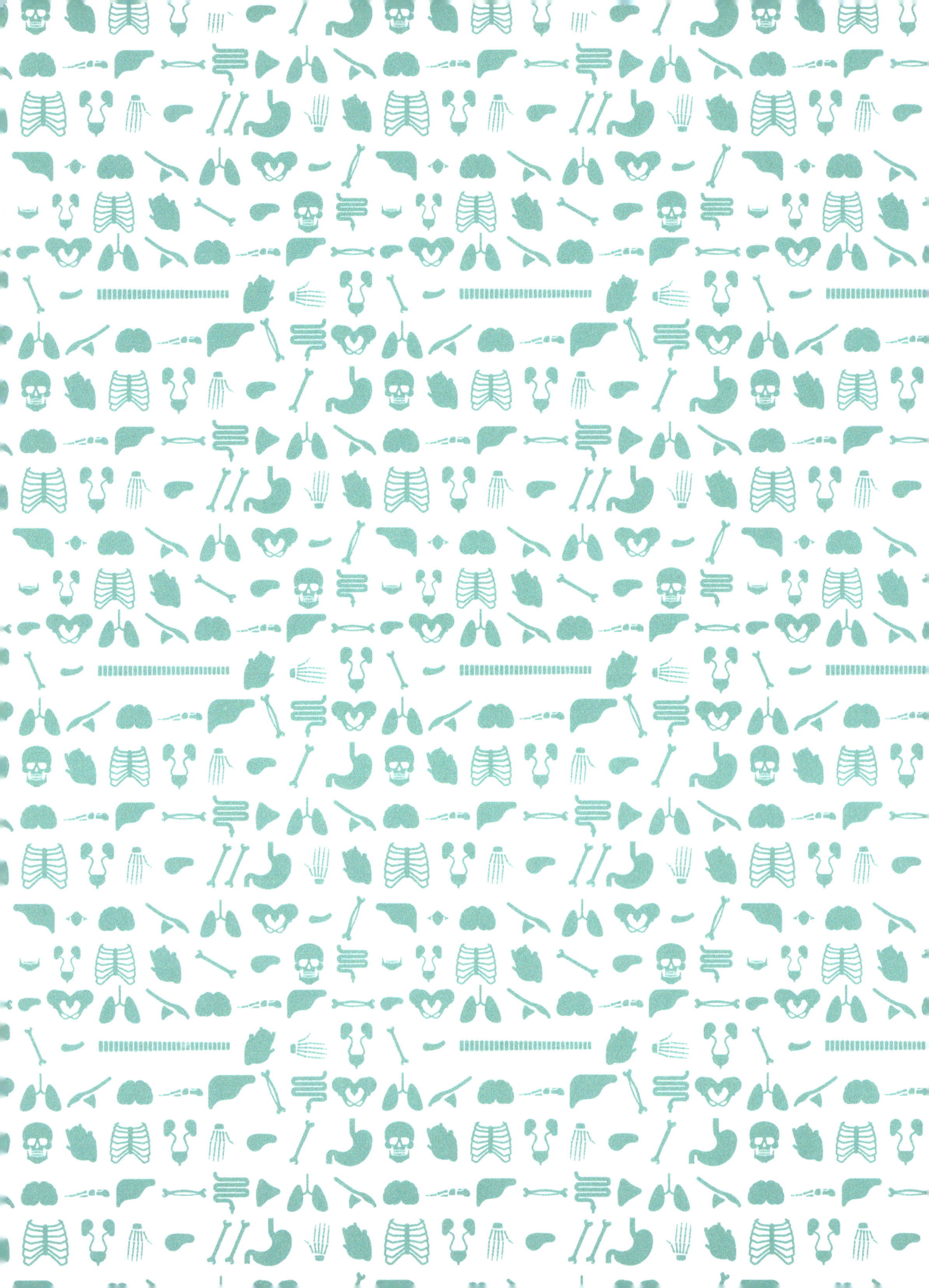

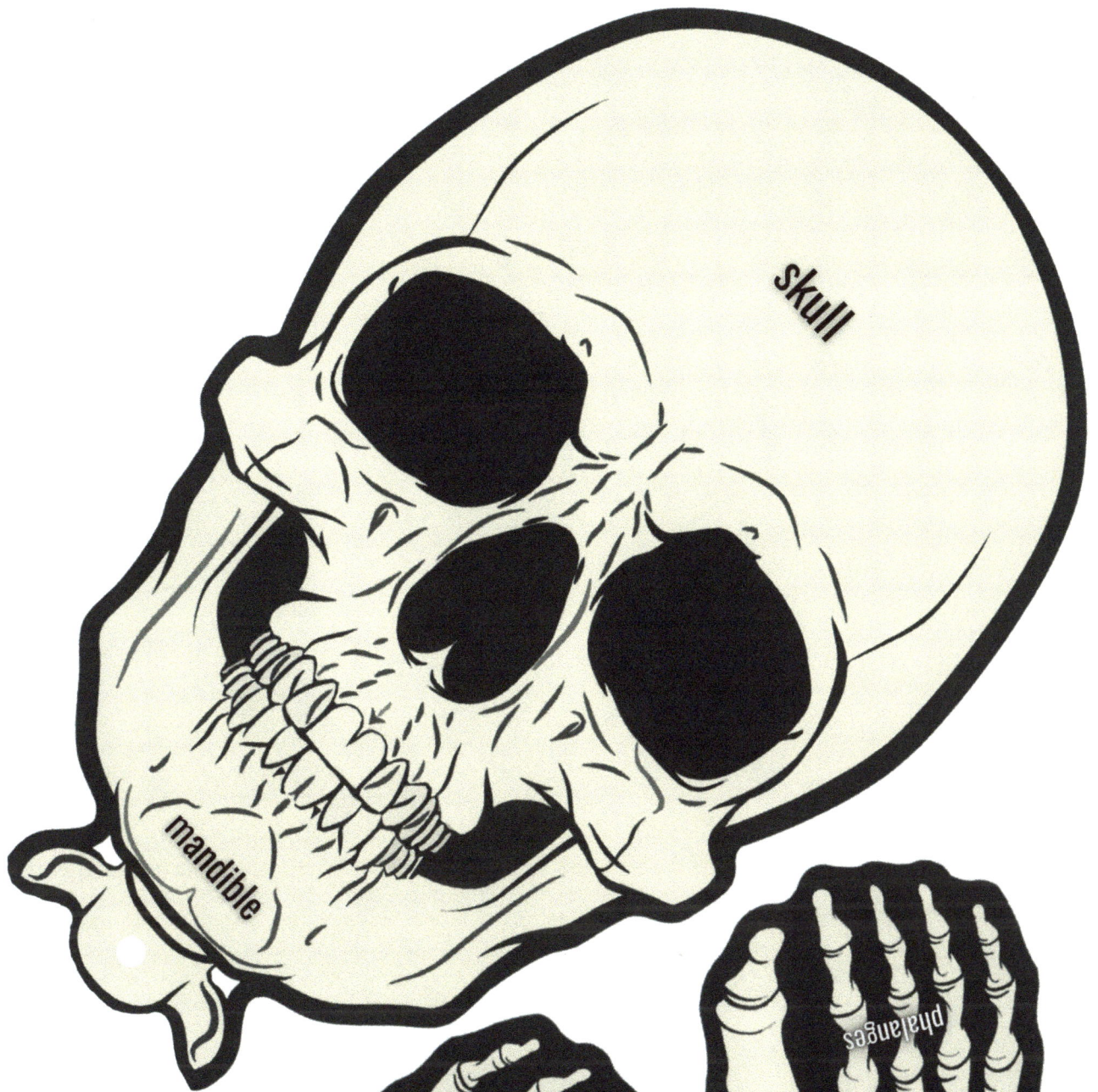

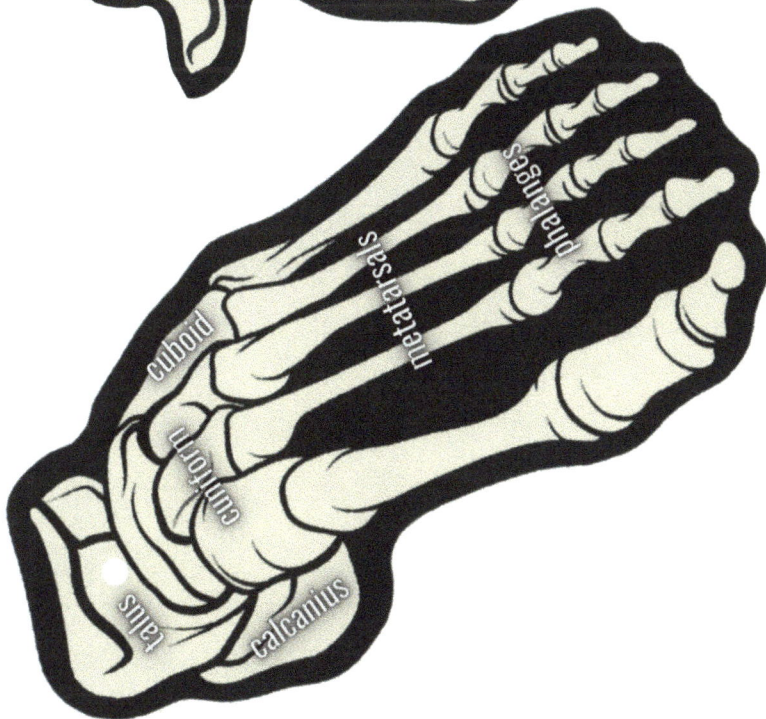

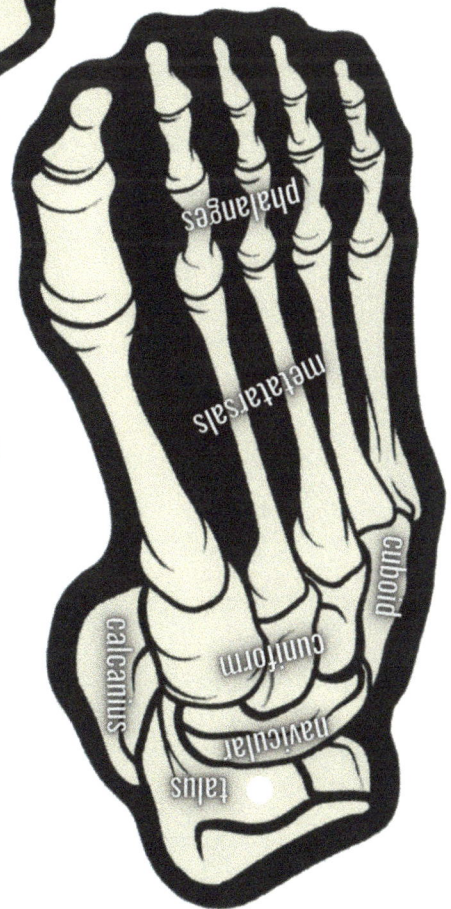

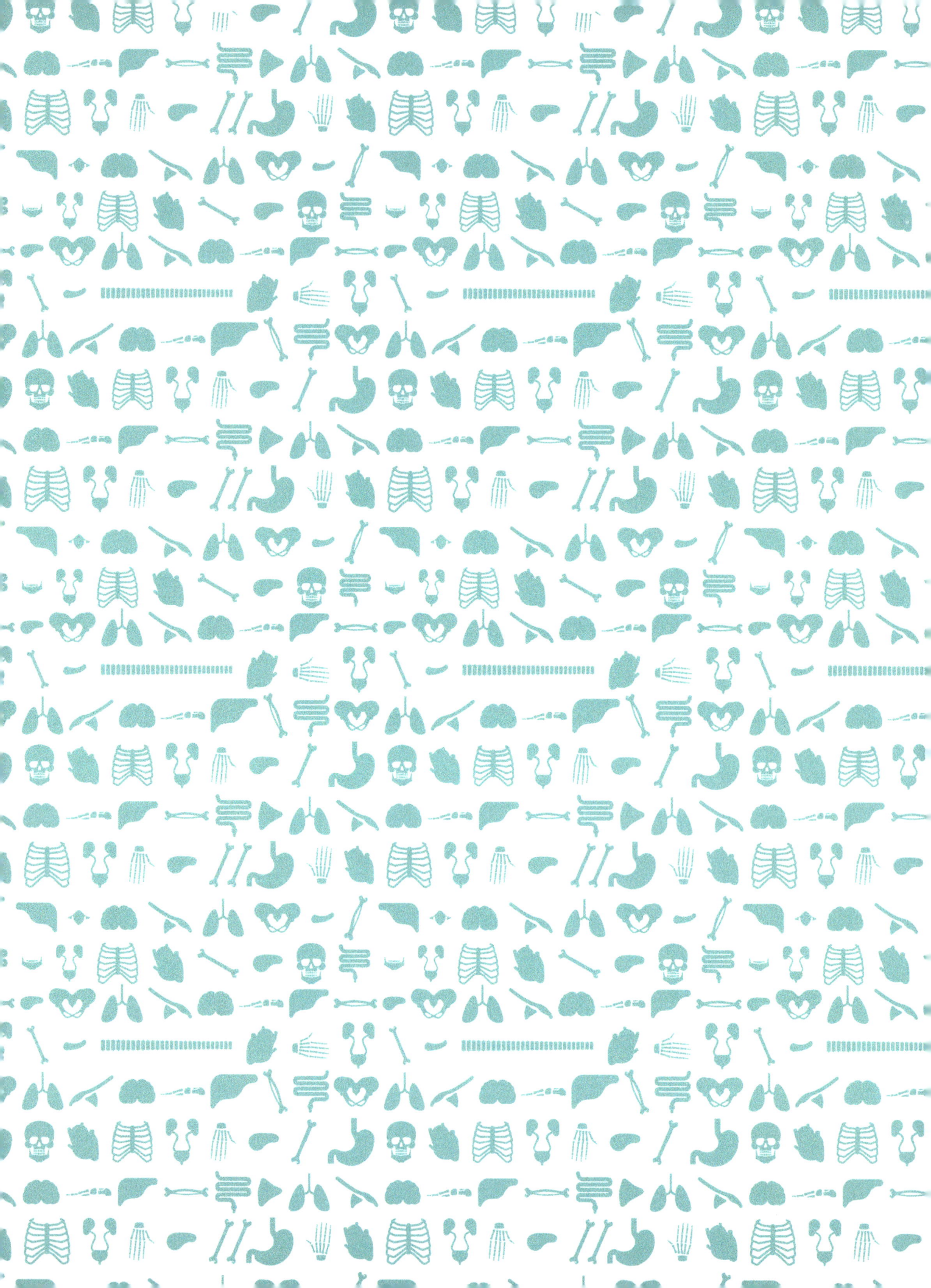

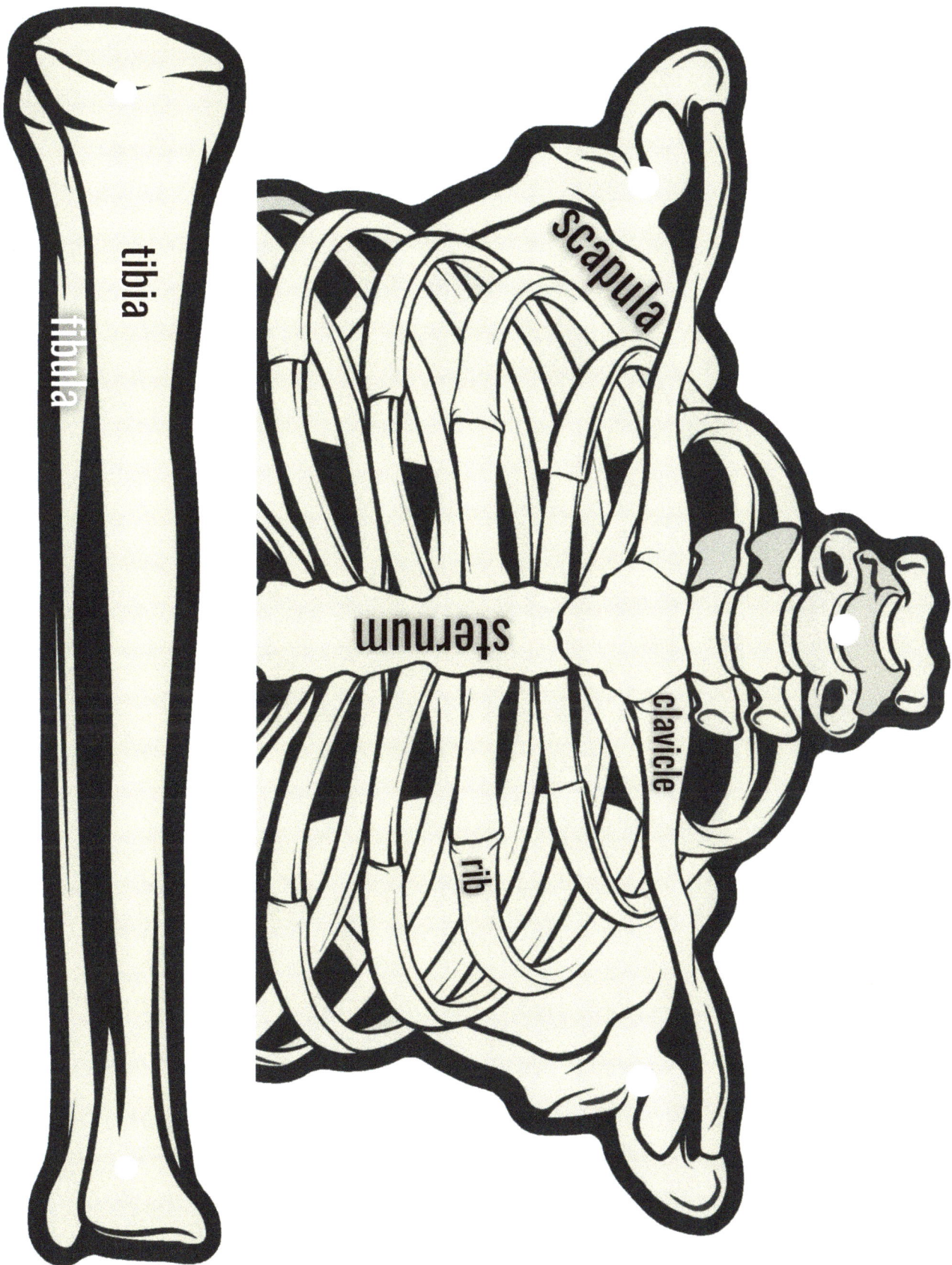

tibia

fibula

scapula

sternum

clavicle

rib

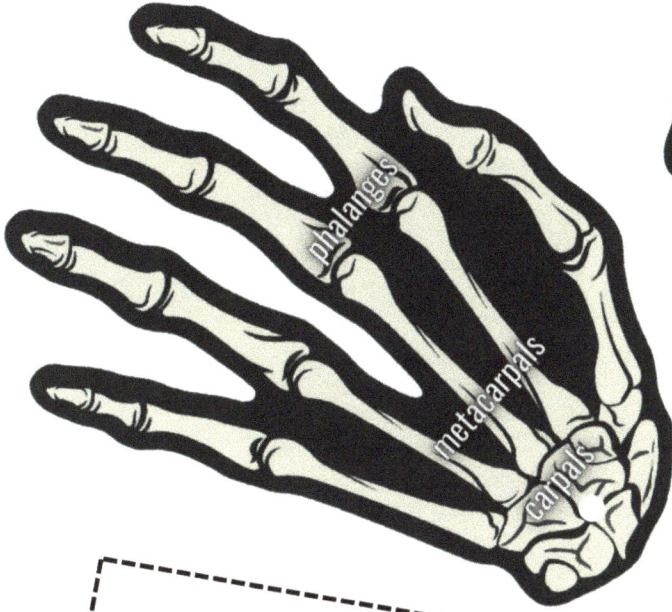

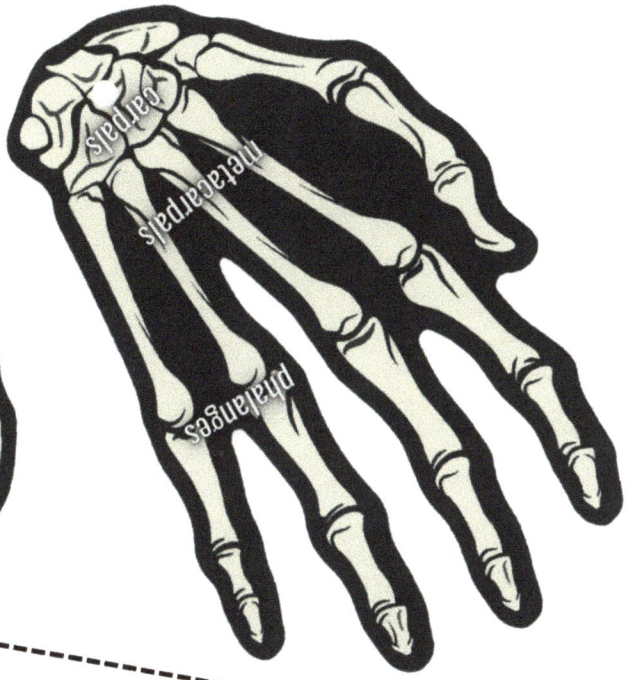

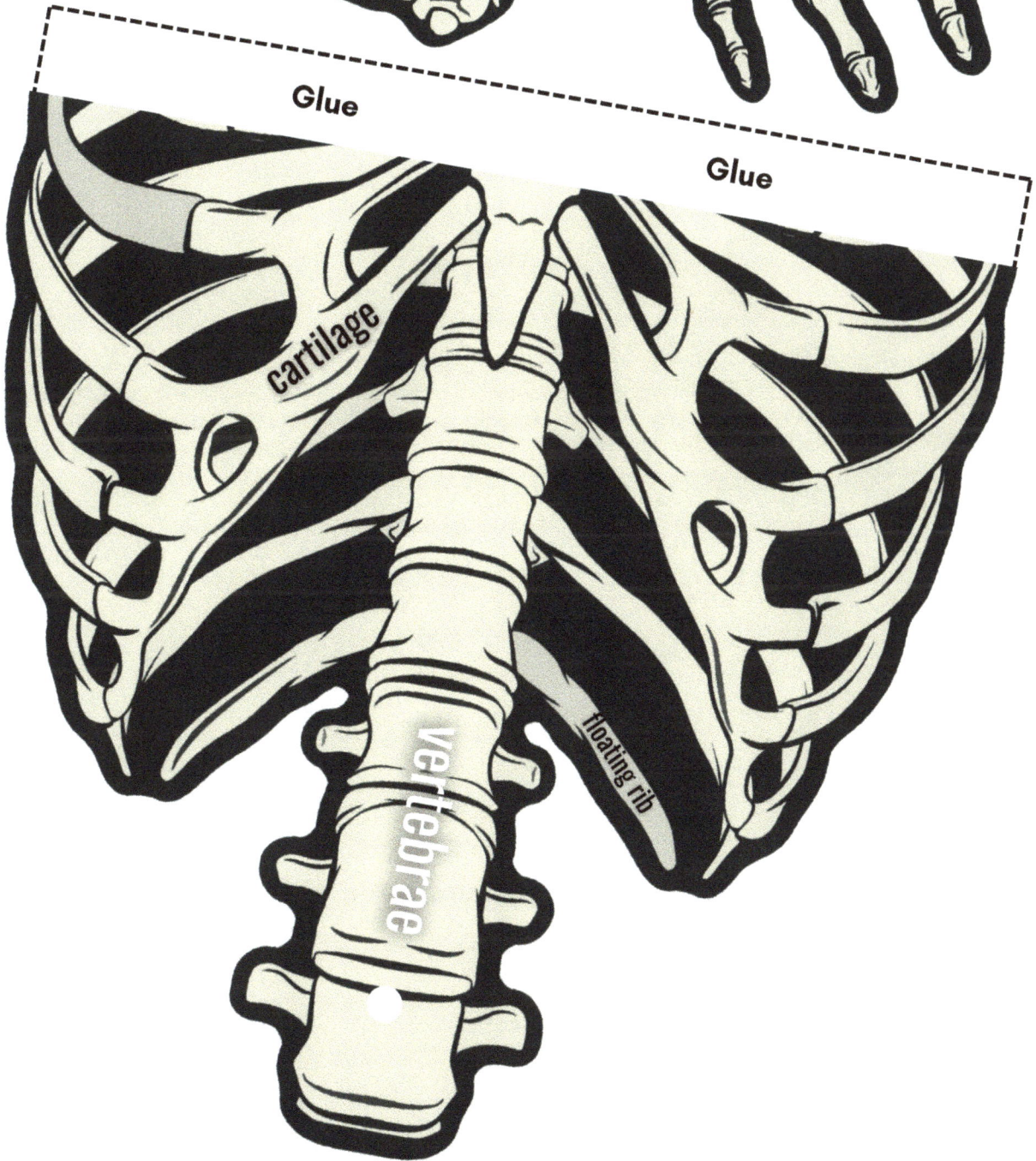

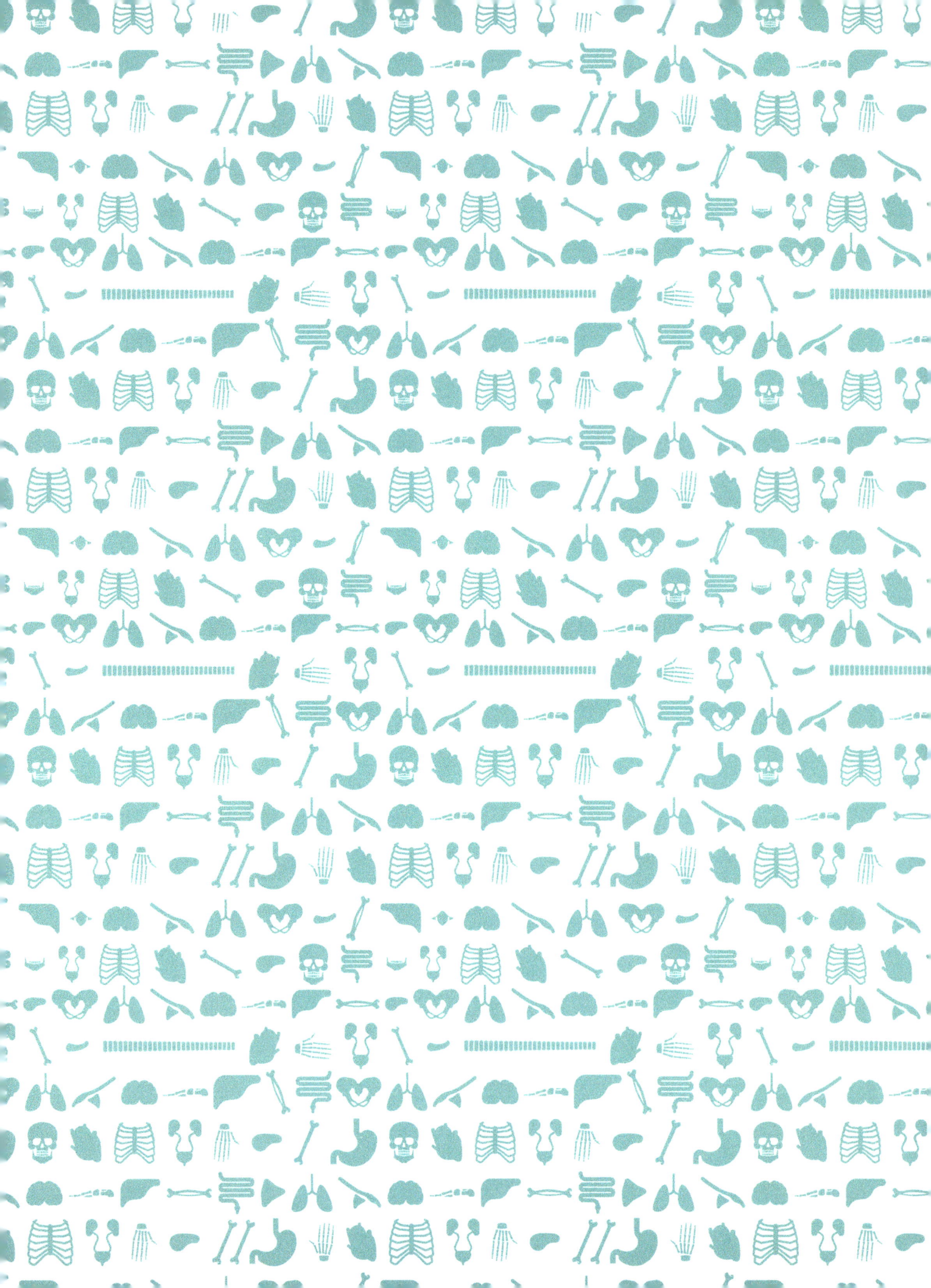

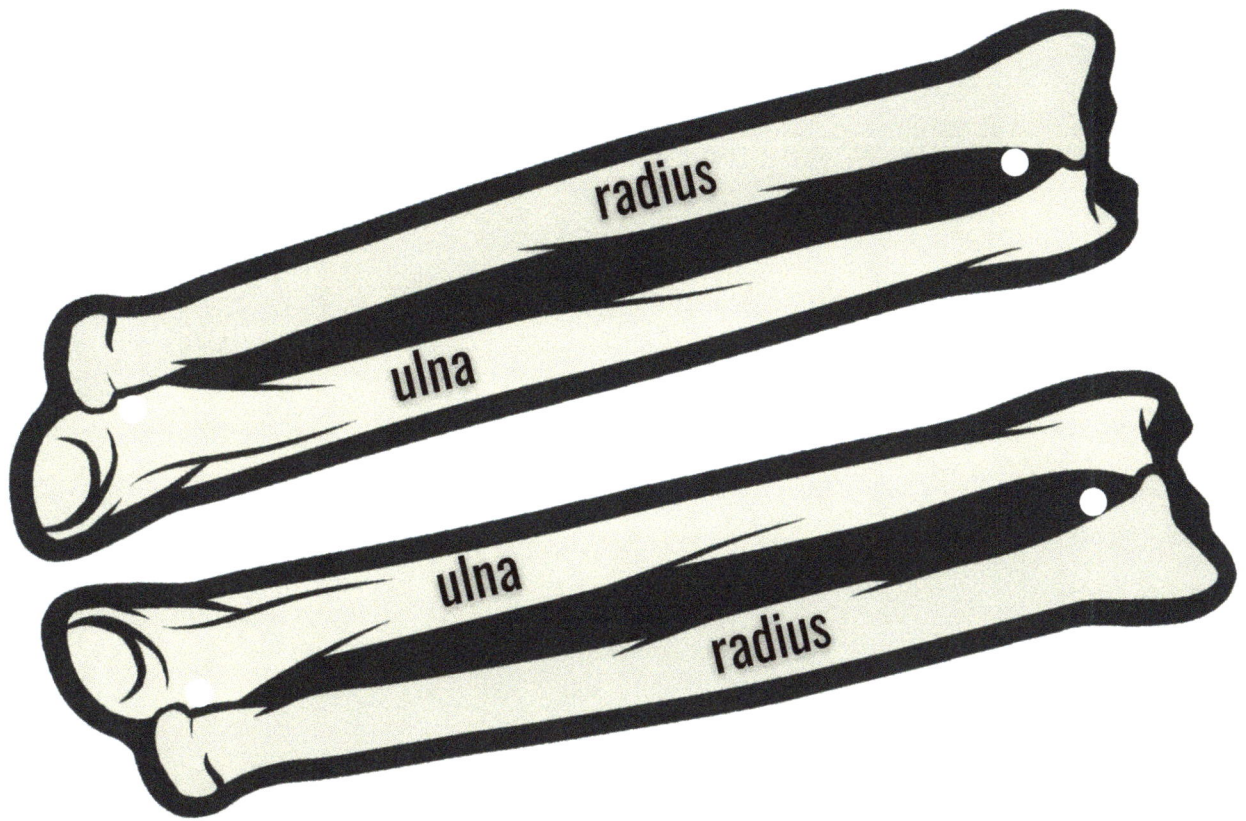

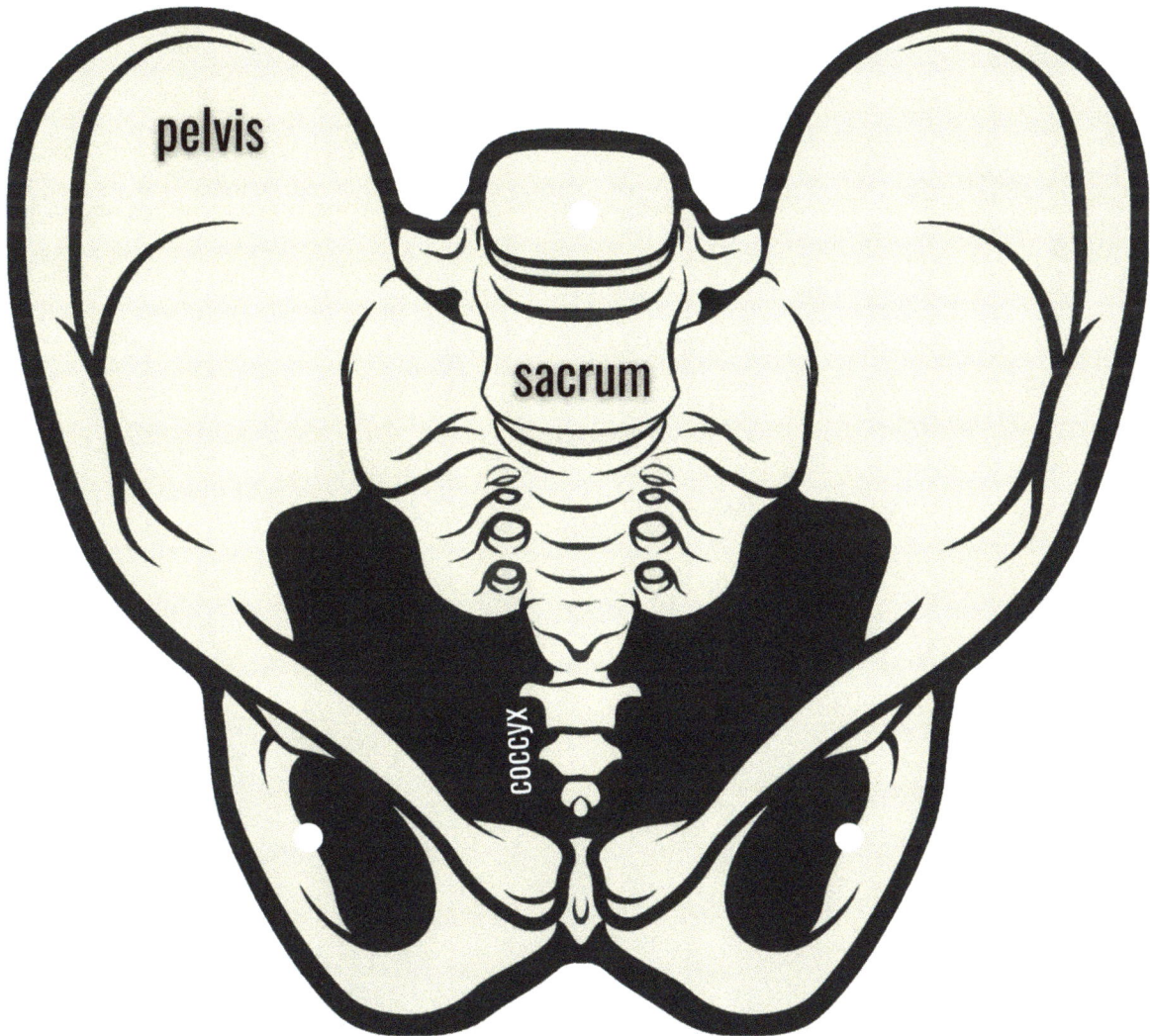

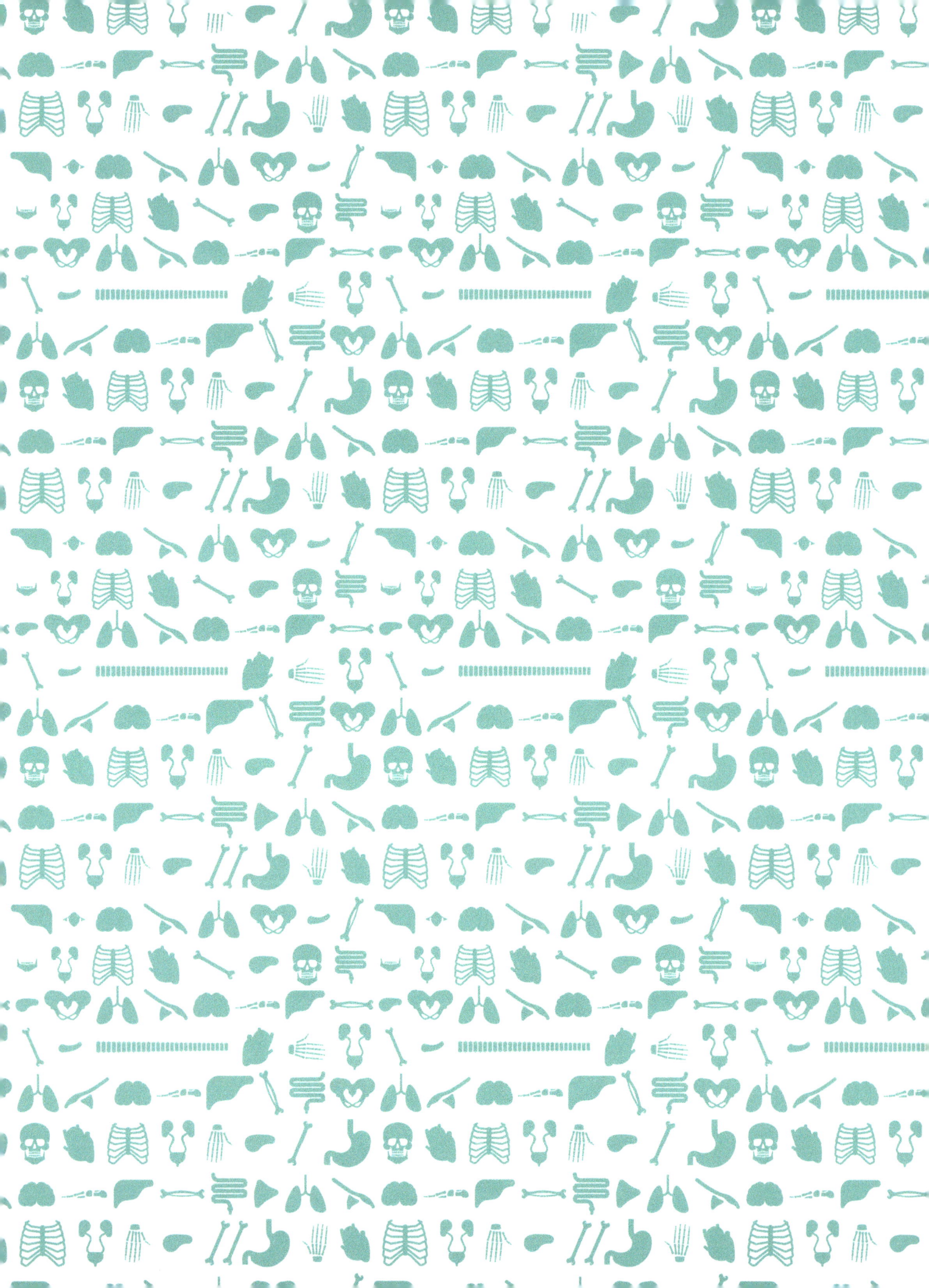

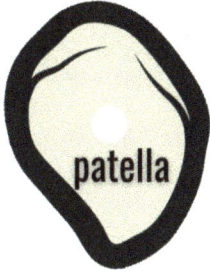

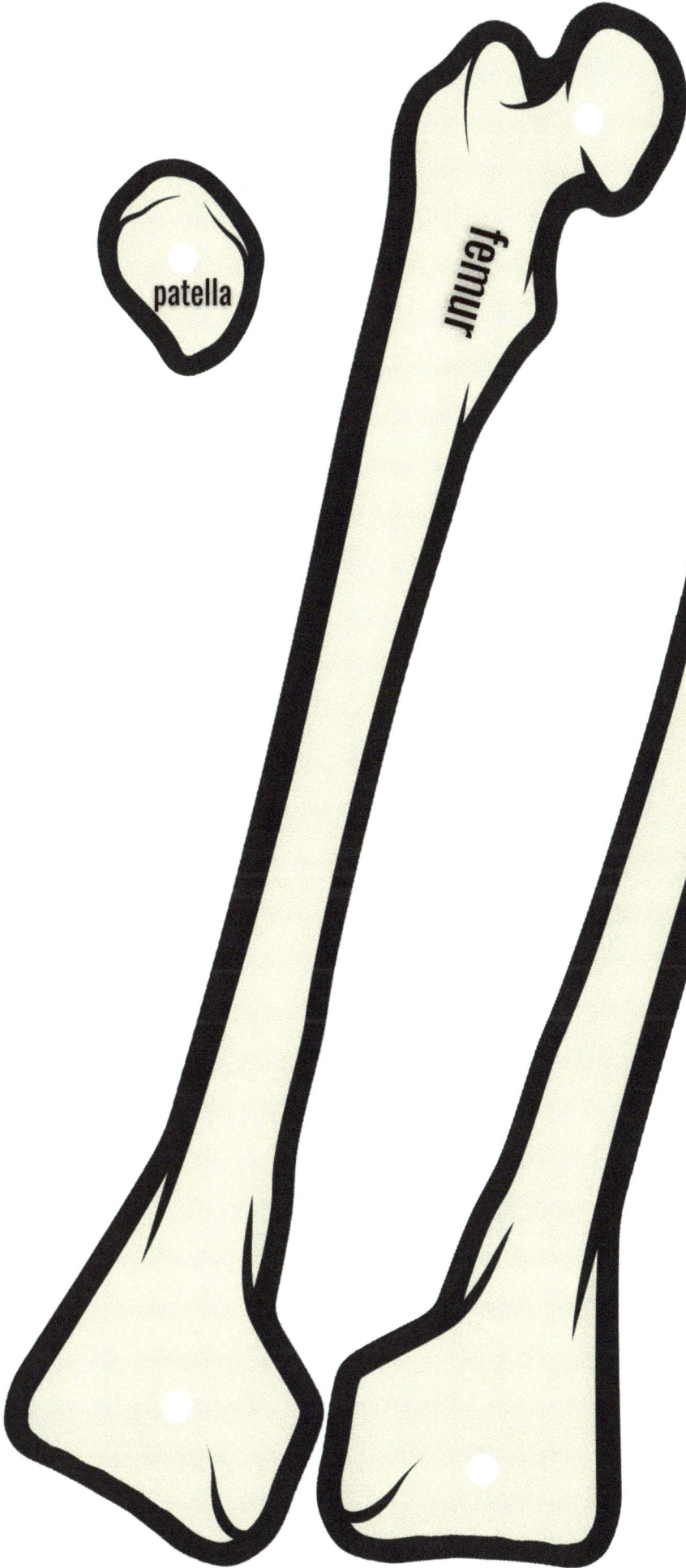

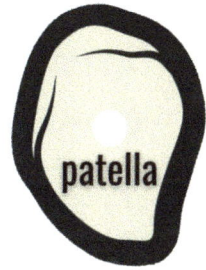

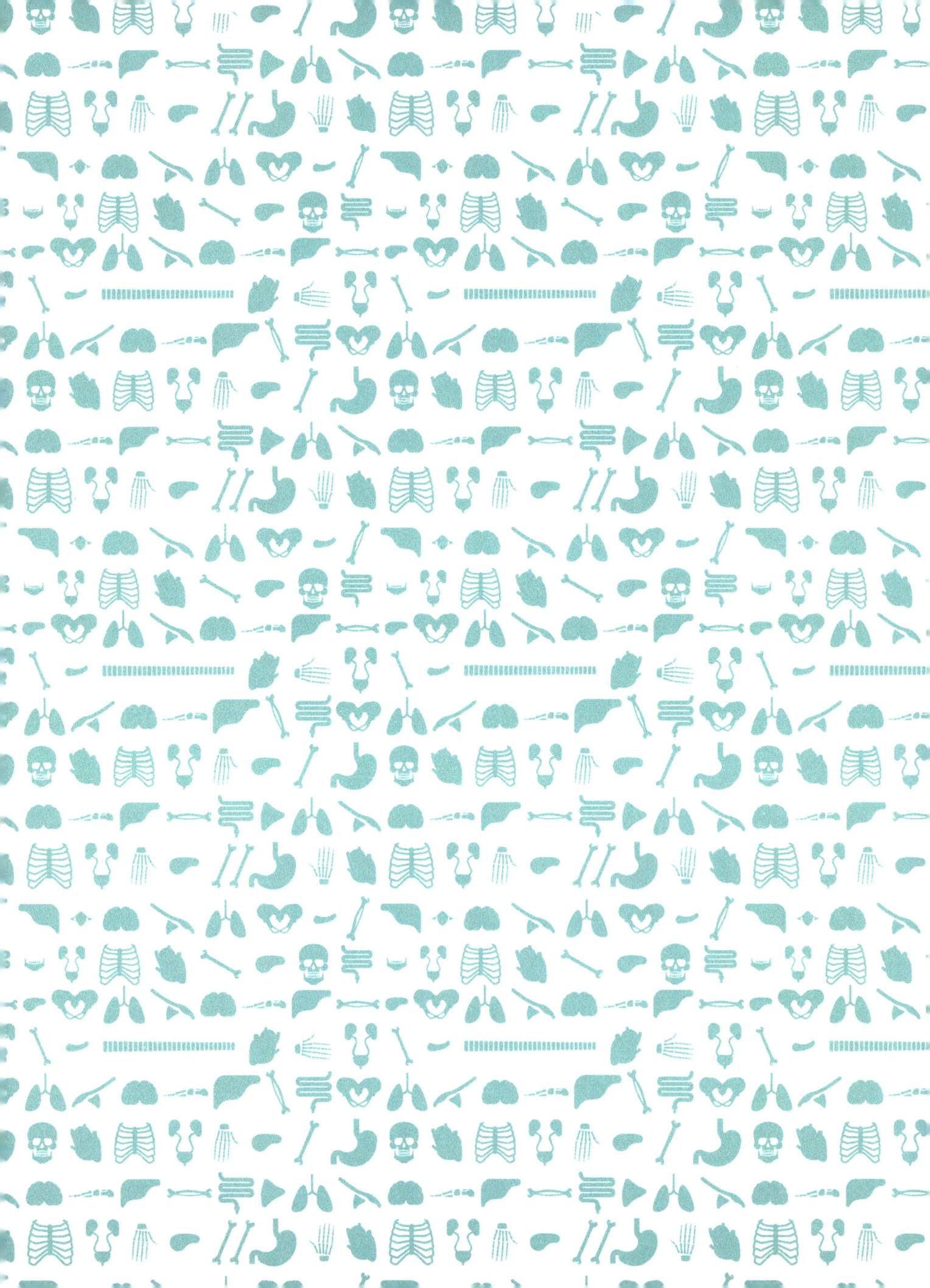

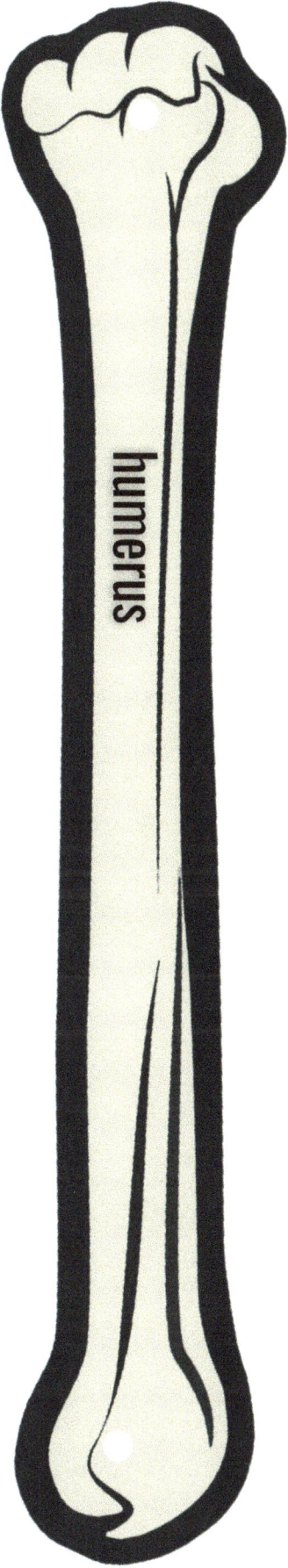

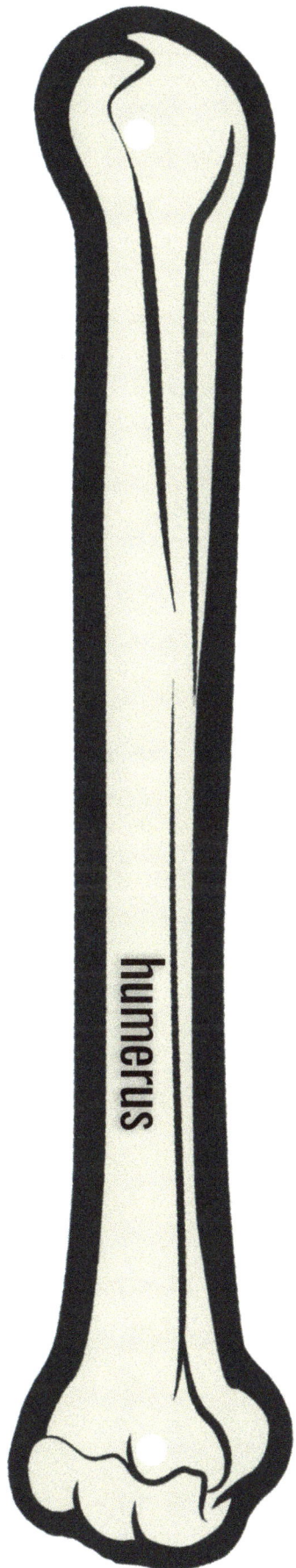

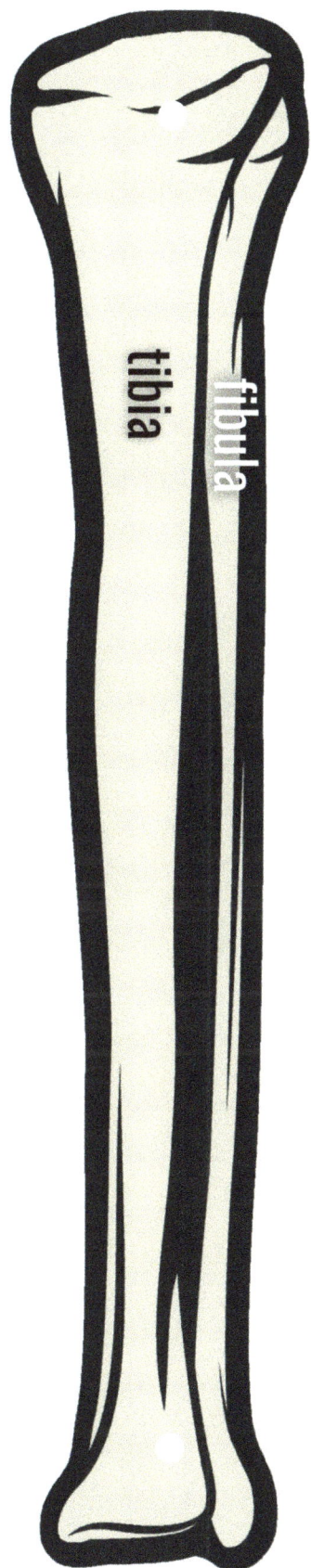

humerus

humerus

tibia

fibula

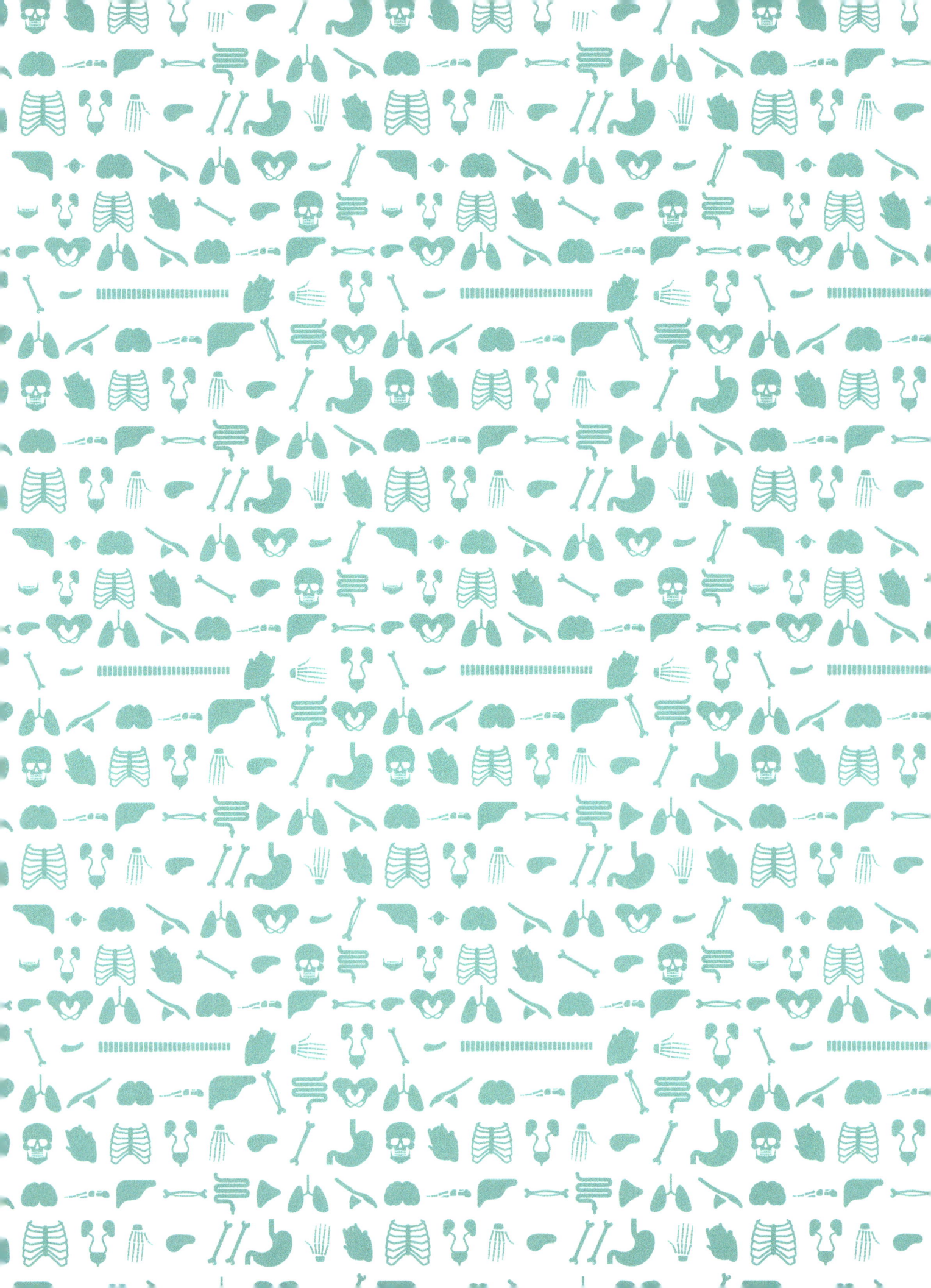

DRY ERASE TEETH BRUSHING

Instructions

Teeth are part of the skeletal system, and perform an important step in digestion. Brushing teeth is important to remove food and plaque, a sticky white film that forms on your teeth and contains bacteria. Most meals contain at least trace amounts of sugar, and the bacteria in plaque produce acids that attack tooth enamel. Over time this can lead to dental cavities, which is the formation of holes on the teeth, a condition that can result in a tooth loss.

Laminate the included teeth template. Cut out if desired. Using a dry erase marker, color in food particles and plaque. Provide the child with illustration and a toothbrush and have them "brush" the plaque and food away. **Discuss:** how important this is to take good care of one's teeth? What happens if you don't brush regularly?

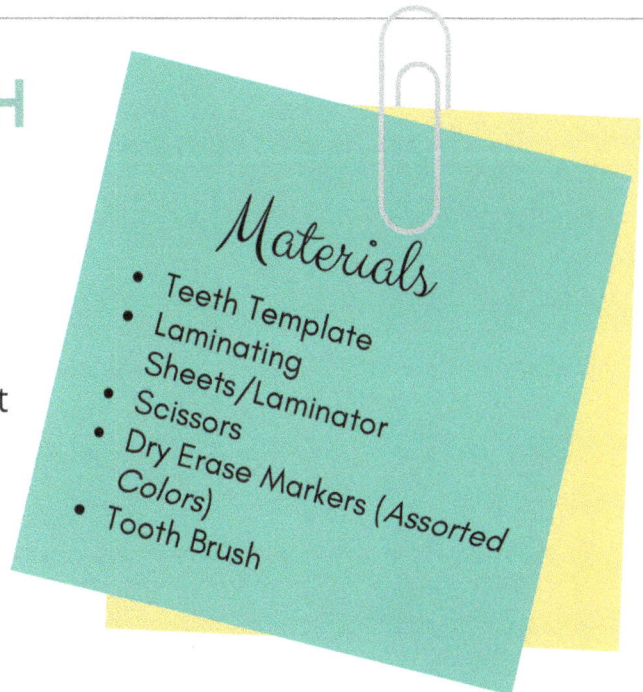

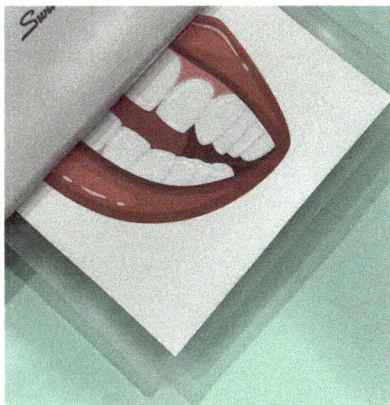

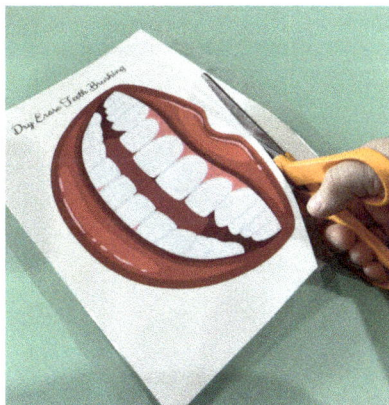

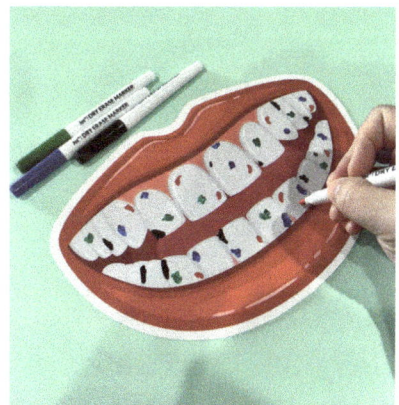

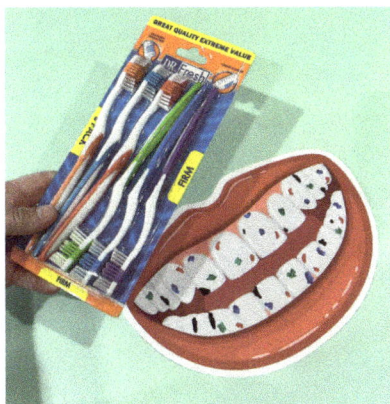

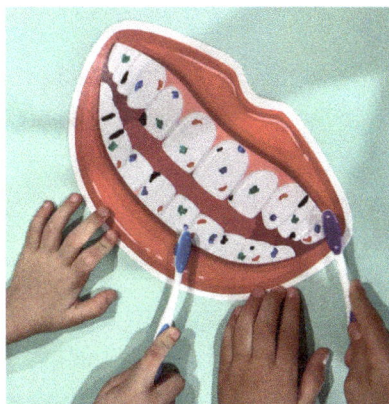

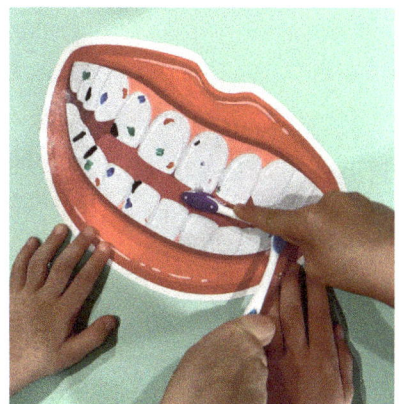

Materials

- Teeth Template
- Laminating Sheets/Laminator
- Scissors
- Dry Erase Markers (Assorted Colors)
- Tooth Brush

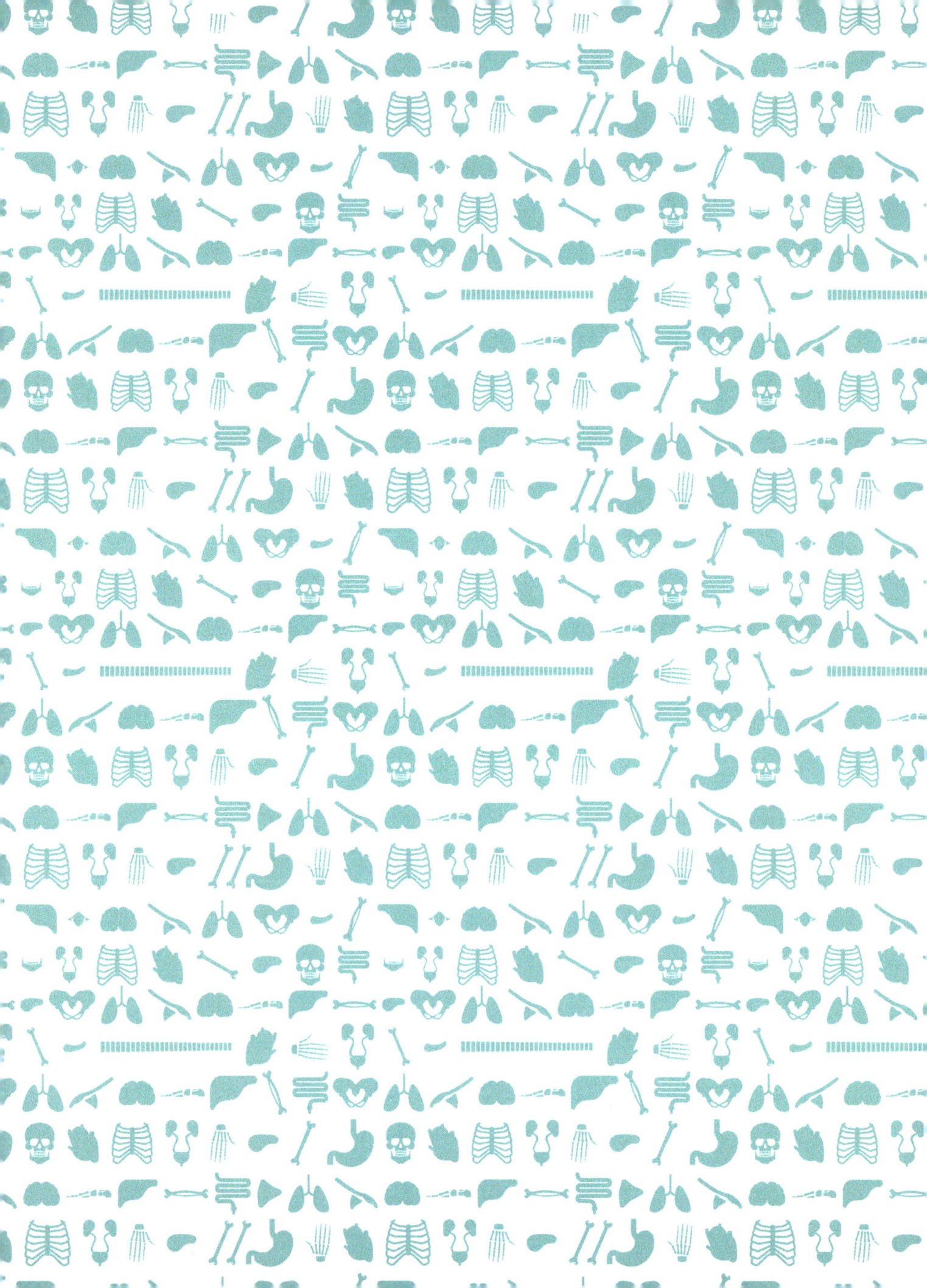

Dry Erase Teeth Brushing

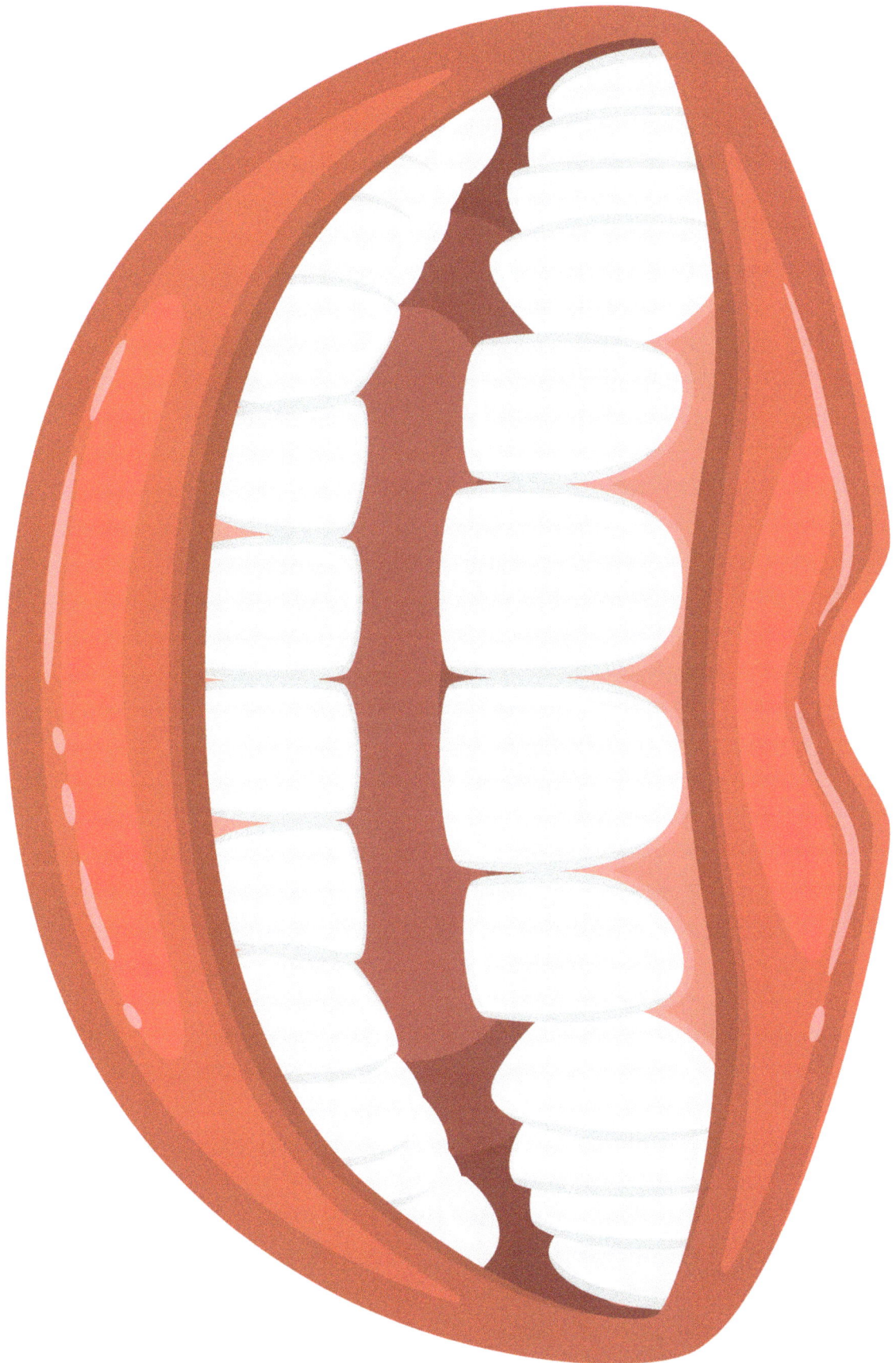

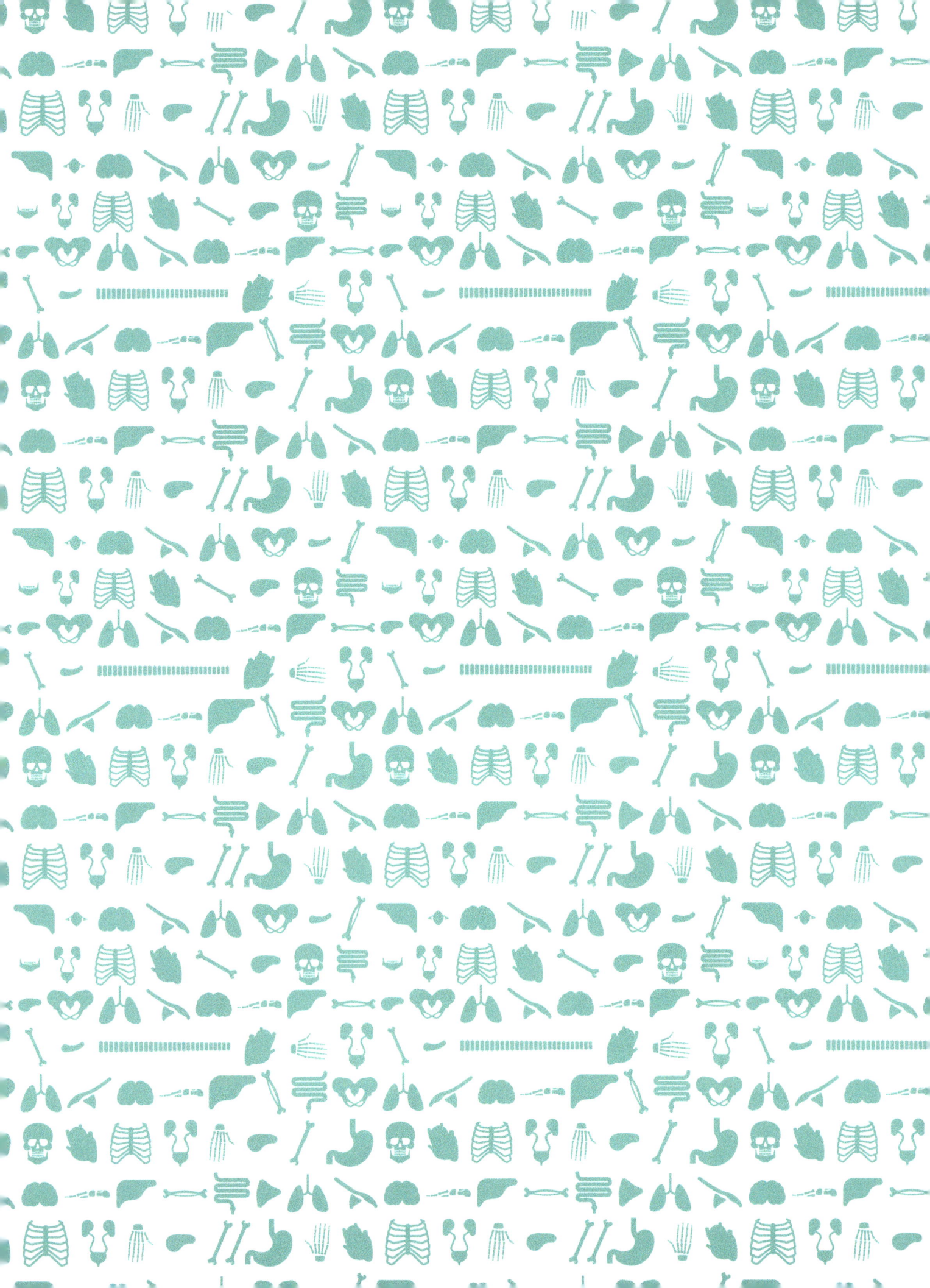

ARTICULATING HAND MODEL

Instructions

The human body has 360 joints. Joints are found between skeletal bones. In the human hand, alone, there 27 joints alone, which provide exceptional movement that allows the hands to move in such diverse ways.

Cut out included hand illustration. Cut 0.5-1" sections of straws and glue pieces as indicated areas along the phalanges and metacarpals of the model. Thread string or yarn through each of these sections and secure by knotting at the end or gluing to the fingertips. Allow to dry completely if gluing before articulating the hand. Pull the bottom of the strings to flex or extend (by releasing) the fingers. Pull all the strings at once to move the fingers all together. Compare with the movement of a real hand. Flex and extend each finger individually. Flex and extend all fingers at once.

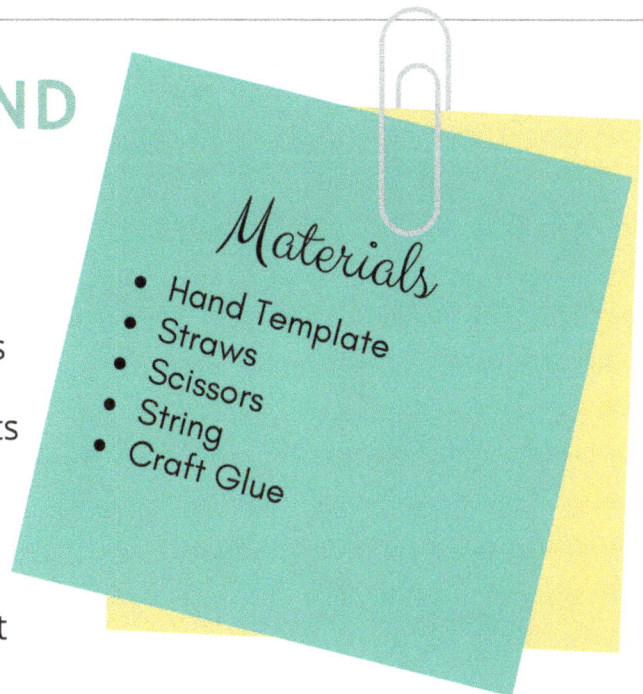

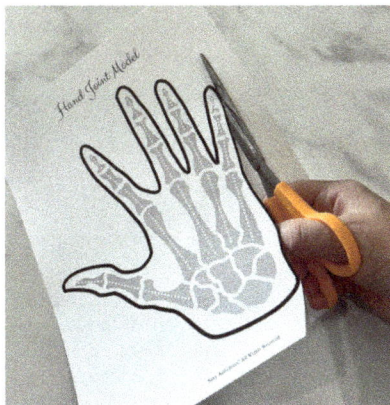

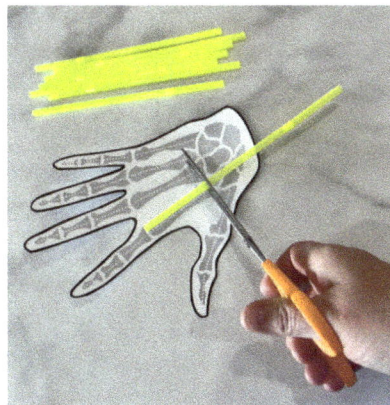

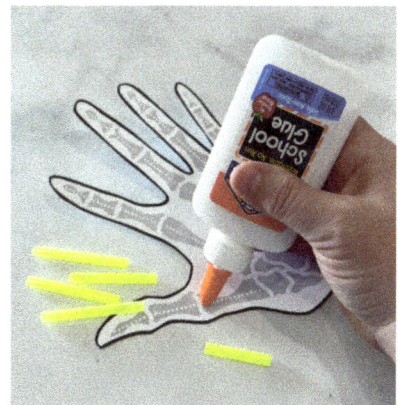

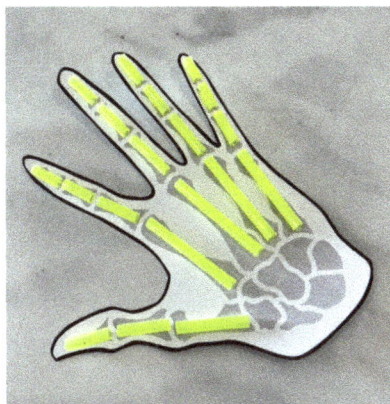

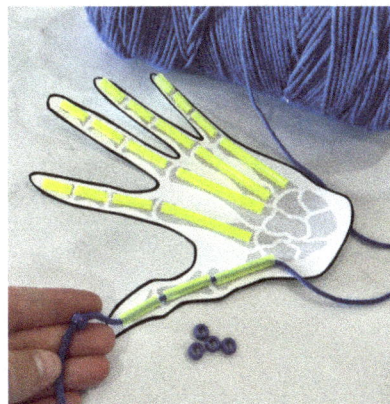

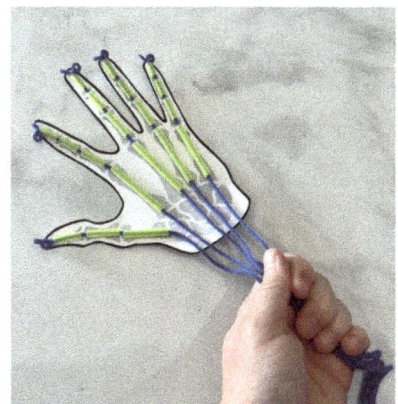

Materials

- Hand Template
- Straws
- Scissors
- String
- Craft Glue

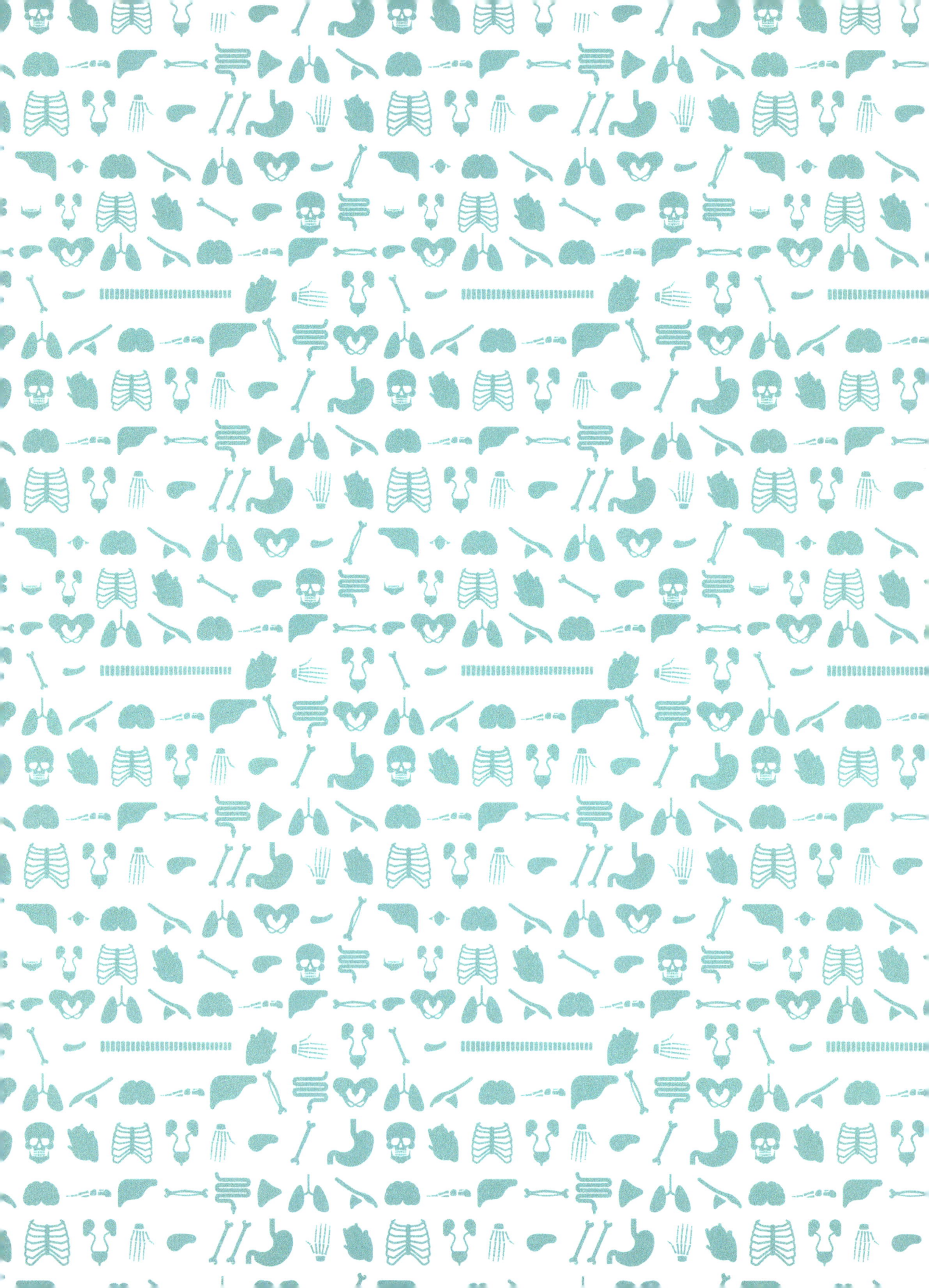

Hand Joint Model

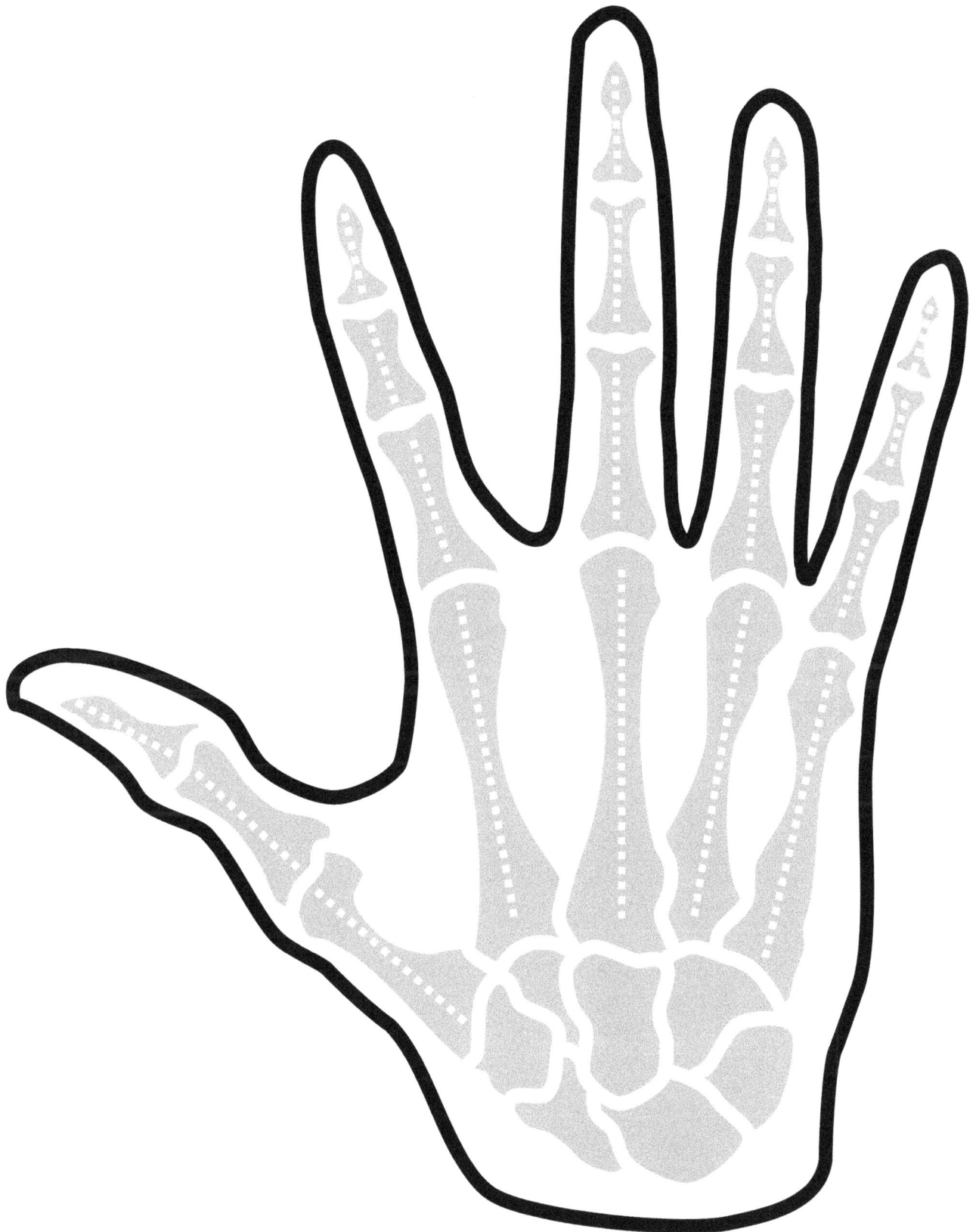

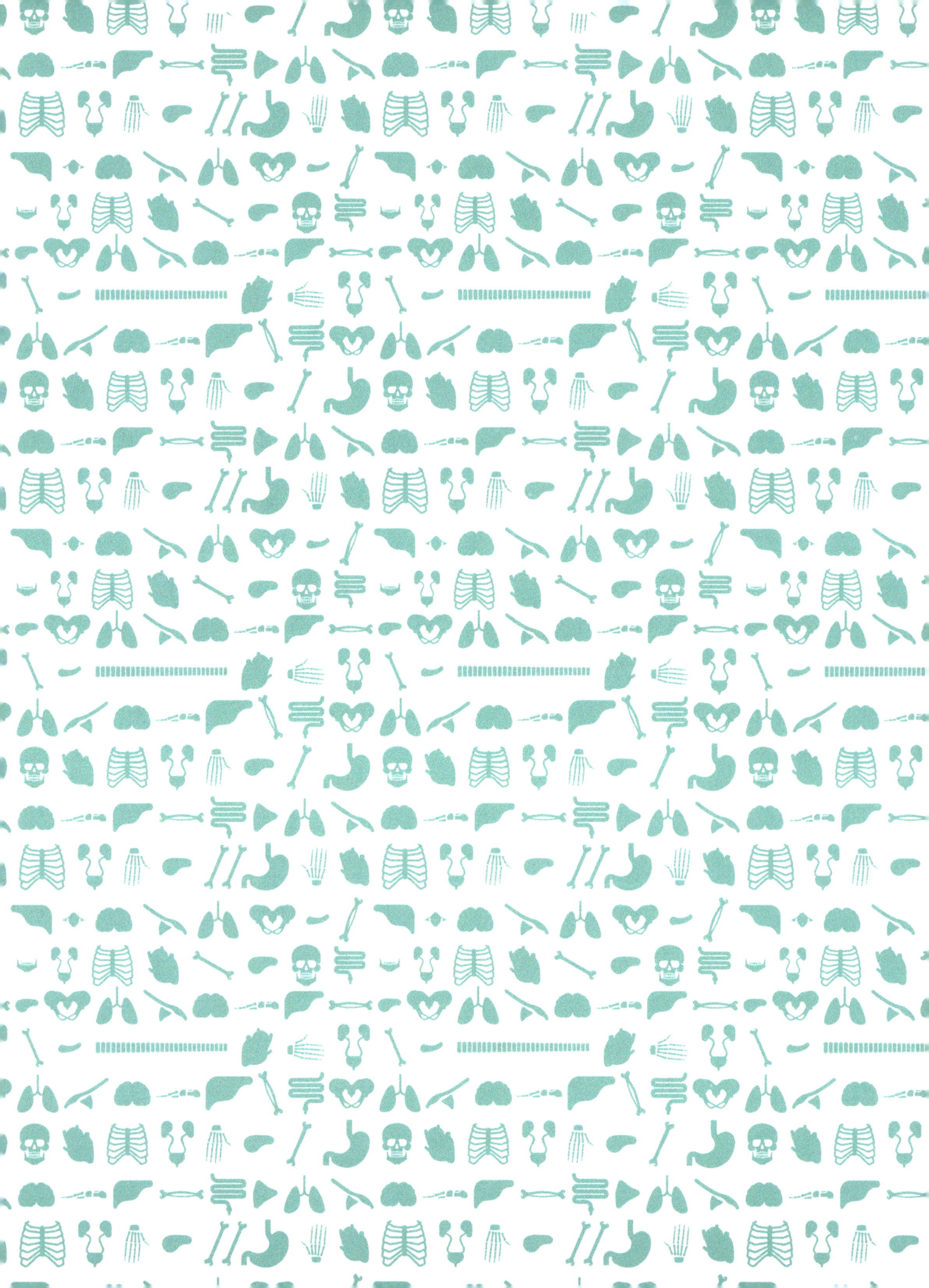

Joint Types Cards

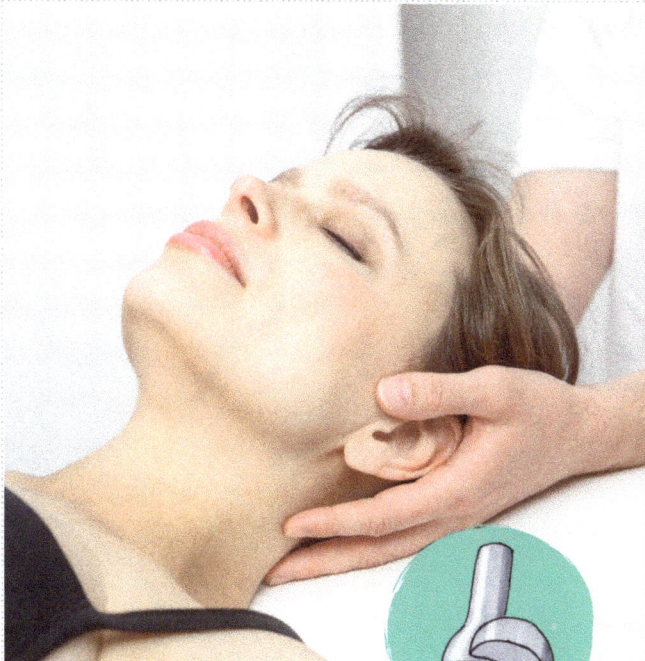
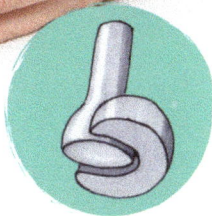

Pivot Joint

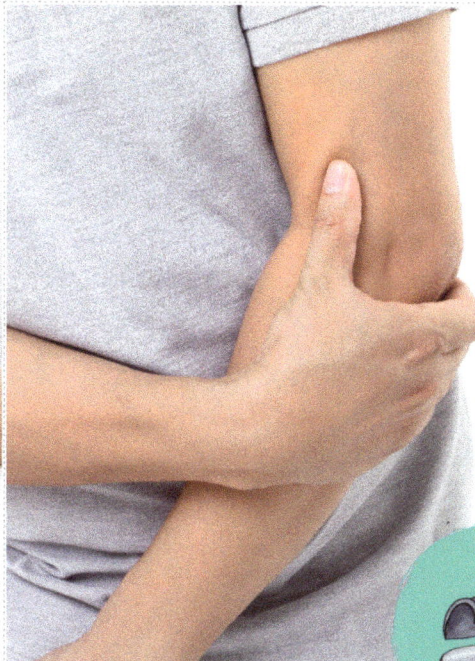
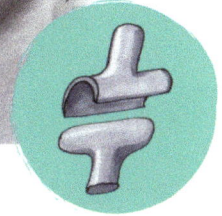

Hinge Joint

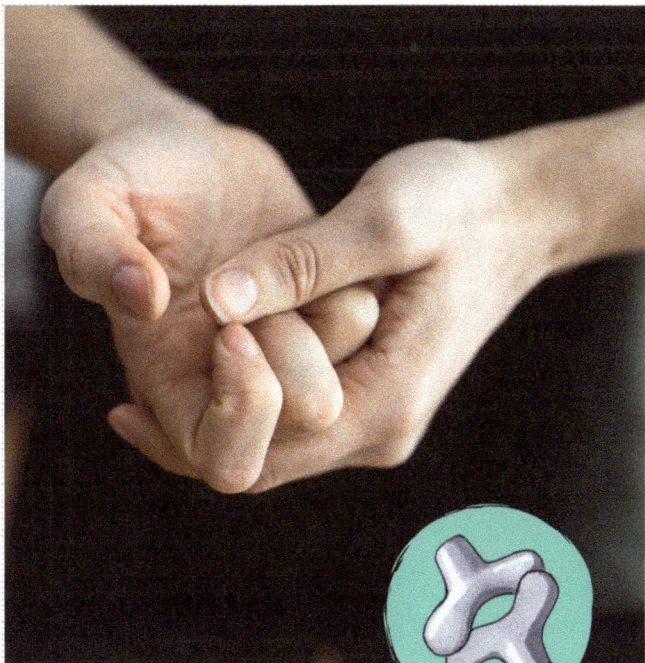
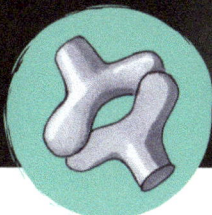

Saddle Joint

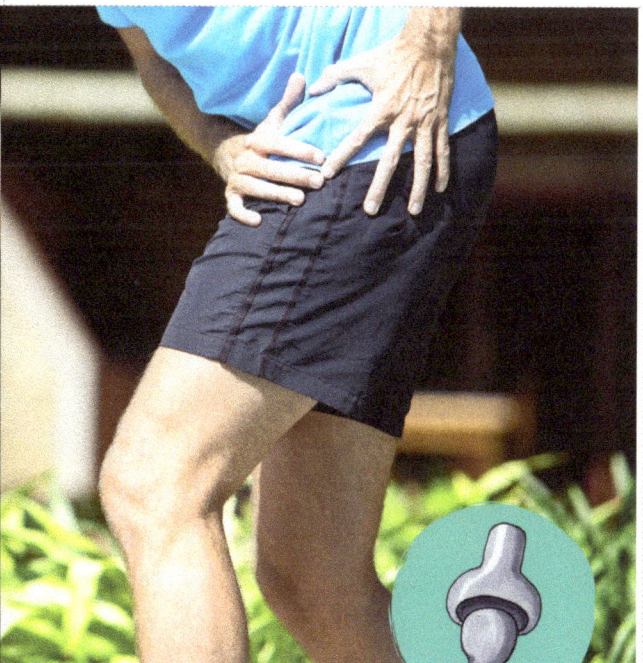
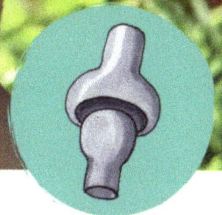

Ball & Socket Joint

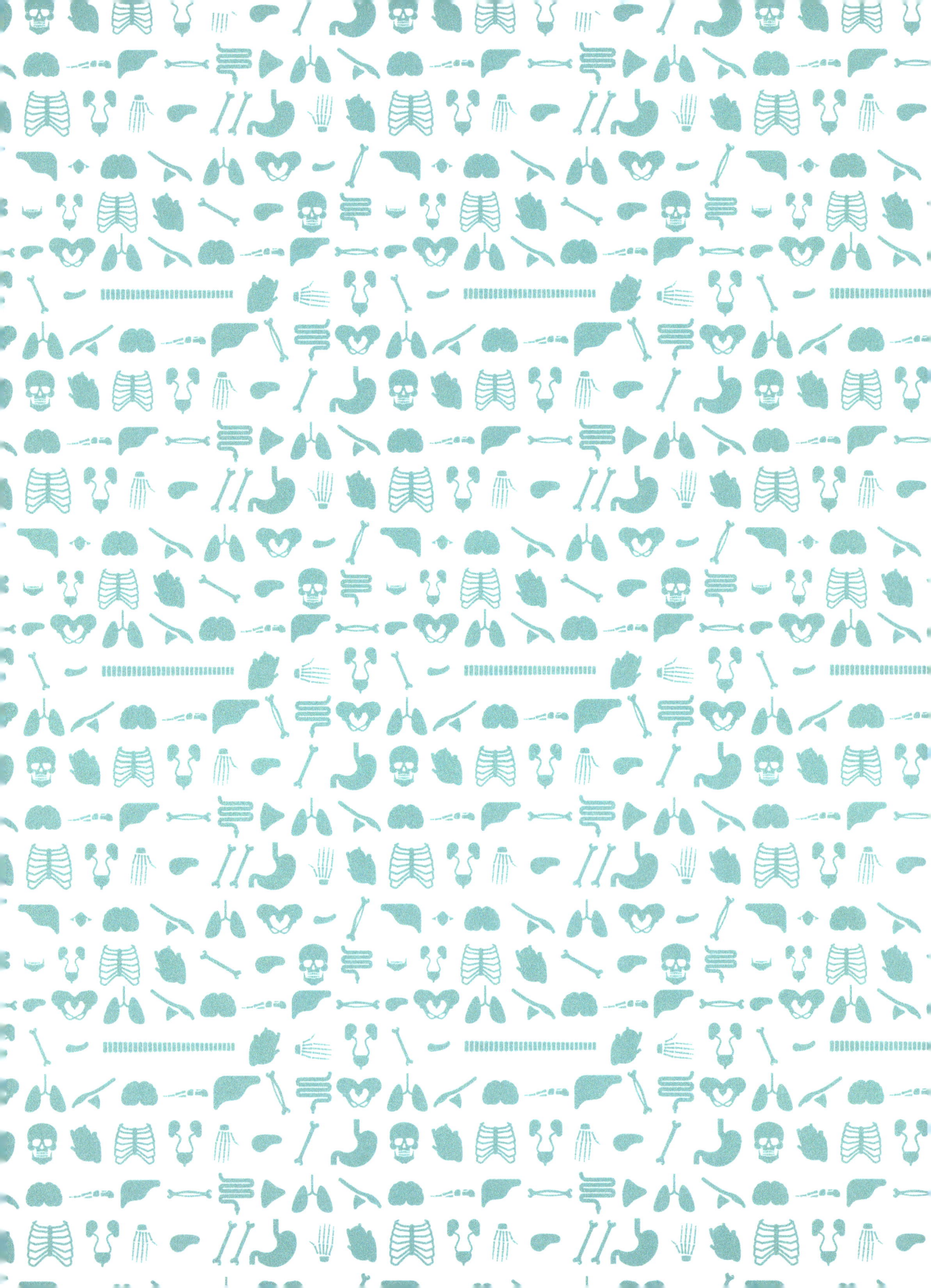

Joint Types Cards

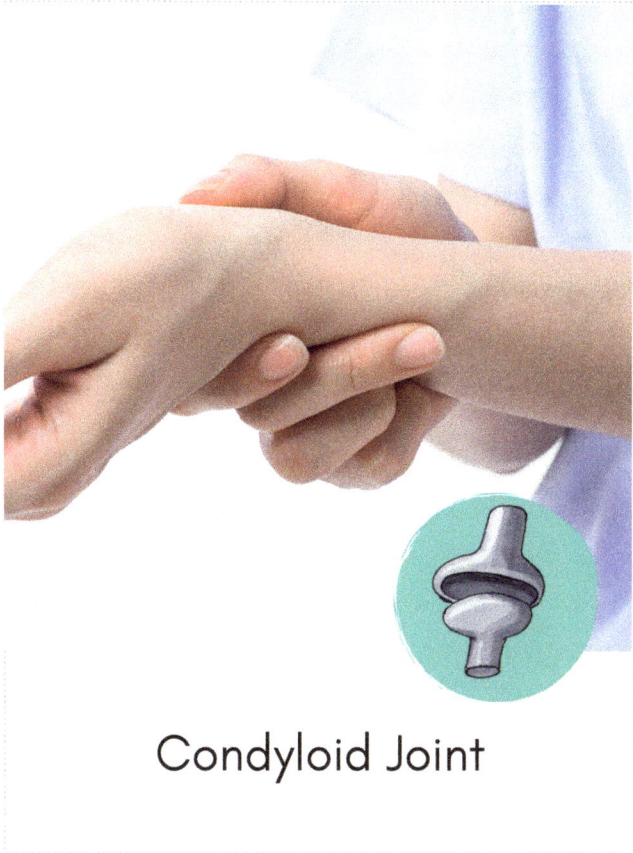

Condyloid Joint

Arm Muscle Model

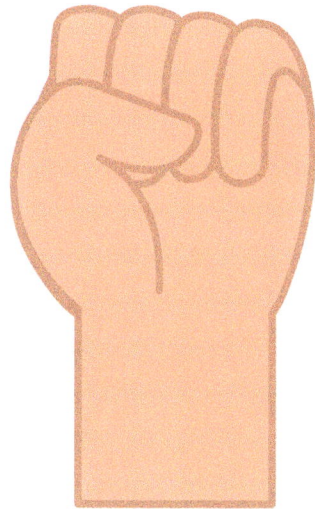

Concentric – Muscle fibers shorten

Eccentric – Muscle fibers lengthen

Isotonic – Muscle fibers remain the same

ARM MUSCLE MODEL

Instructions

The muscular system provides the ability to move throughout the human body. Muscles are attached to the bones of the skeletal system and make up roughly half of a person's body weight. Muscles provide both contraction and resistance during movement. During concentric movement, the muscle fibers shorten as it contracts and alternatively, during eccentric movement, the muscle fibers lengthen as the muscle elongates.

Materials

- Hand Template
- Craft Sticks
- Two Long Balloon (Rubber Band Works too)
- Drill
- Brad

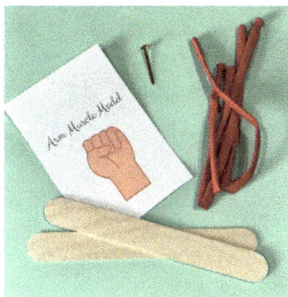

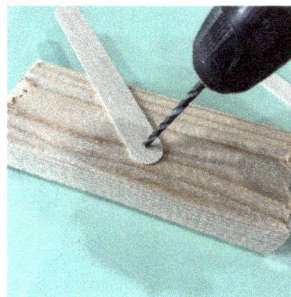

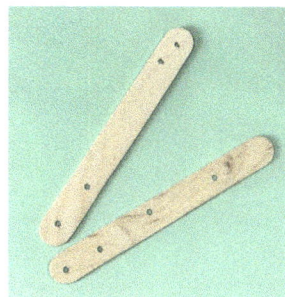

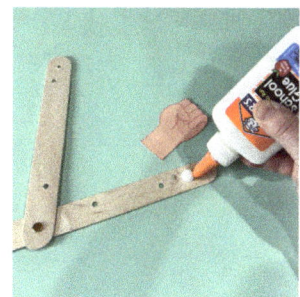

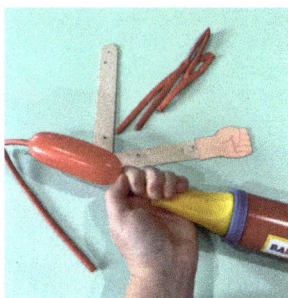

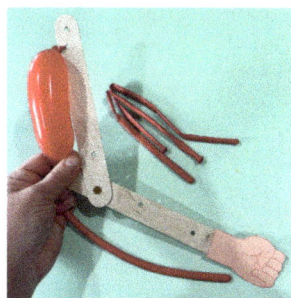

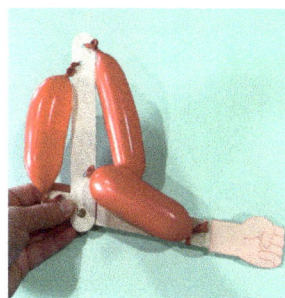

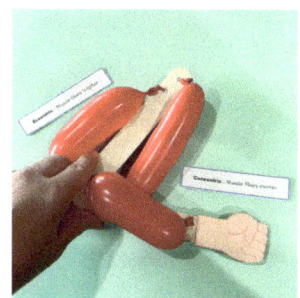

Drill holes as indicated in large craft sticks. Each stick should have four holes as indicated. Make sure to drill against a hard surface so the stick doesn't split down the middle. Attach sticks together with a metal brad. This lever illustrates the elbow. Use the hand template and glue to the end of the bottom stick. Blow up three long balloons - just enough to have a "muscle bump" but provide some tension when the "elbow" is moved. Attach one balloon to the back of the "arm" and connect to the bottom stick - this becomes the triceps brachii muscle. Tie the balloon securely and cut off excess. Repeat with muscle connecting the vertical stick with the horizontal stick - this becomes the bicep brachii muscle. Lastly connect a balloon on the lower hole of the vertical stick to the hole just before the fist. This becomes the brachioradialis muscle. Move the arm and watch the balloon "muscles" - do they contract or lengthen? What positions do the "muscles" have concentric movement? Eccentric movement?

MECHANISMS OF BREATHING

Instructions

The mechanism of breathing involves two main processes: inspiration and expiration. Inspiration occurs when the diaphragm and the external intercostal muscles contract. This changes the volume of the lungs, in turn changing the pressure inside the lungs, causing air to move into the lungs down the pressure gradient. Expiration occurs when the diaphragm and the intercostal muscles relax, causing air to move out of the lungs.

Drill two holes in the bottom of the cup. Push straws through holes and cover the inside end with two balloons, securing them with small rubber bands - these represent the lungs and the bronchus. Cut the bottom of a balloon off with scissors and cover the ribbed opening of the cup leaving the knotted end on the outside. This will be the "handle" to manipulate the diaphragm. Use craft glue to glue the respiratory model template to back of the cup to complete the model. Allow to dry completely. Pull on the knotted handle of the diaphragm - watch the balloon "lungs" fill up with air. Release the handle and watch the lungs deflate.

Materials

- Clear Plastic Cup w/Rim
- Drill & Bit
- Three Large Balloons
- Two Straws
- Two Small Rubber Bands
- Scissors
- Respiratory Model Template
- Craft Glue

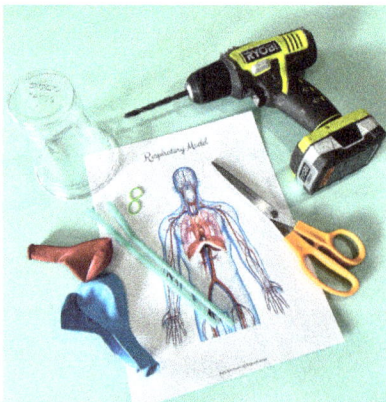

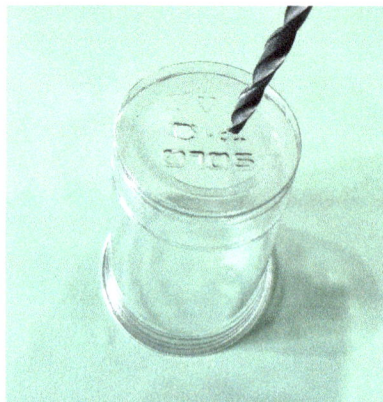

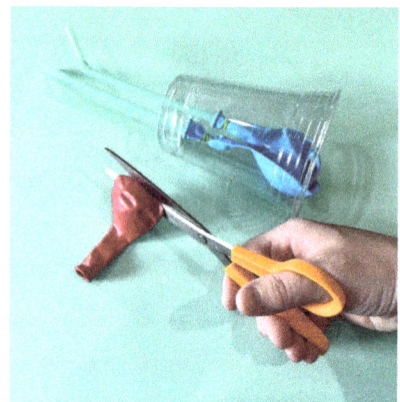

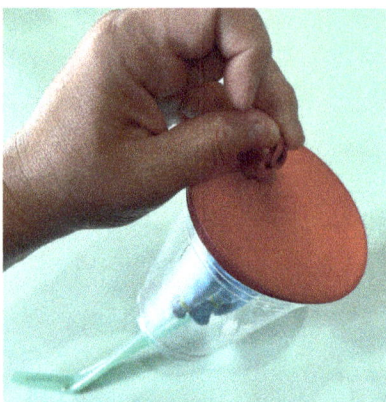

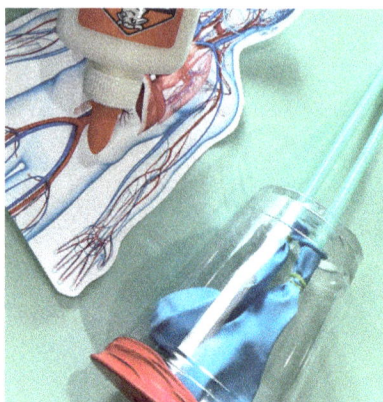

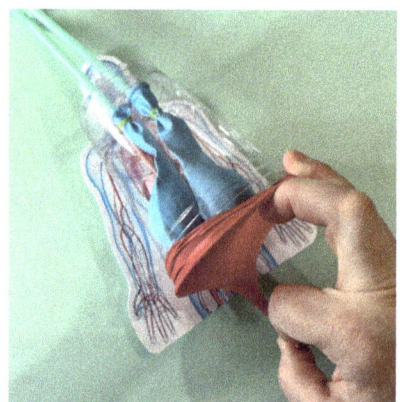

Respiratory Model

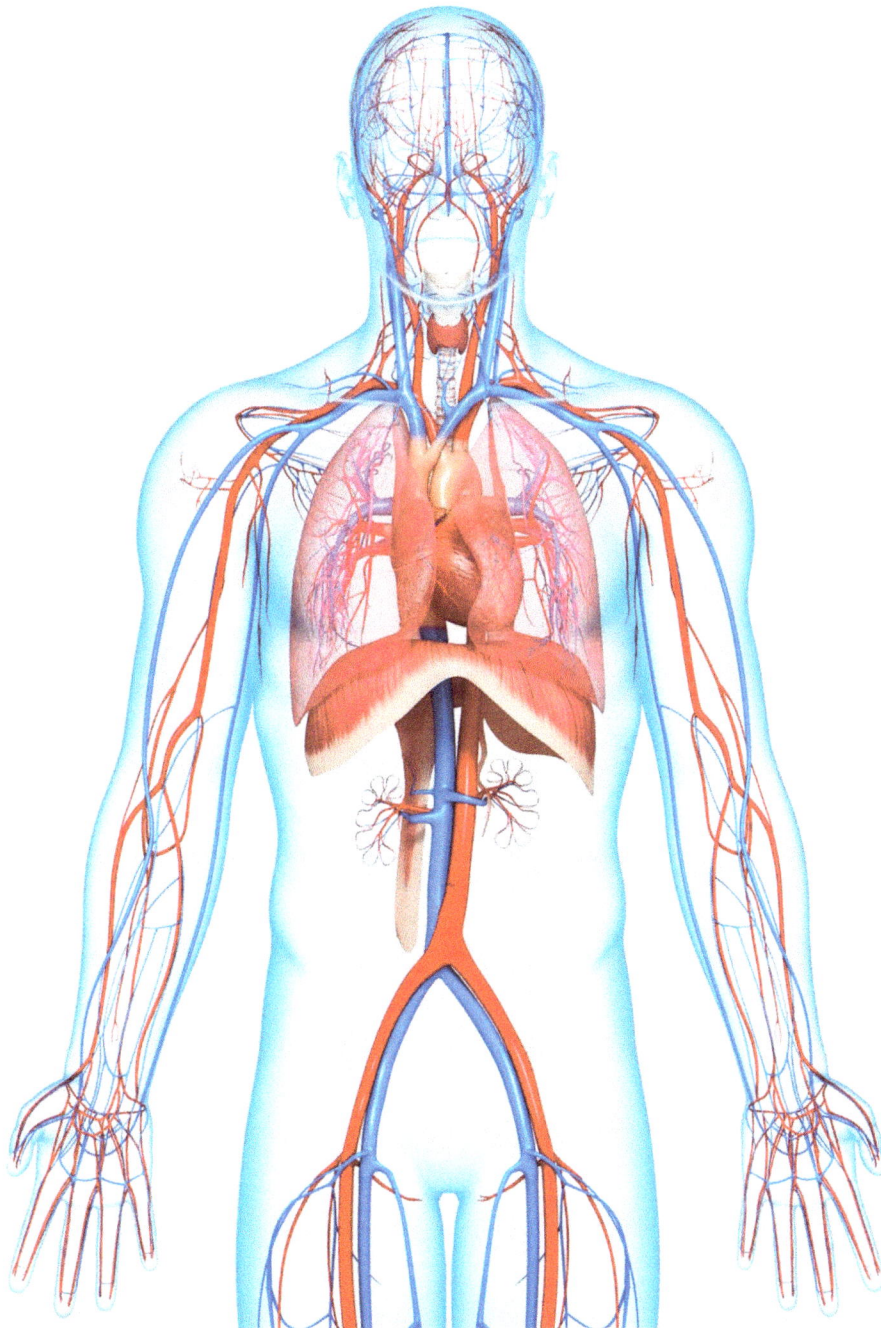

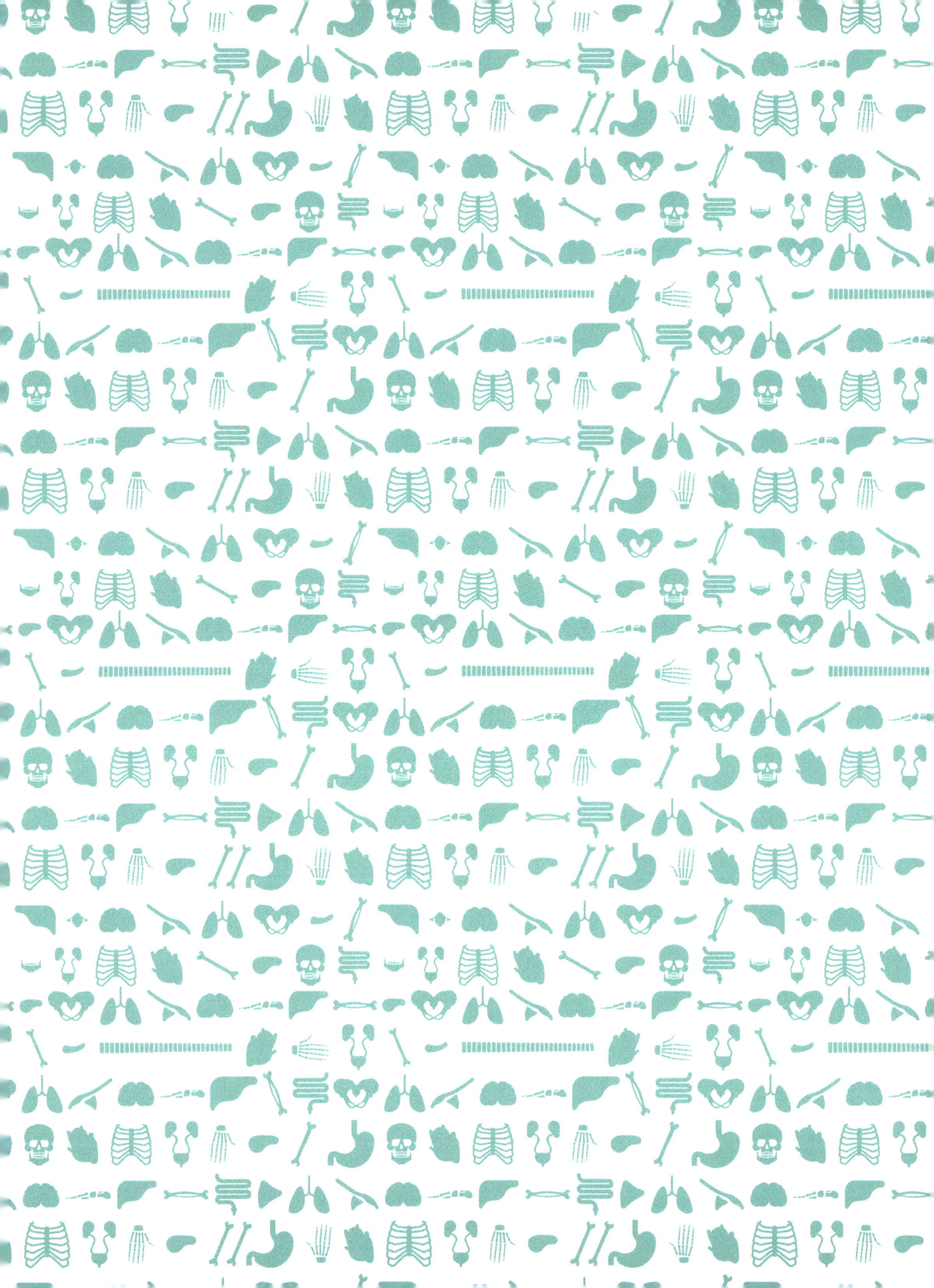

Anatomy of the Heart

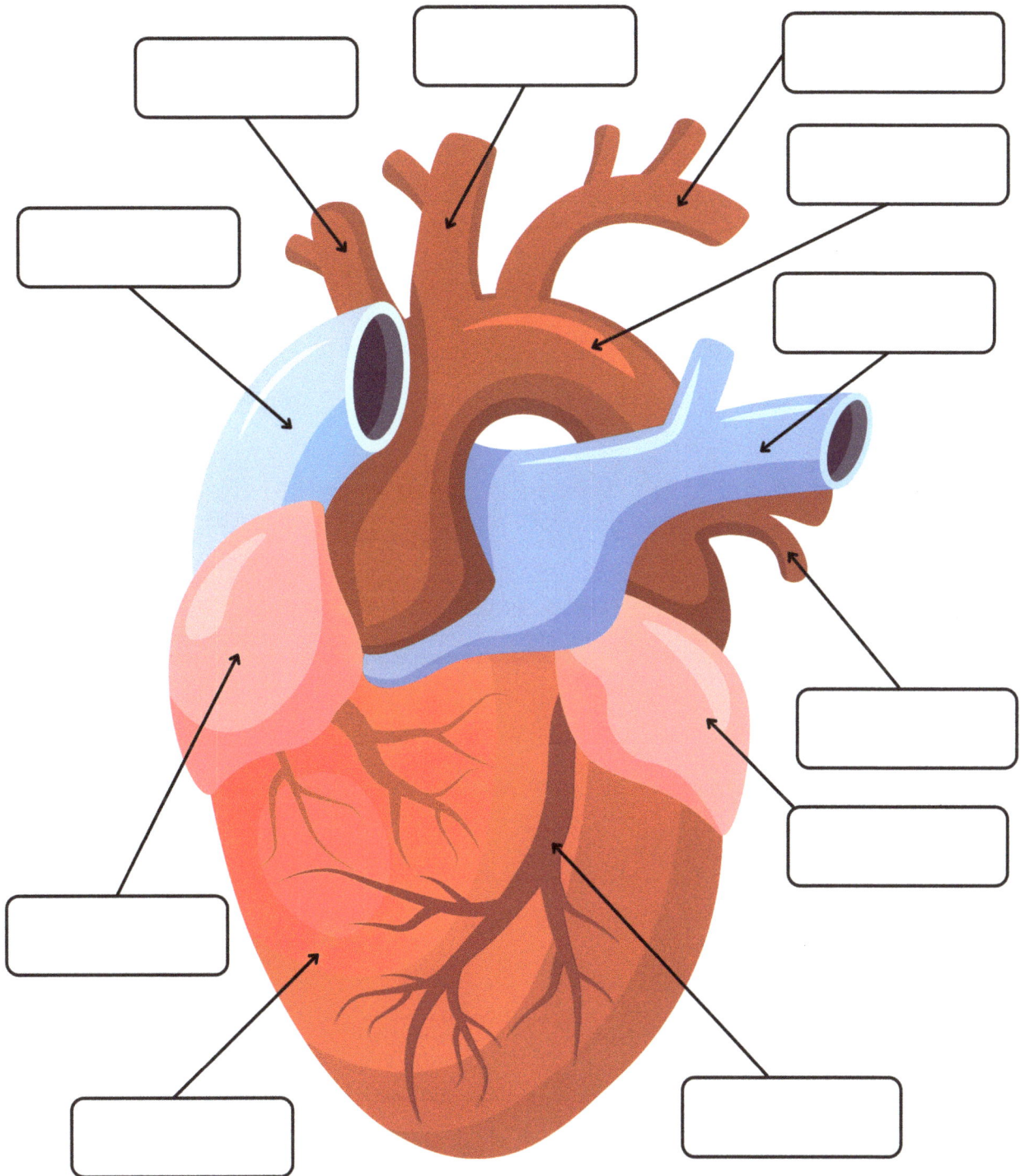

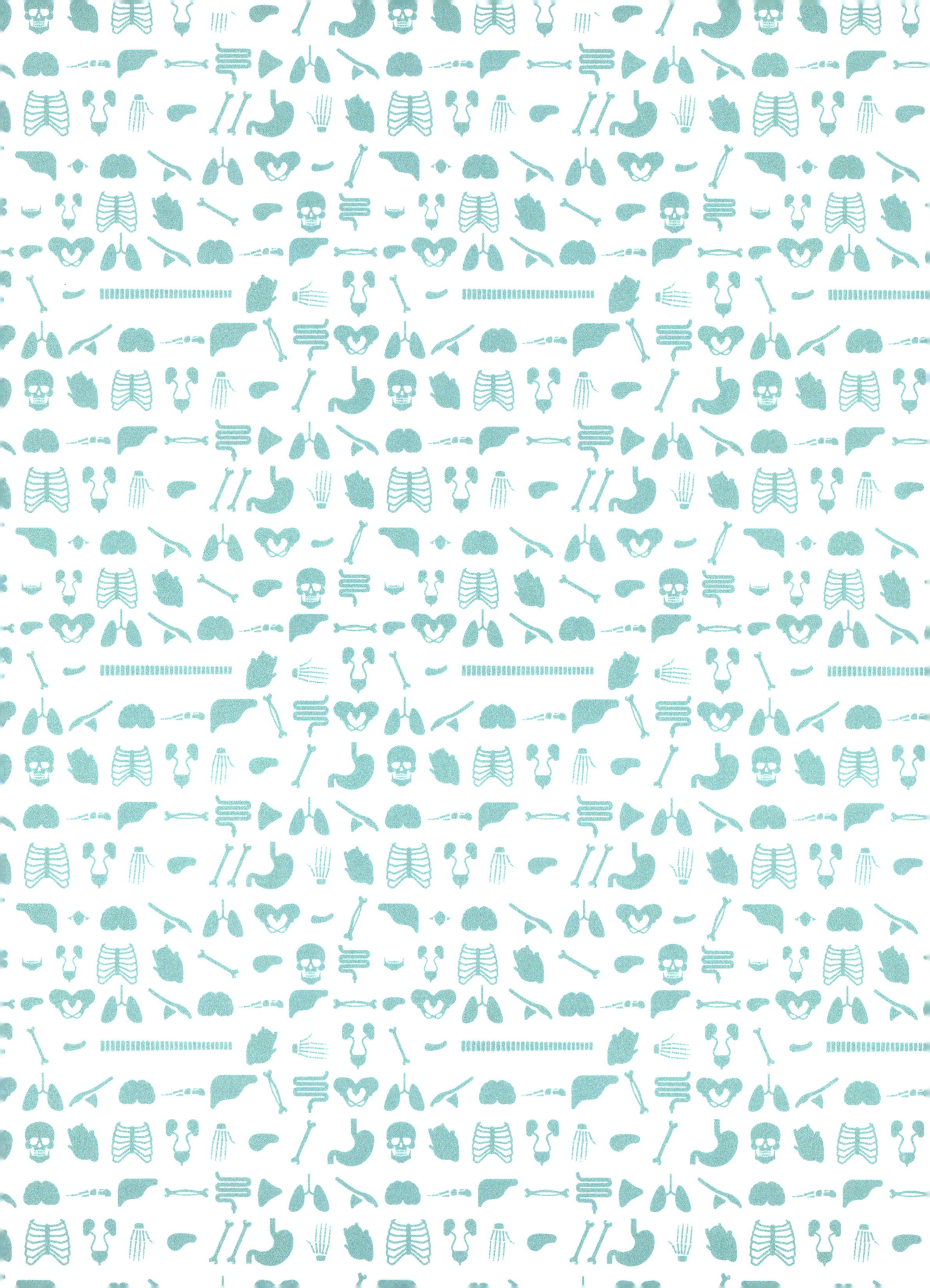

Anatomy of the Heart

Bracheocephalic Artery	Left Common Carotid Artery	Left Subclavian Arterty	Coronary Artery
Superior Vena Cava	Aortic Arch	Pulmonary Artery	Myocardium
Right Atrium	Left Atrium	Pulmonary Vein	

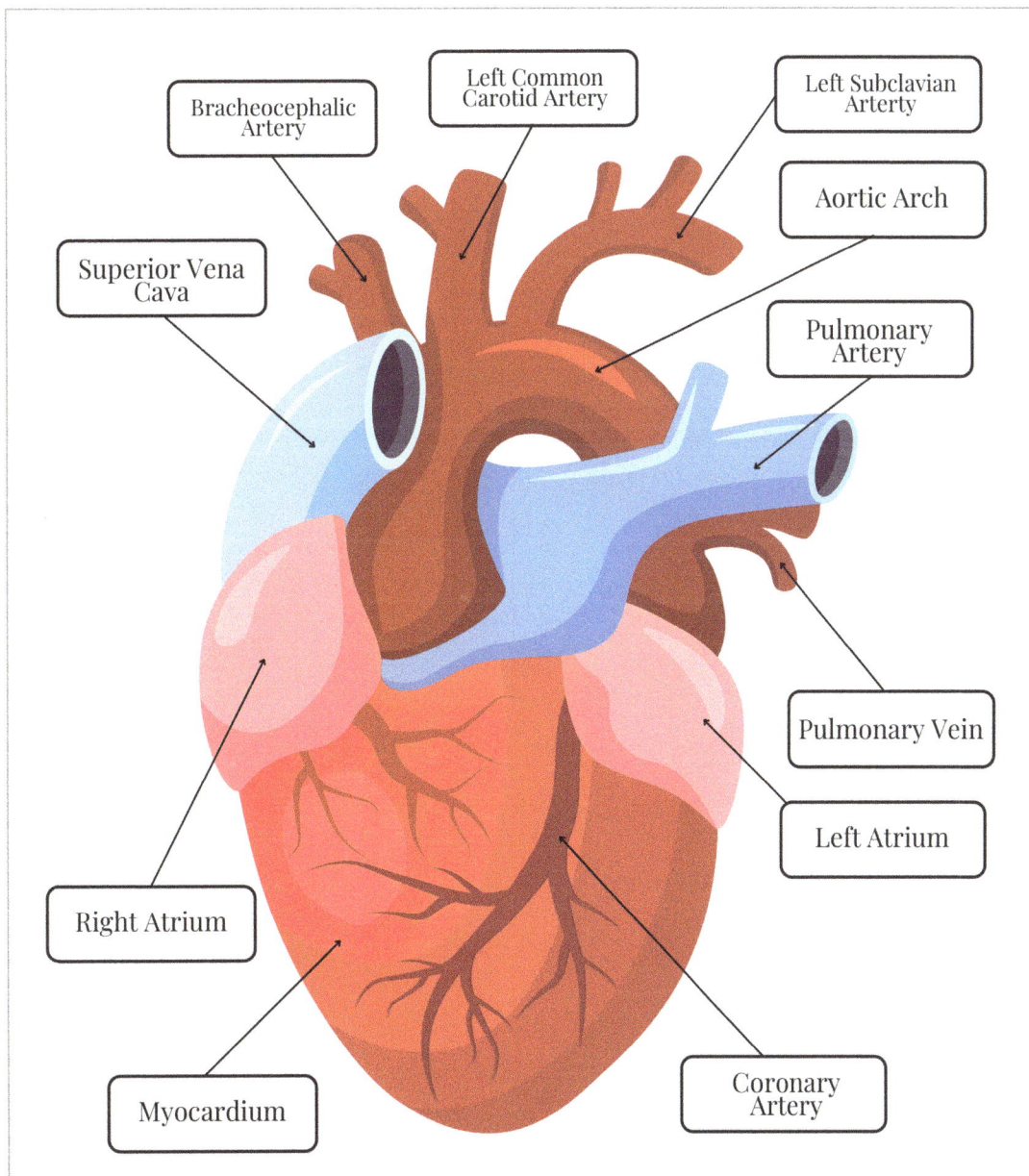

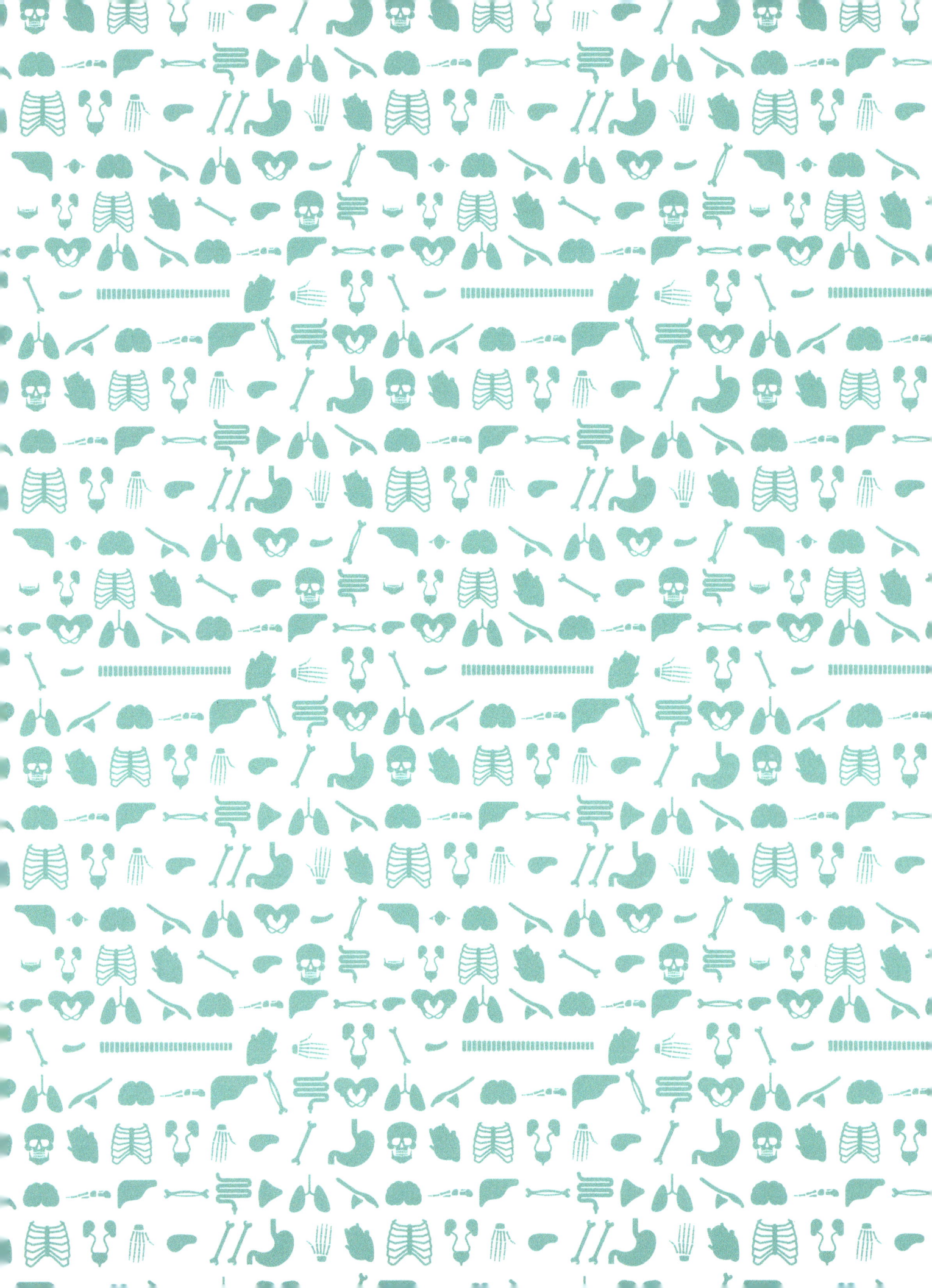

BLOOD SENSORY TRAY

Instructions

The blood is made up of four main components - plasma, which is the straw-colored liquid portion of blood, and the red blood cells which carry oxygen and nutrients to the entire body. It also includes white blood cells (which actually are clear, not white), the main component of the immune system and protects the body against pathogens, and platelets, which allow the blood to clot when needed. Place the jumbo clear beads and regular red water beads in one bowl and the regular clear beads in another bowl. Add yellow food coloring to the clear beads in the second bowl and allow to absorb the water - overnight usually works. Squish the clear beads in the yellow liquid - this becomes the plasma and the platelets. Place into display tray. Add the jumbo clear beads and the red beads, which are the red & white blood cells, respectively. Compare to images of real blood under the microscope. Have the child identify the different components.

Materials

- Clear Jumbo Water Beads
- Red & Clear Regular Water Beads
- Yellow Food Coloring
- Water
- Display Tray

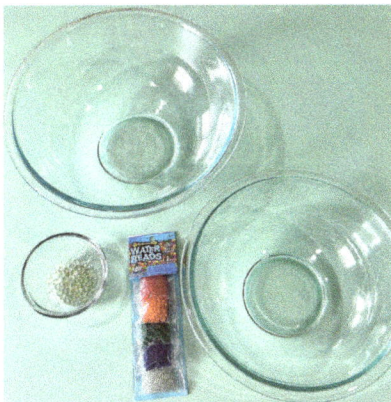

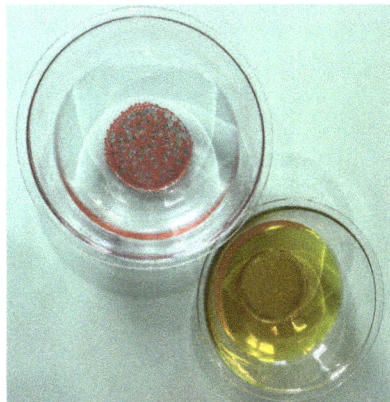

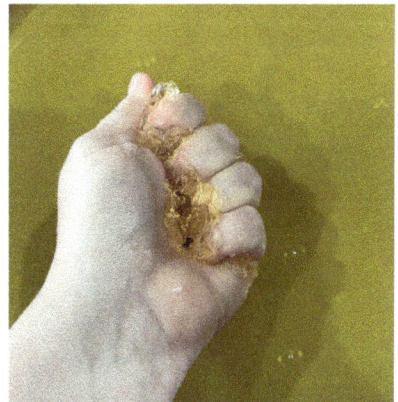

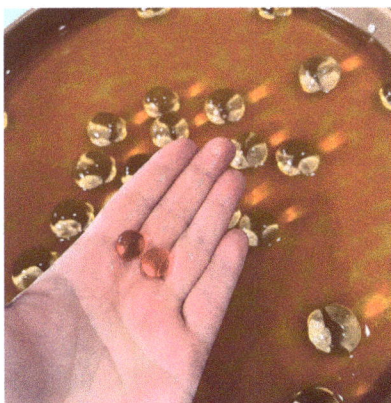

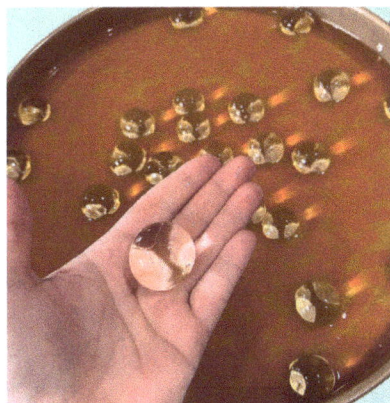

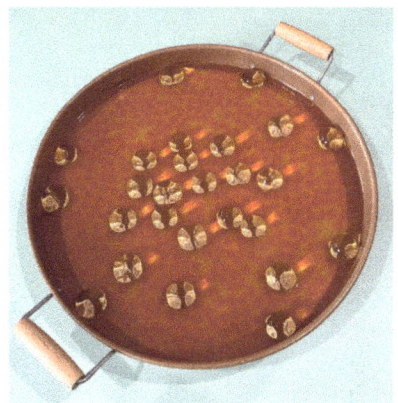

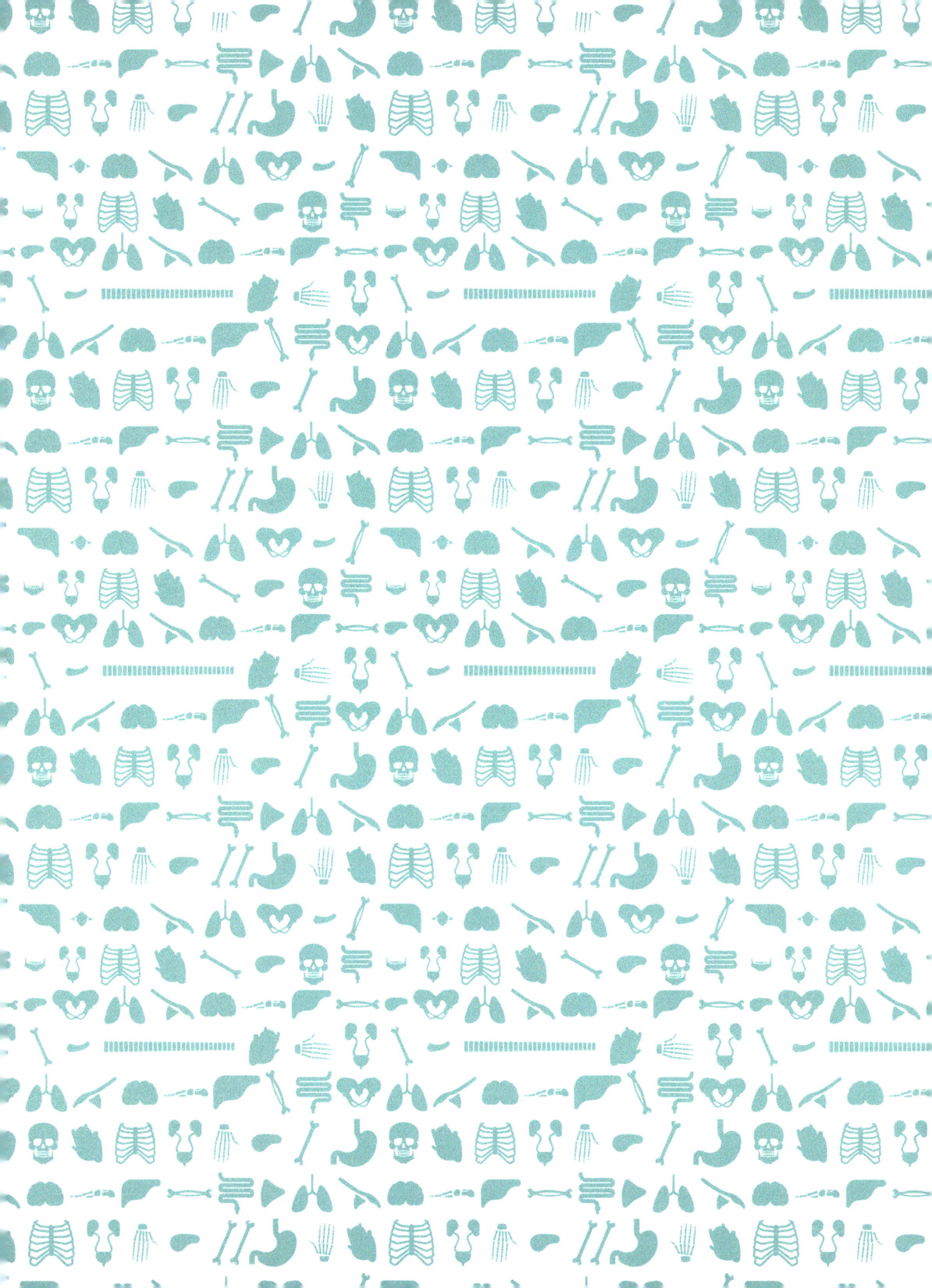

Components of Blood Slides

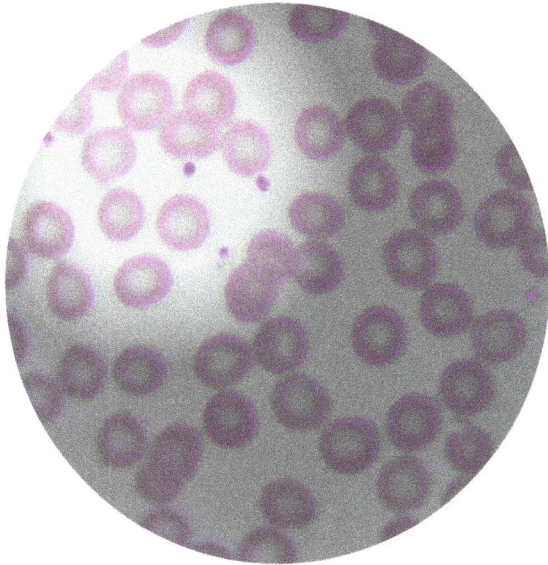

Red Blood Cells
Light Microscope

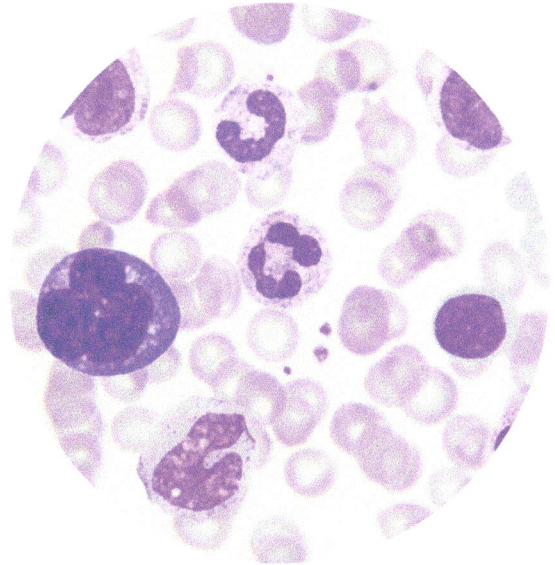

White Blood Cells
Light Microscope

Plasma
Light Microscope

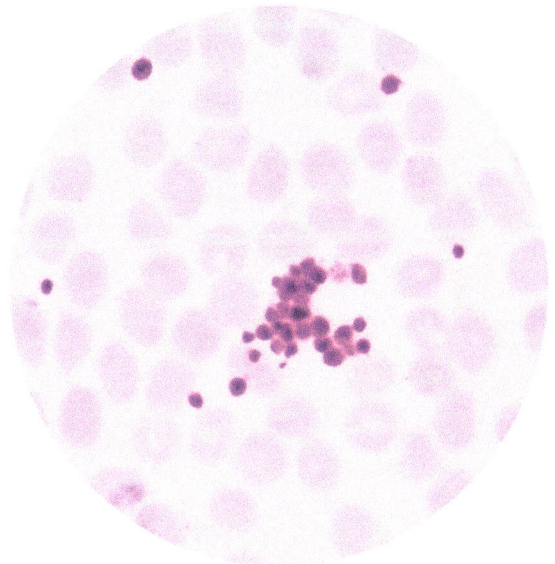

Platelets
Light Microscope

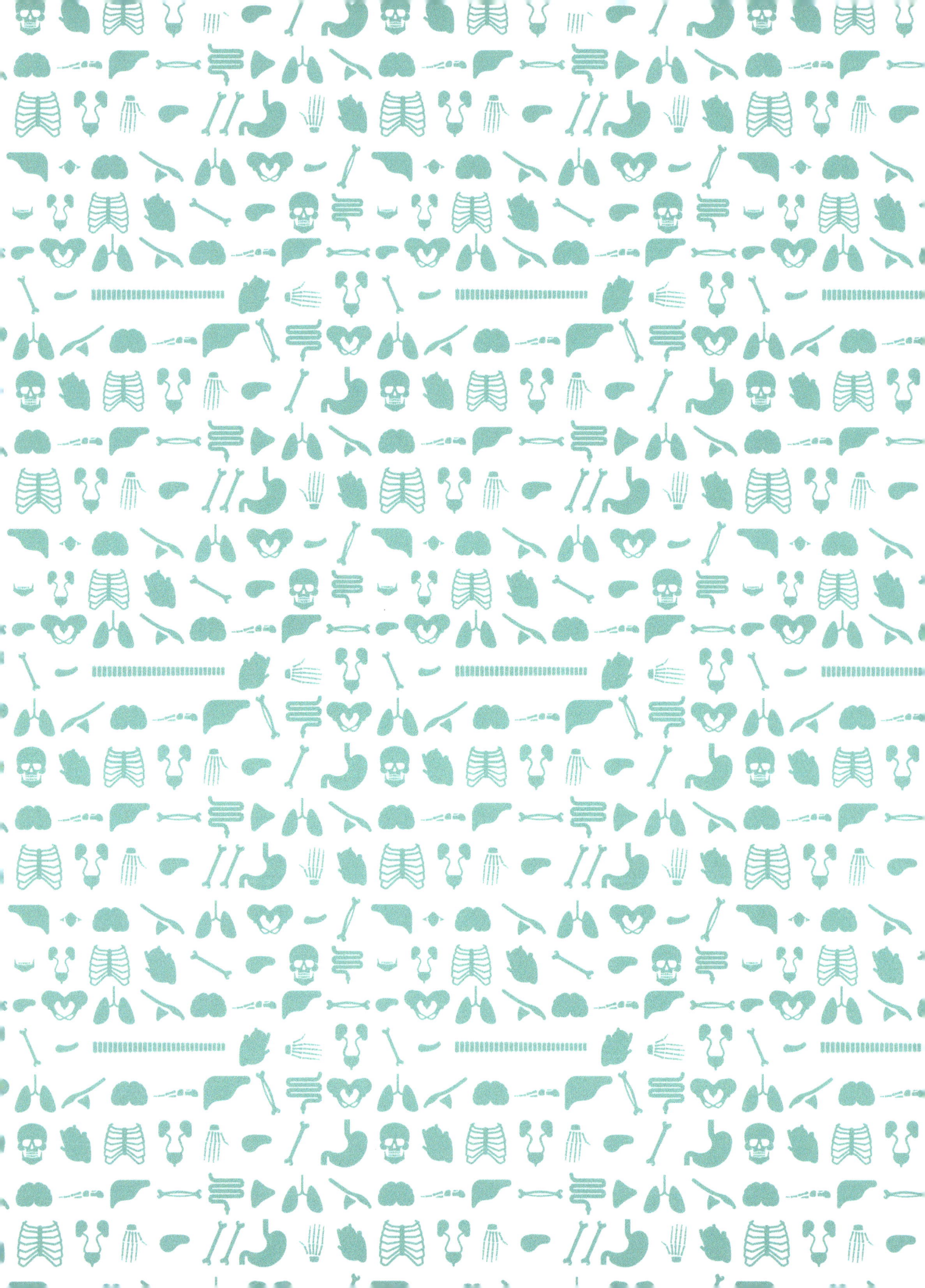

Cardiopulmonary Circulation

Identify which areas contain oxygen rich versus oxygen poor blood by coloring these areas either blue or red.

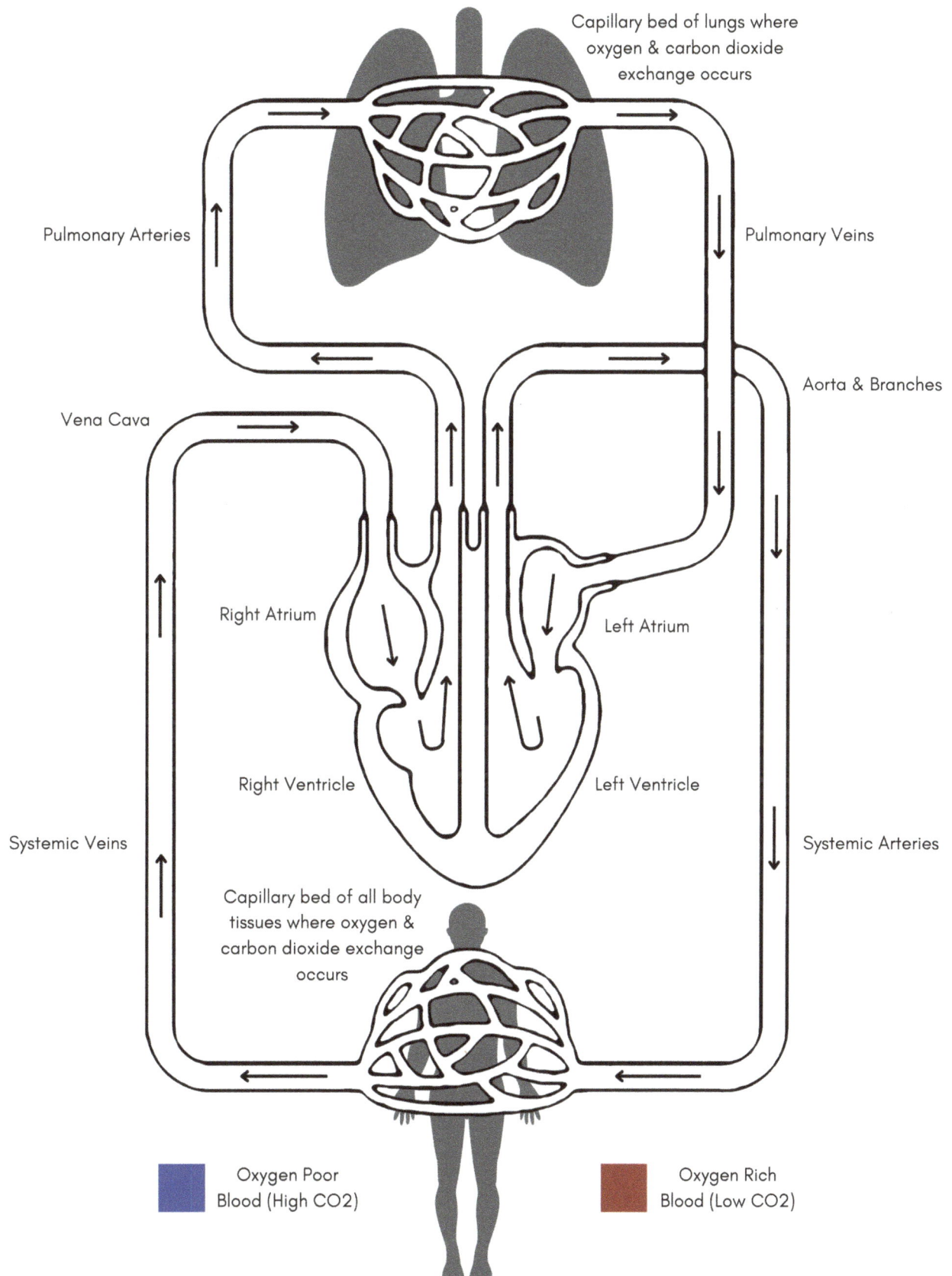

Capillary bed of lungs where oxygen & carbon dioxide exchange occurs

Pulmonary Arteries

Pulmonary Veins

Aorta & Branches

Vena Cava

Right Atrium

Left Atrium

Right Ventricle

Left Ventricle

Systemic Veins

Systemic Arteries

Capillary bed of all body tissues where oxygen & carbon dioxide exchange occurs

Oxygen Poor Blood (High CO2)

Oxygen Rich Blood (Low CO2)

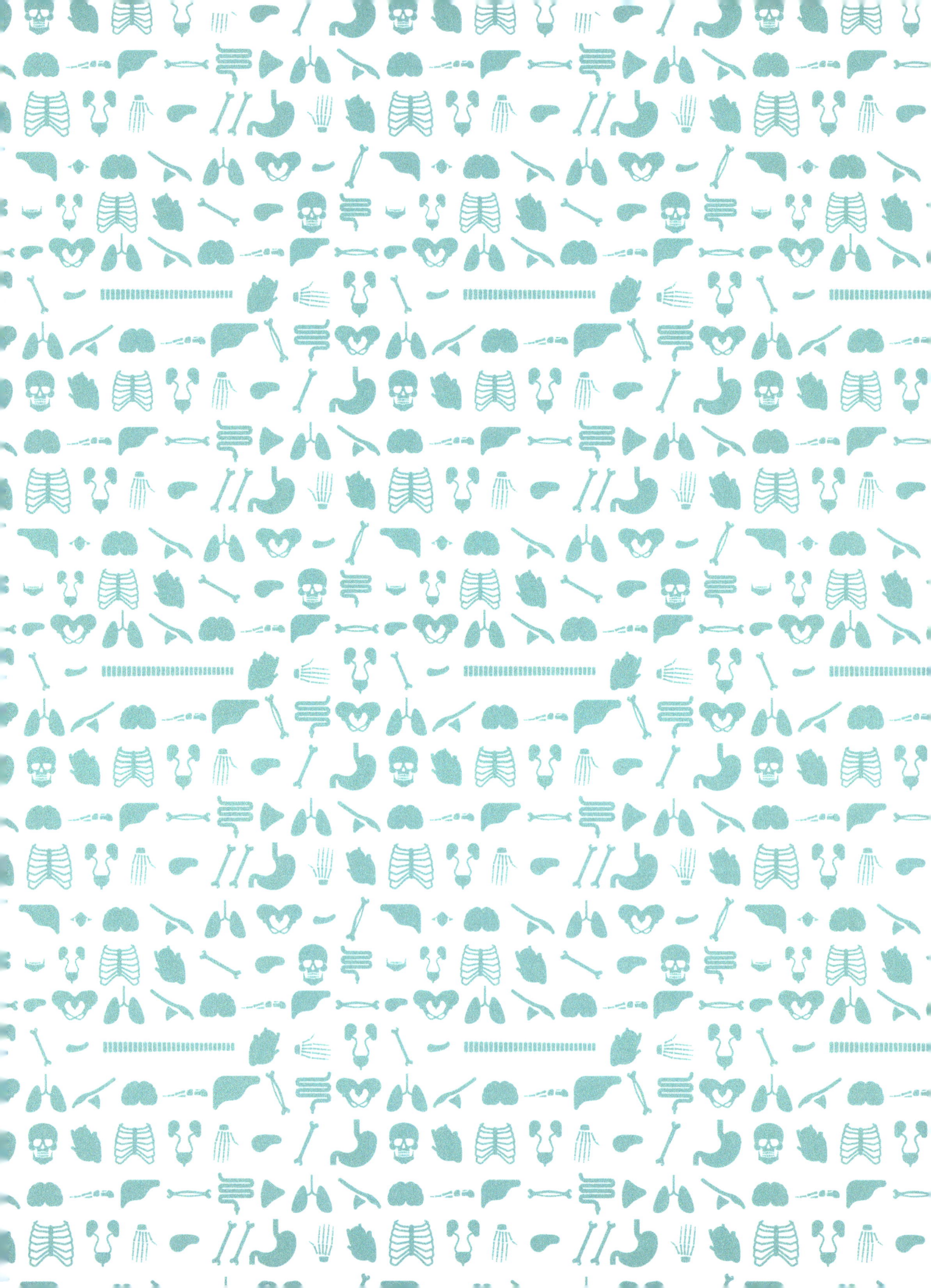

COFFEE FILTER KIDNEY

Instructions

The kidney's job is to filter out waste products from the body as well as balance the body's fluid volume. The kidney is able to filter the blood by a semi-permeable membrane which allows excess fluid and waste products to be removed as urine.

Materials

- Blood Components Sensory Tray
- Funnel
- Coffee Filter
- Two Cups

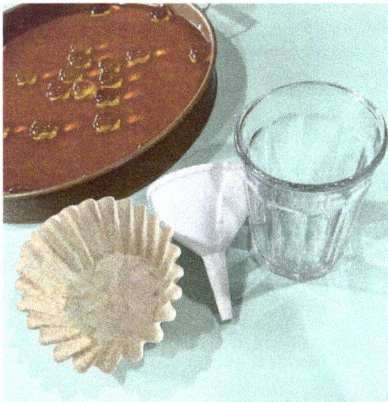

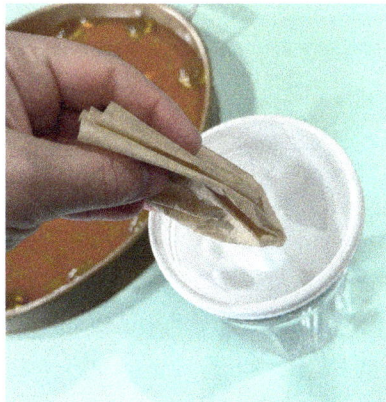

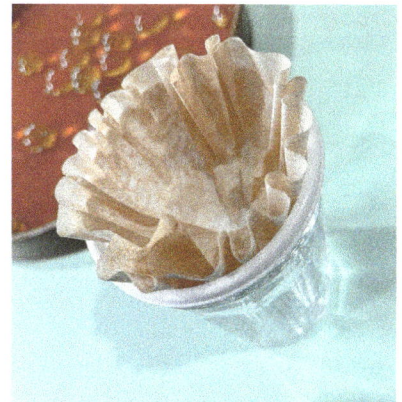

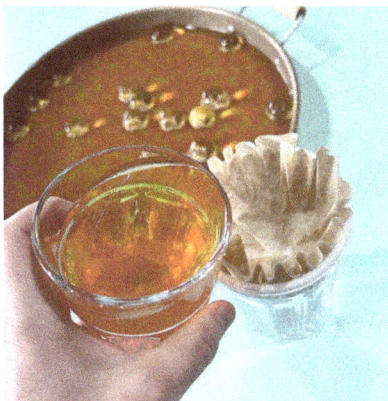

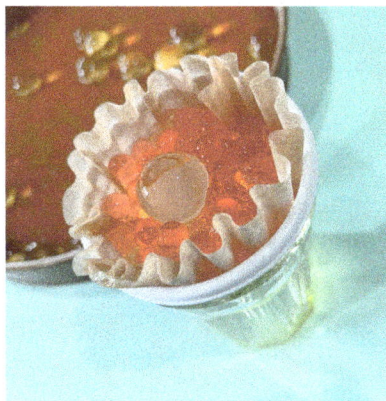

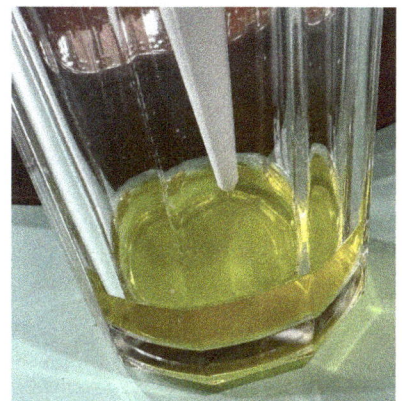

Using the blood components sensory tray, line a funnel with a coffee filter, which demonstrates the semi-permeable membrane. Pour a cupful of the tray's contents into the coffee filter. The water beads (red & white blood cells, platelets) will be trapped inside the coffee filter. The "plasma" will filter through the coffee filter and fill the bottom of the cup with "urine" Discuss the color of the urine. If you add more water to the "urine" in the cup, does it change in color? Does the amount of water consumed affect the color of the child's urine?

POM-POM LYMPH NODE CRAFT

Instructions

Lymph nodes filter substances that travel through the lymphatic fluid, and they contain white blood cells that help the body fight infection and disease. There are hundreds of lymph nodes found throughout the body and they are connected to one another by lymph vessels. During sickness, lymph nodes get larger when more blood cells come to fight off an invading infection. They all essentially pile in, causing pressure and swelling. This is why medical professionals often feel around the neck (cervical) area to check for enlarged lymph nodes as this is a sign the body is fighting an infection.

Color the included template. Glue on green (or other color) pom poms to represent lymph nodes. Imagine if these were on the outside of the body - how funny would that look?

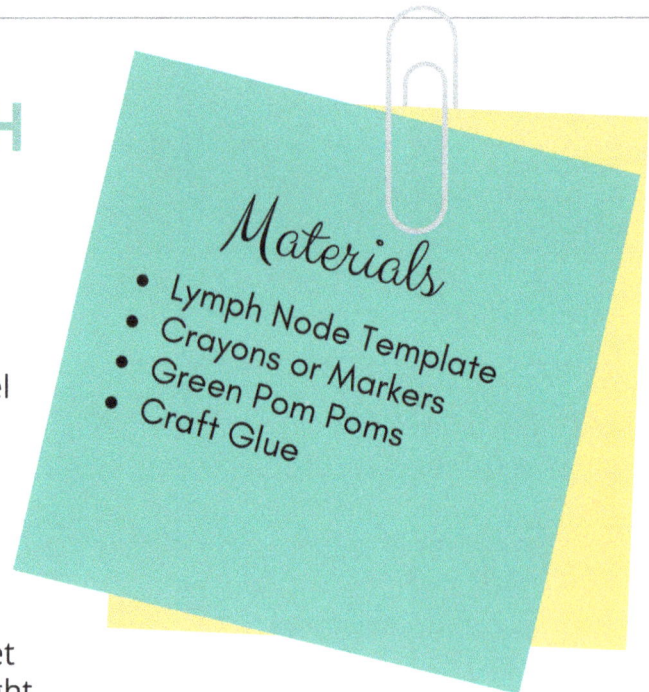

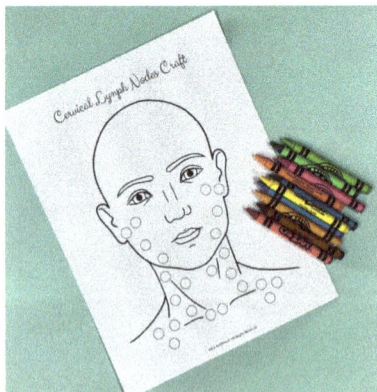

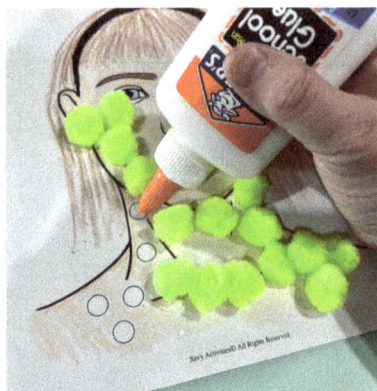

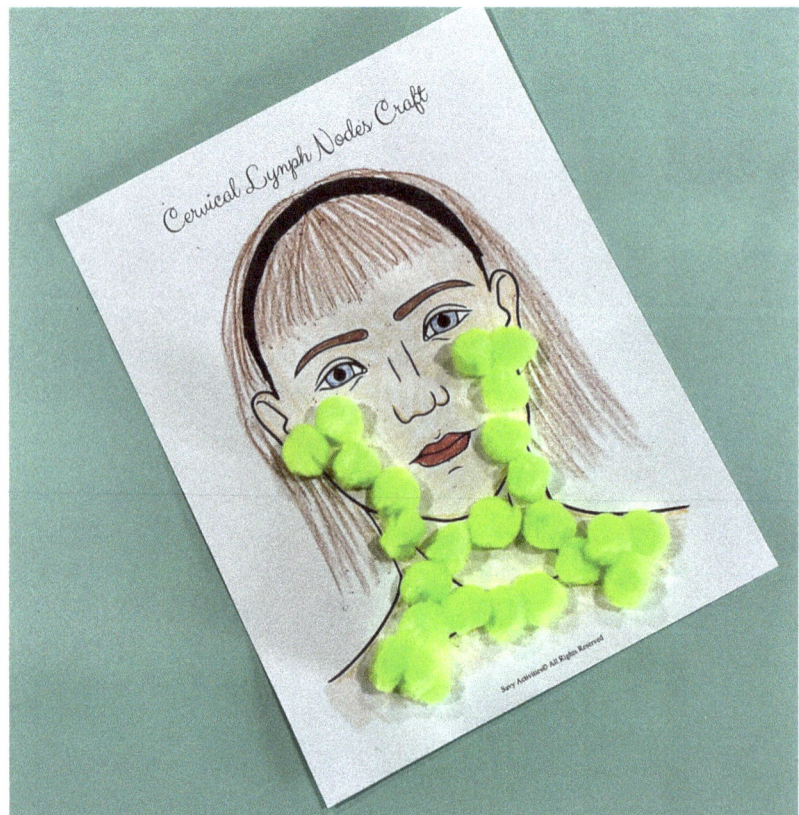

Cervical Lymph Nodes Craft

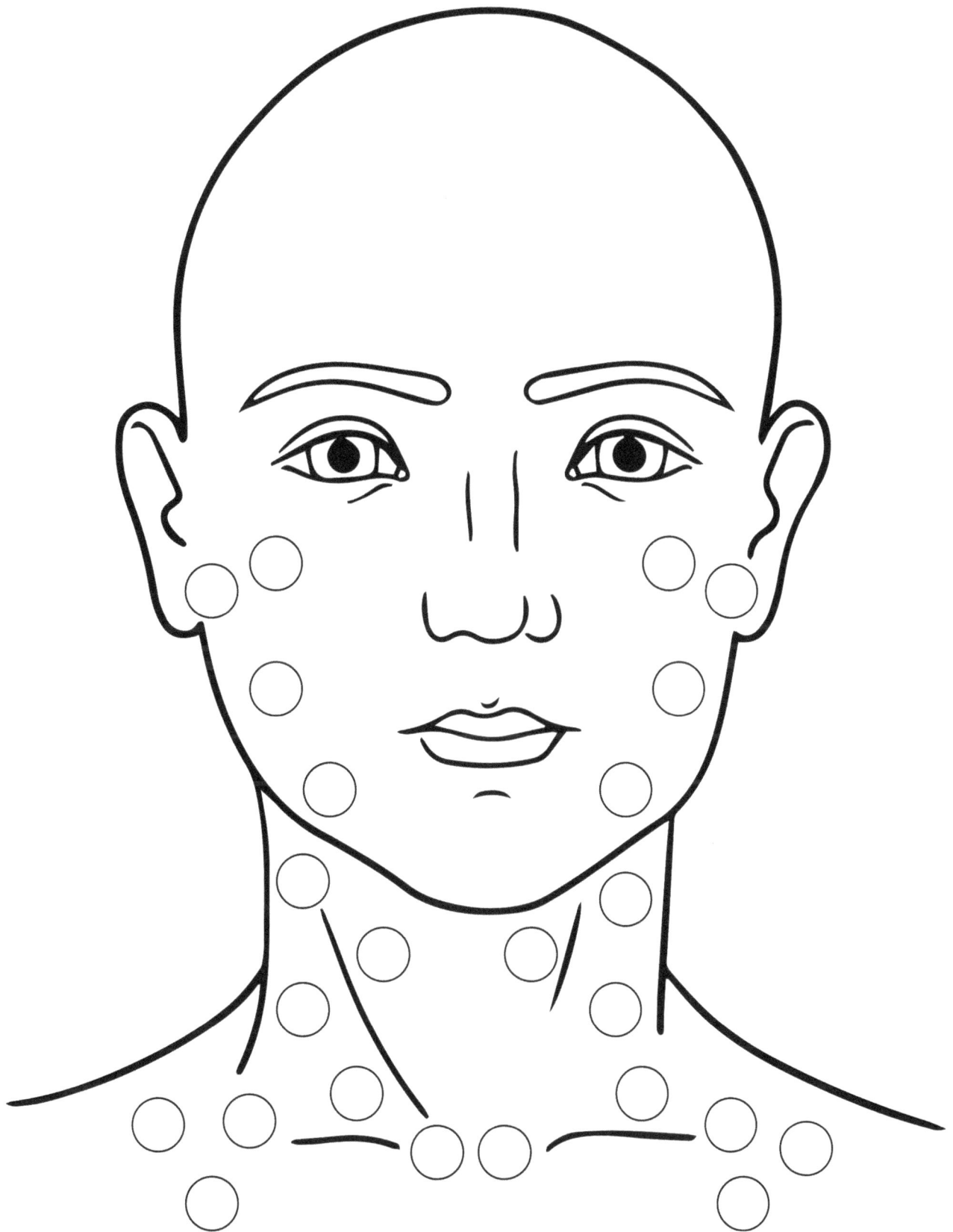

Immune Cells Cards

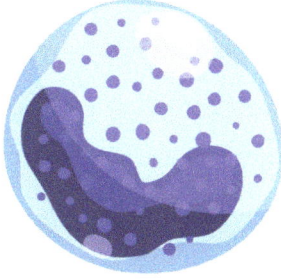

Basophil

Helps detect and destroy some early cancer cells. Releases histamine during an allergic reaction or asthma attack.

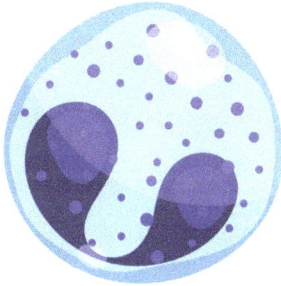

Eosinophil

Involved in inflammatory processes like allergic reactions, and controls inflammatory responses.

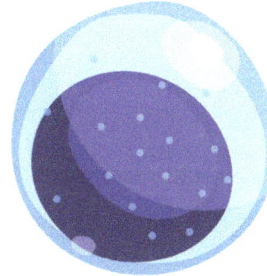

Lymphocyte

Involved in both innate and adaptive immunity. Determines the specificity of the immune response to infectious microorganisms and other foreign substances.

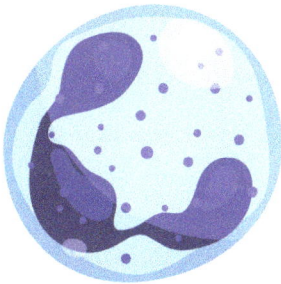

Neutrophil

First responders of the innate immune system. Communicates with other immune cells.

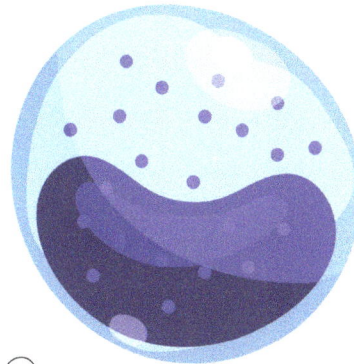

Monocyte

Largest white blood cell. Kills microorganisms, ingests foreign material, removes dead cells, and boosts immune responses.

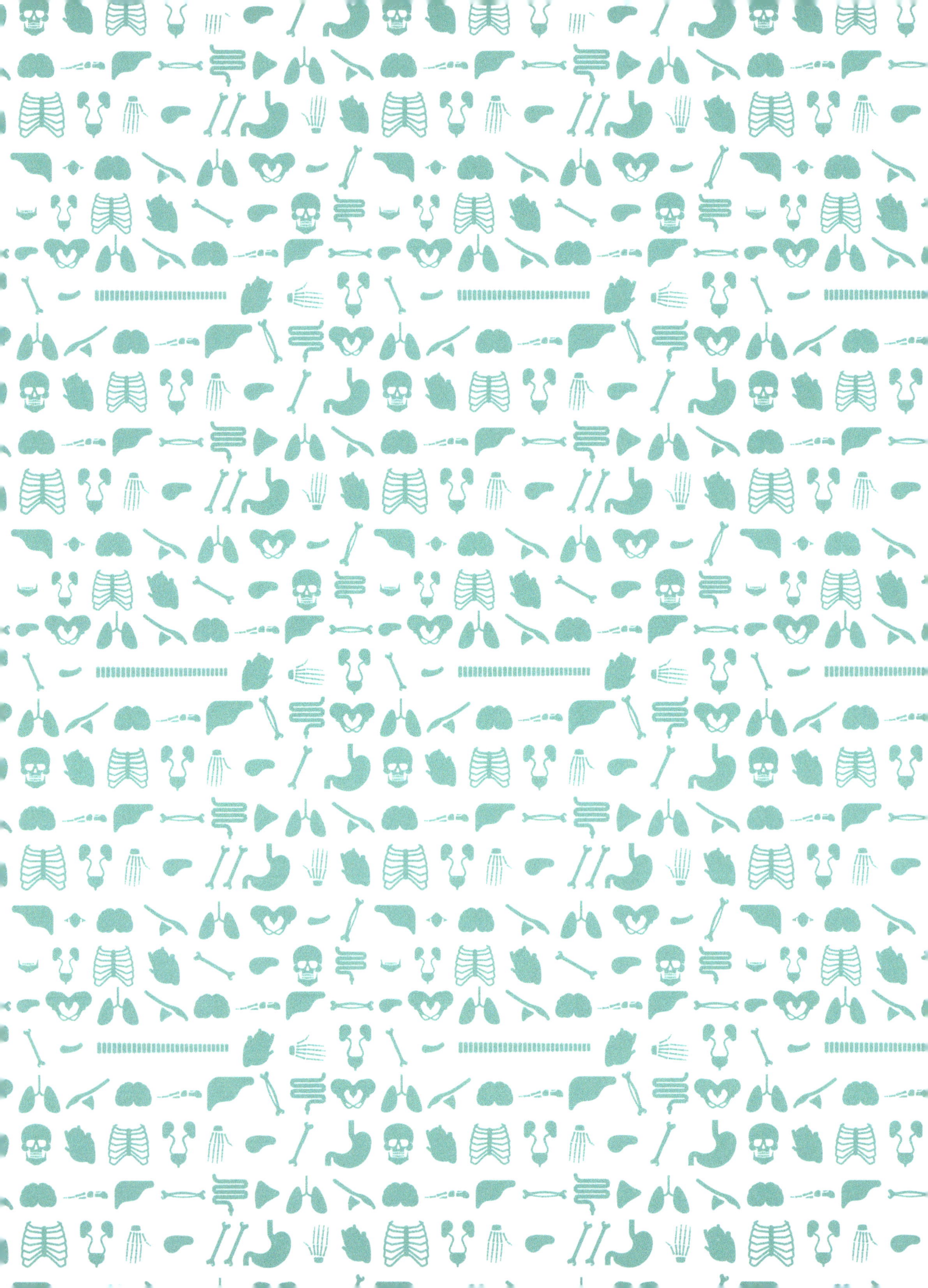

Immune Response Cards

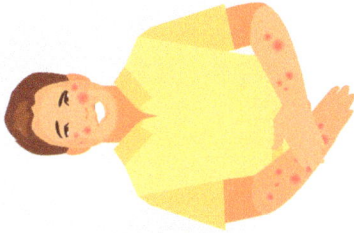

Swelling

Swelling is the result of the increased movement of fluid and white blood cells into the area of infection or injury.

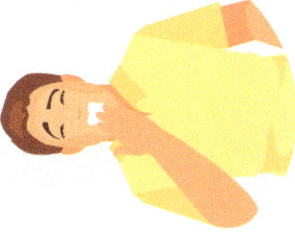

Tired

During an immune response, the body is under a lot of stress. Rest can allow the body to focus on fighting the infection.

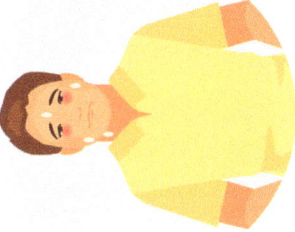

Warmth

Warmth is caused by increased blood flow to the area of infection or injury. With systemic infections, the body may have a fever, which makes it harder for pathogens to replicate.

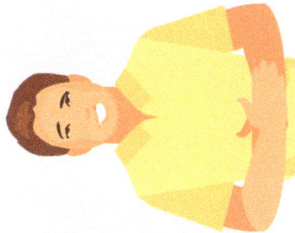

Chills

Chills often occur at the start of an infection, and most associated with a fever. Caused by rapid muscle contraction and relaxation, which is the body's way of warming itself.

Redness

Redness is caused by increased blood flow to the areas of infection or injury, bringing white blood cells, which attack pathogens.

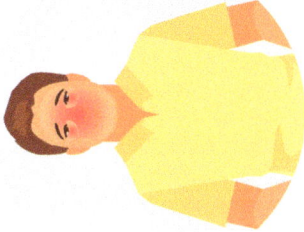

Pain

Pain during an immune response can be caused by swelling due to additional blood flow, irritation from the inflammation or because touch receptors are injured.

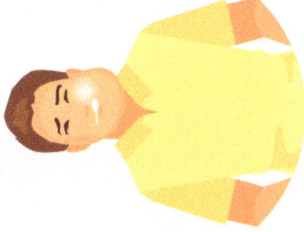

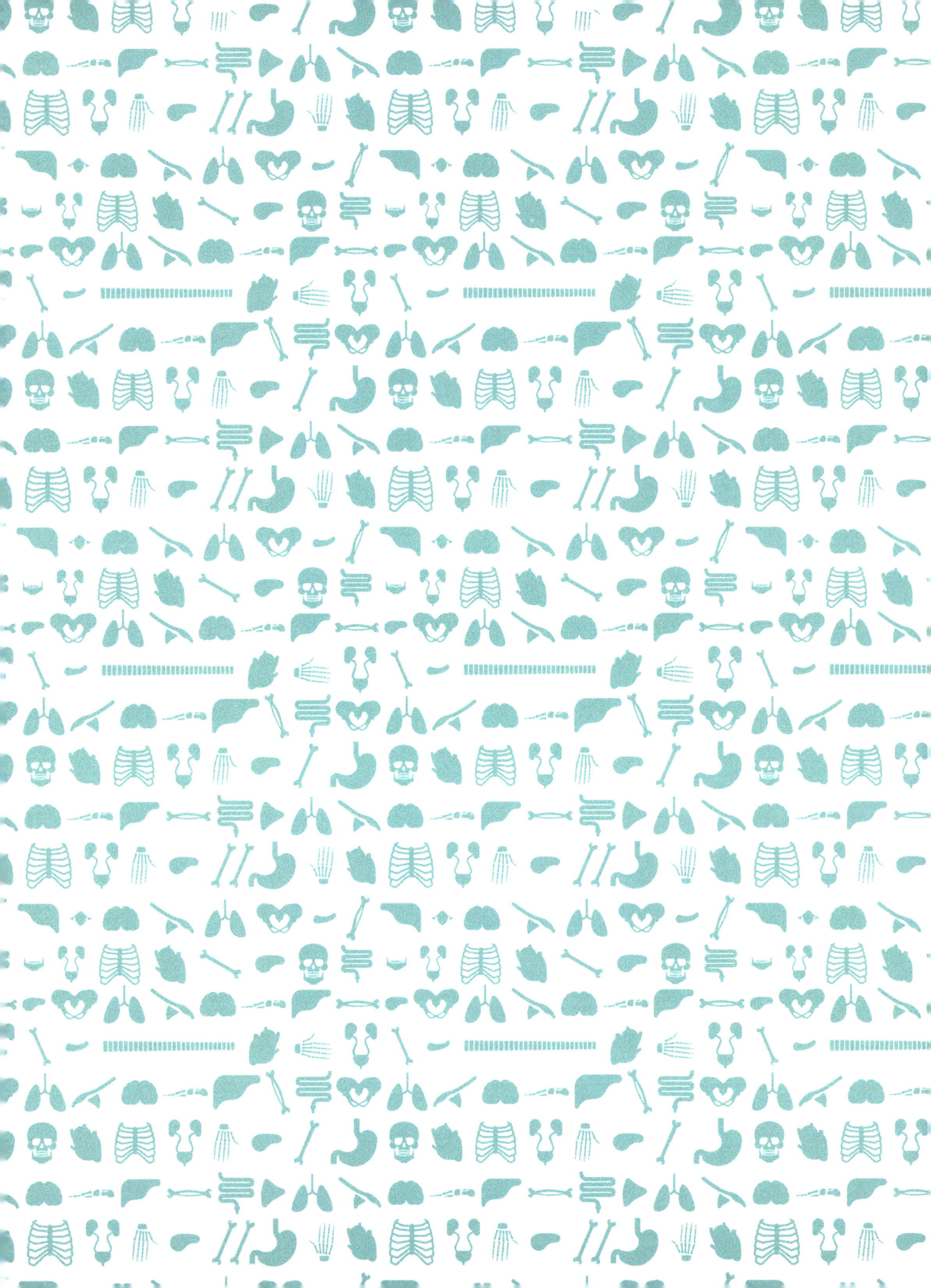

Better Choice Cards

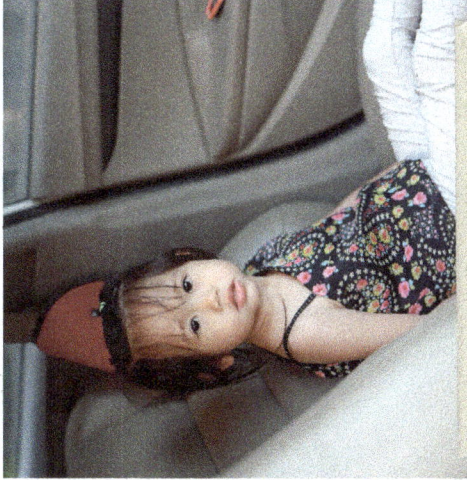

No seatbelt

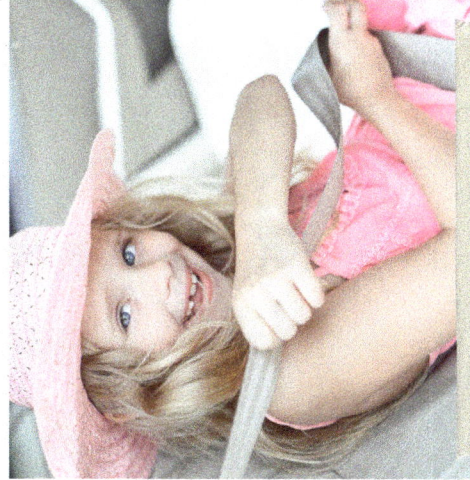

Wears seatbelt

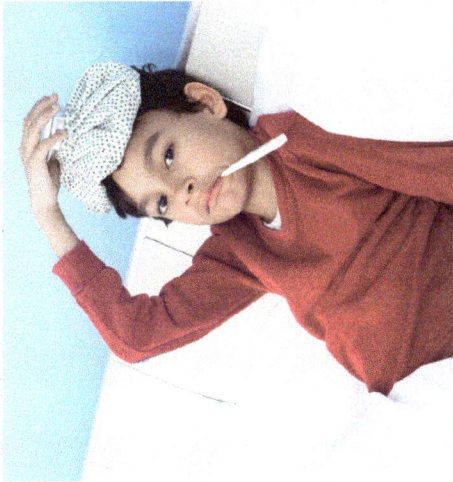

No preventative care

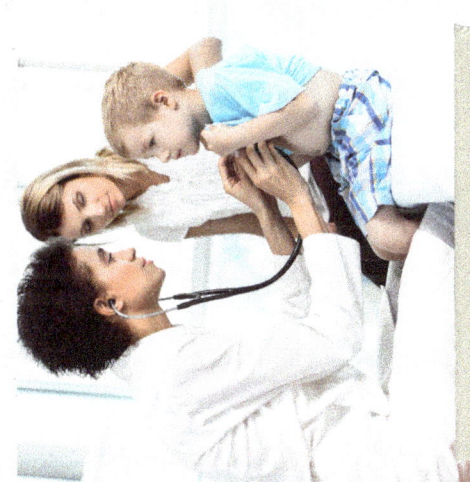

Gets regular checkups

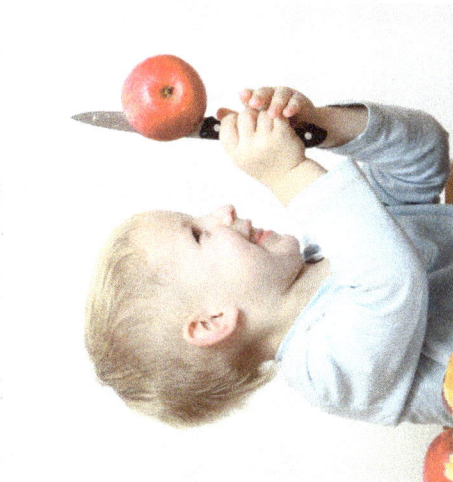

Uses dangerous items without supervision

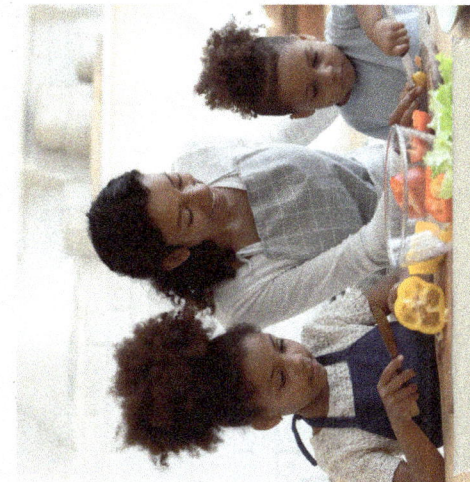

Has adult supervise while using dangerous items

Better Choice Cards

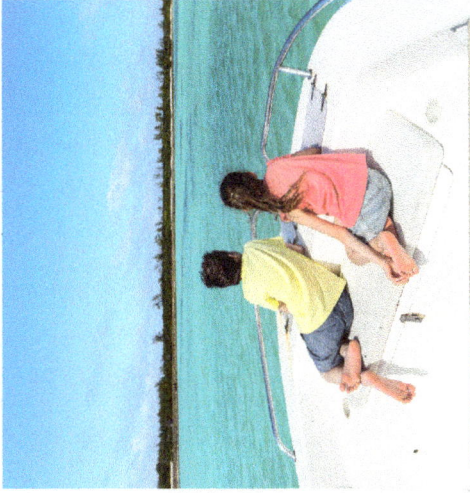
No water safety

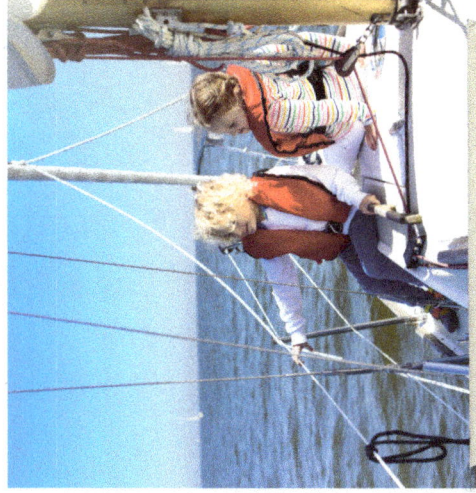
Water safety

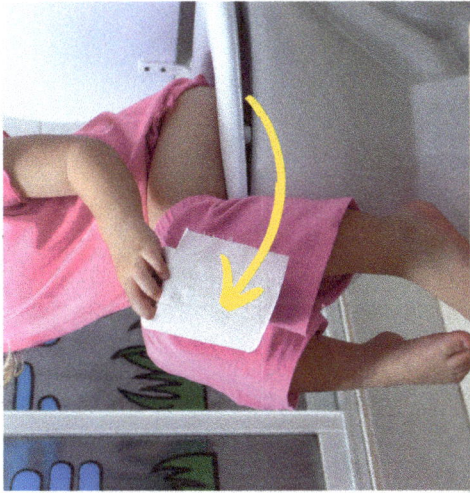
Wipes back to front after toilet

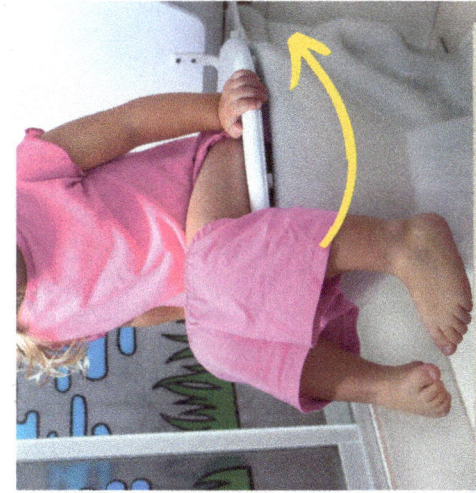
Wipes front to back after toilet

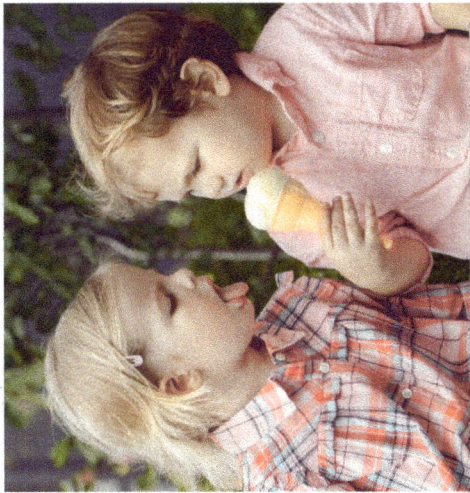
Shares germs

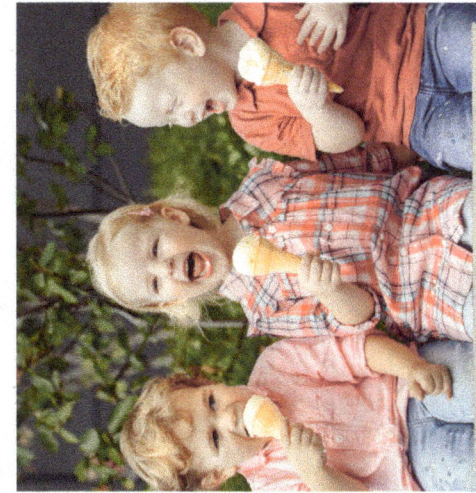
Avoids sharing germs

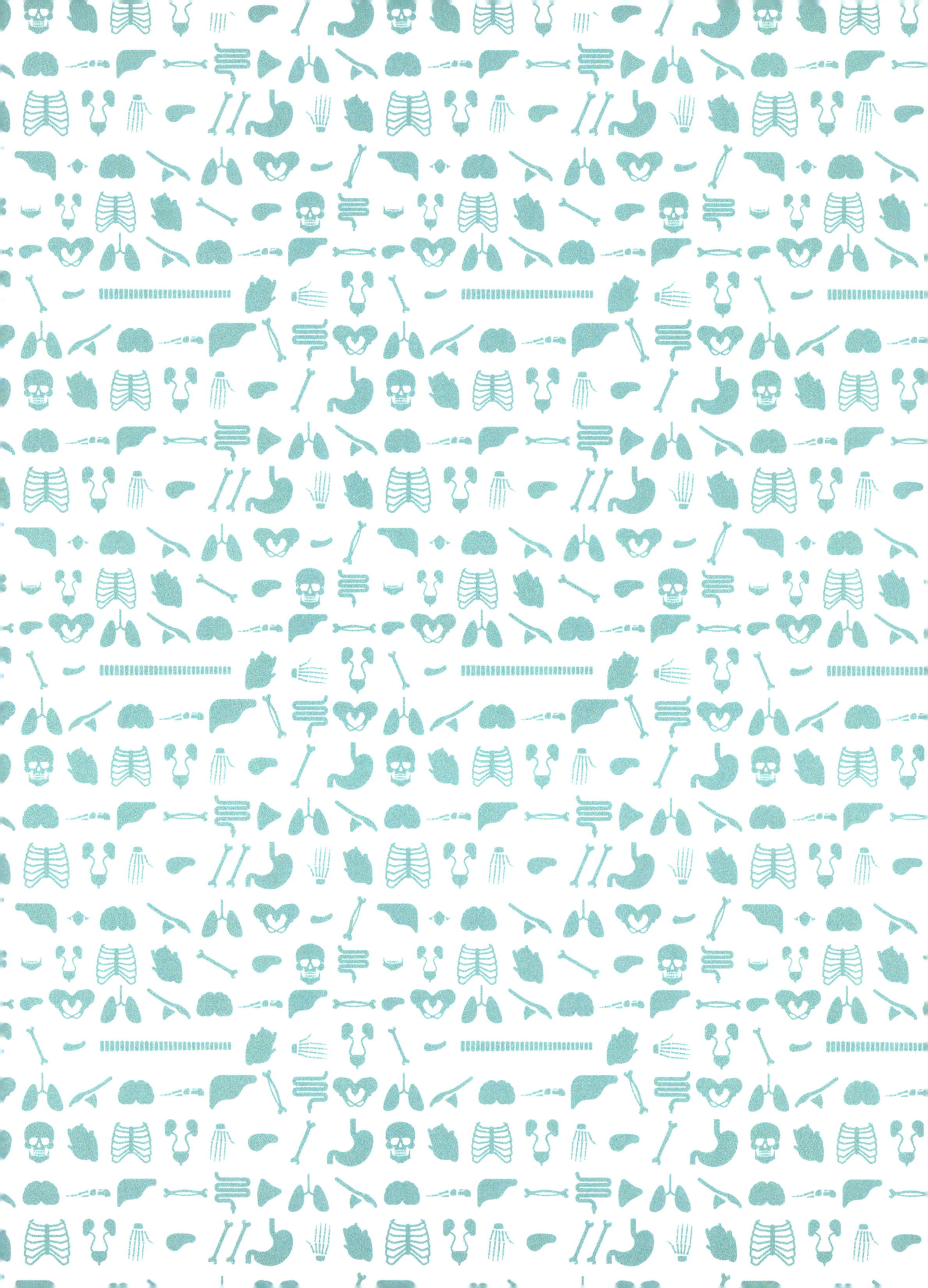

Better Choice Cards

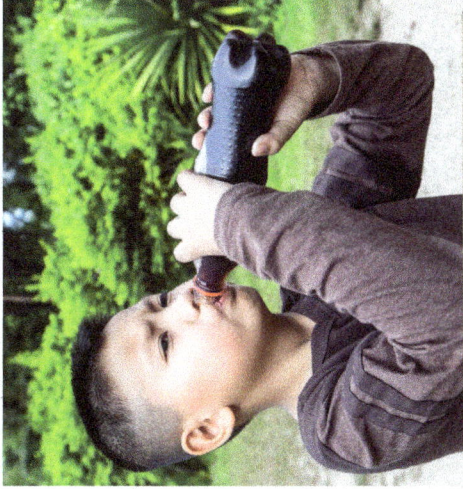
Drinks sugary beverages

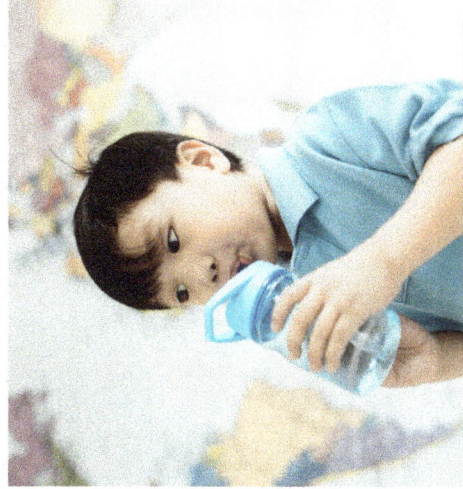
Drinks water

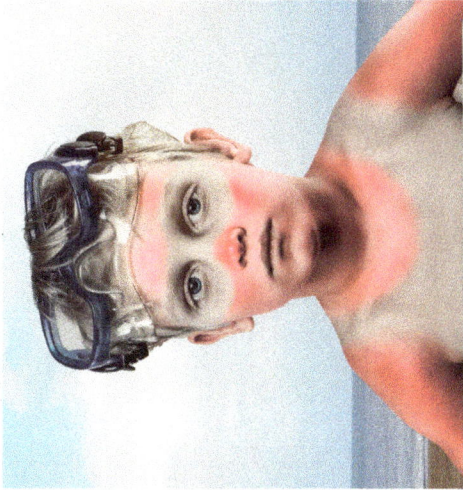
Doesn't wear sunscreen

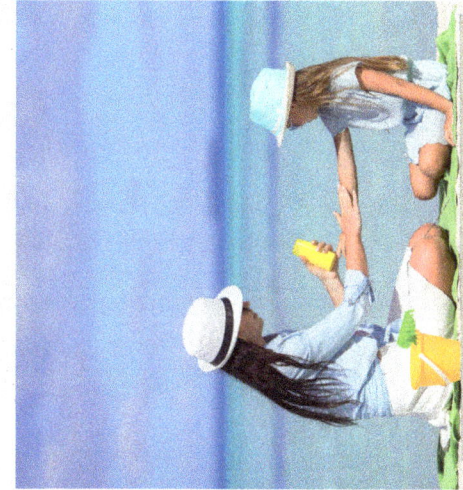
Wears sunscreen and sun protection

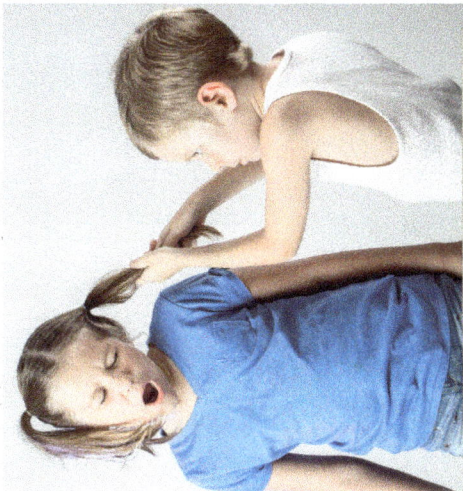
Uses bad touch

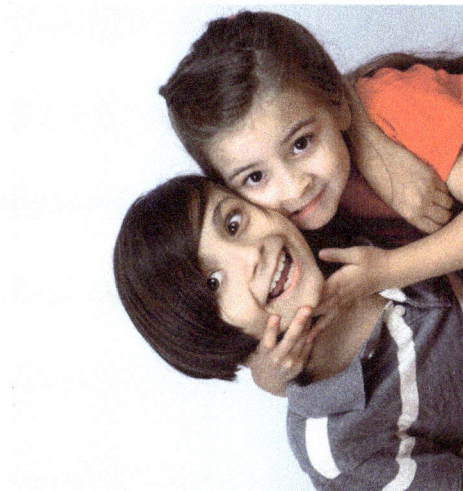
Uses good touch

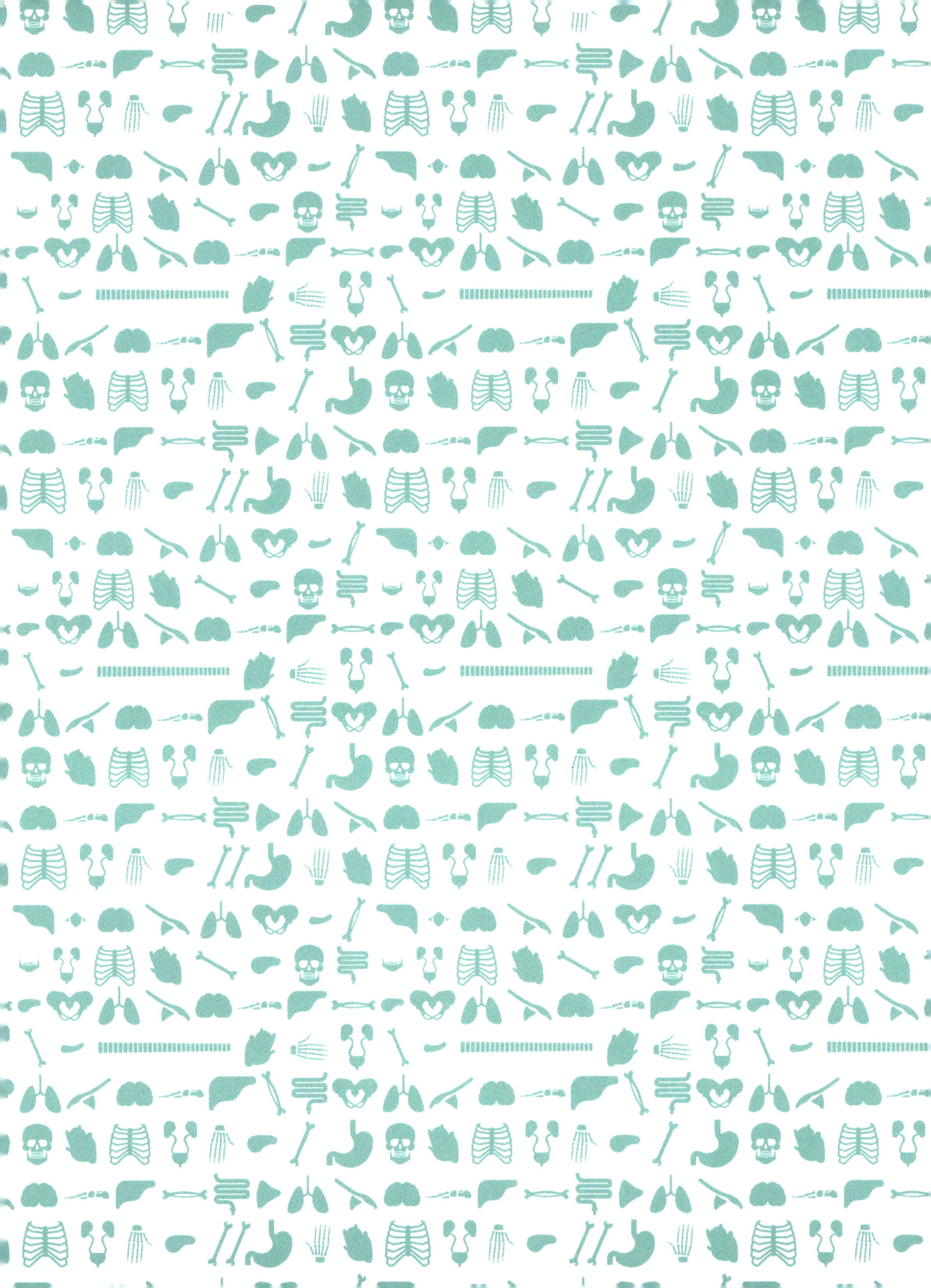

Better Choice Cards

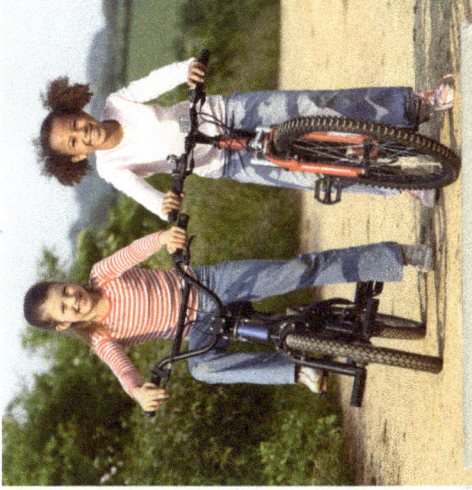
Does not wear helmet

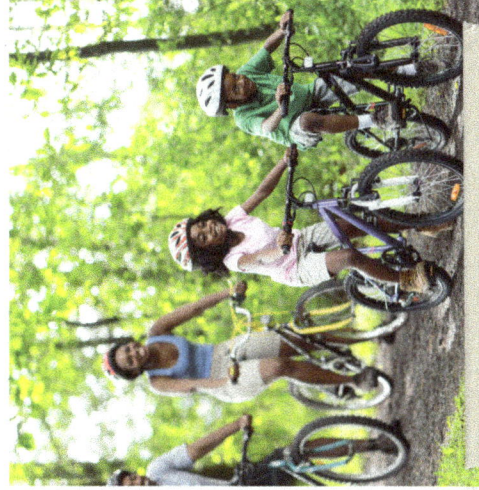
Wears helmet

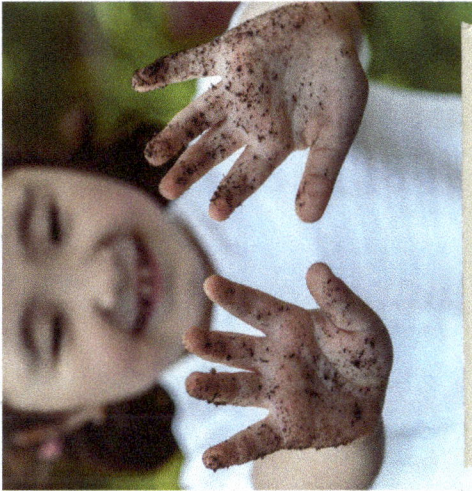
Dirty hands

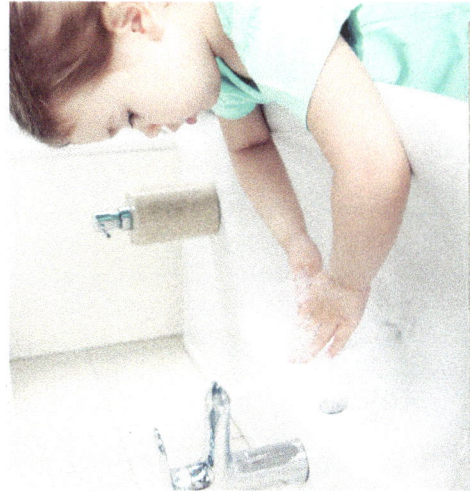
Washes hands often

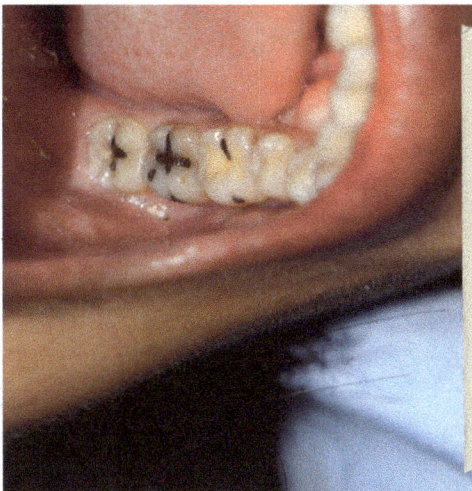
Dirty teeth

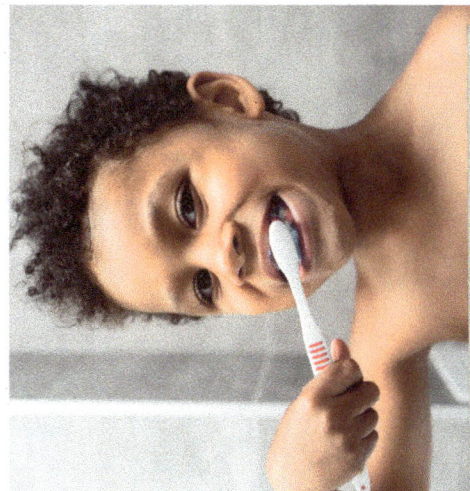
Brushes teeth

Better Choice Cards

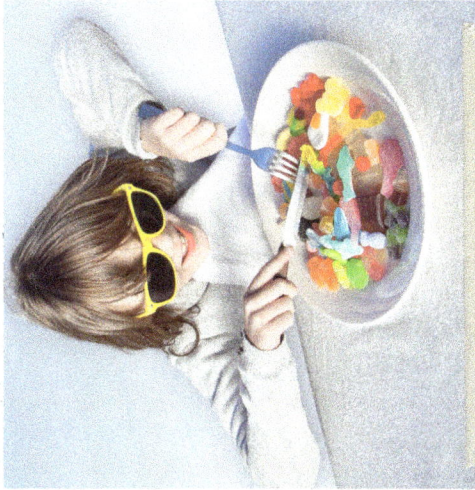
Eats unhealthy food

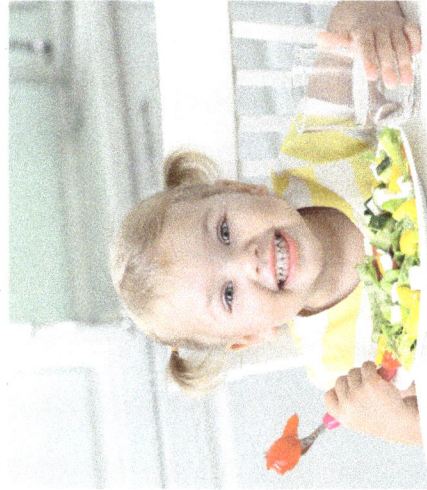
Eats healthy food

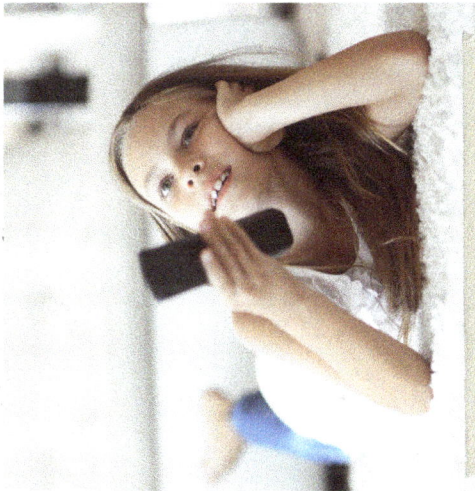
Frequent screen time

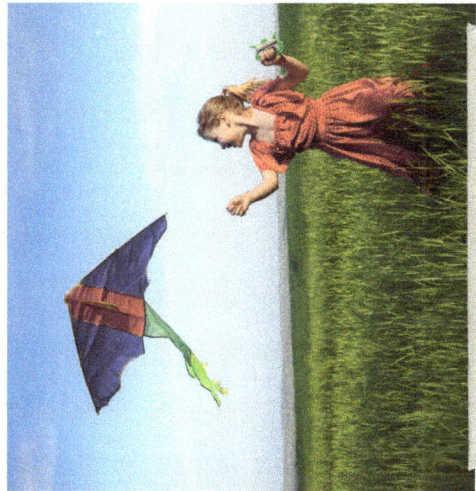
Frequent outdoor time

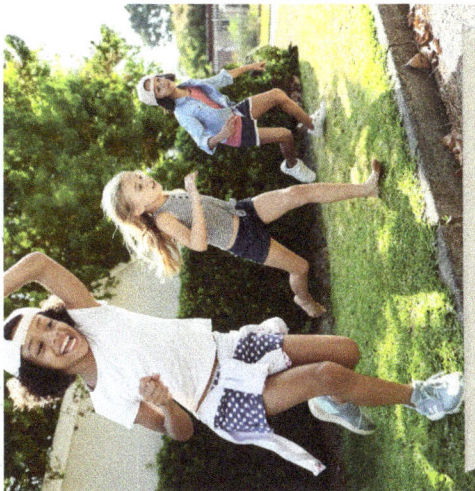
Crosses street without looking

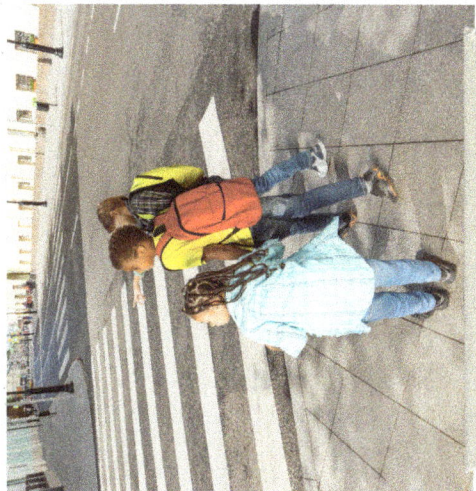
Looks both ways before crossing street

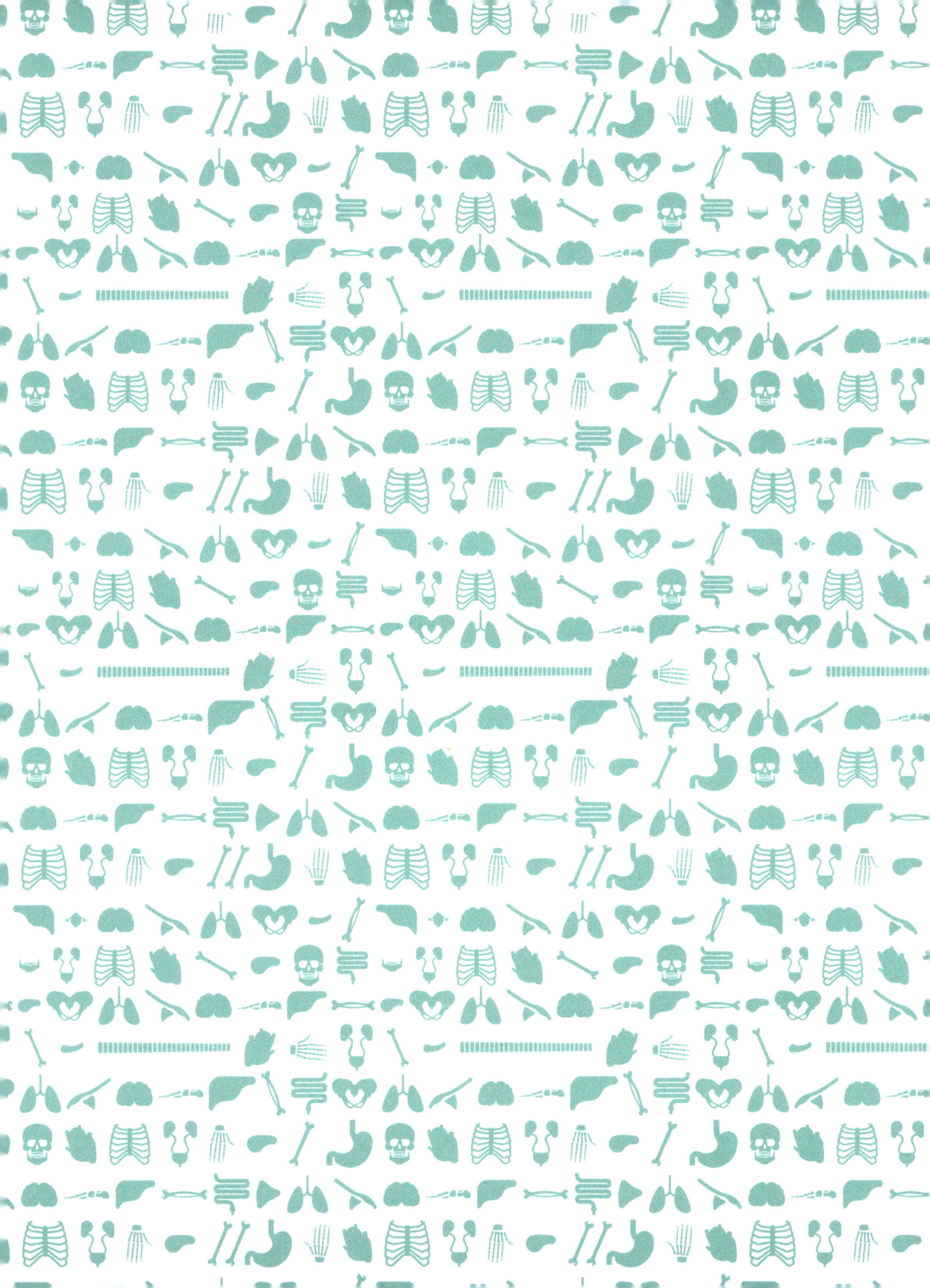

Better Choice Cards

Use with better choice cards. Show the child two cards and have them pick the safer option and place a blue ribbon on the better choice. Discuss.

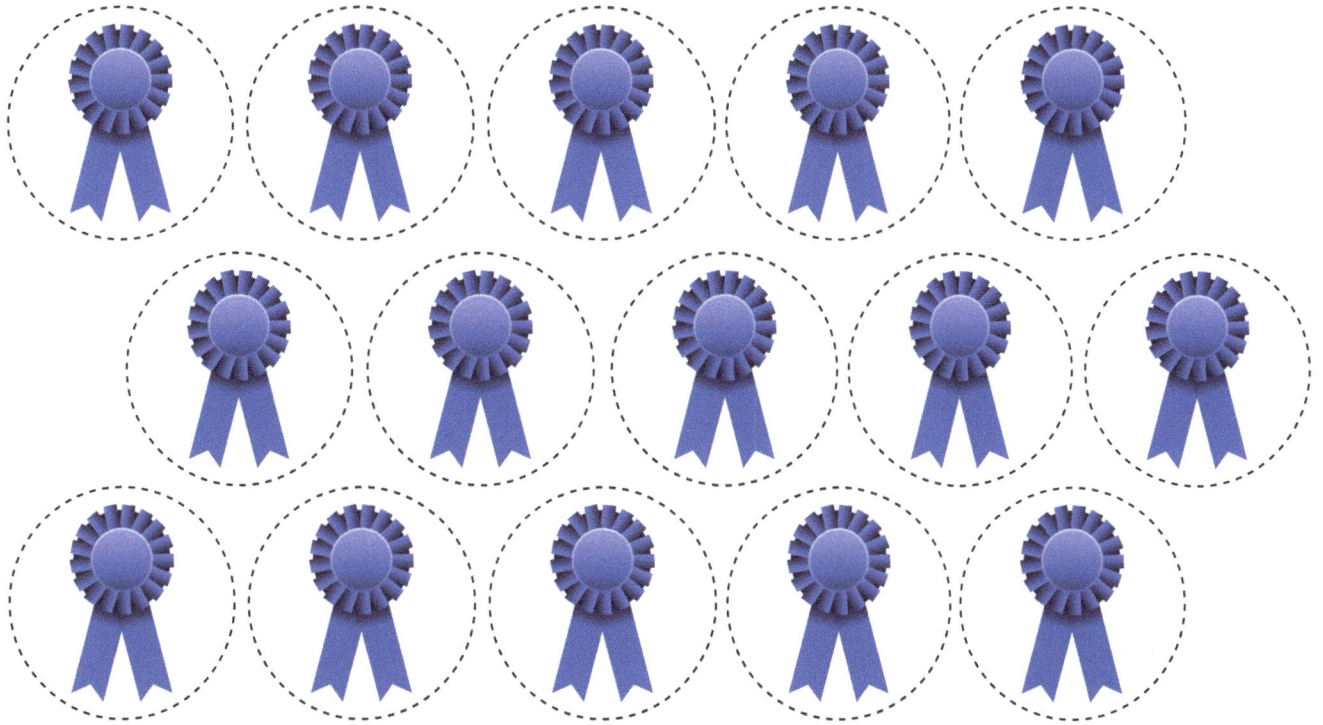

Abdominal Cavity	Fallopian Tube	Ovary	Vertebrae
Uterus	Rectum	Pubic Bone	Bladder
Labia	Bladder	Urethra	Seminal Vesicle
Prostate	Vertebrae	Pubic Bone	Abdominal Cavity
Urethra	Testis	Epididymis	Scrotum
Rectum	Vas Deferens	Penis	

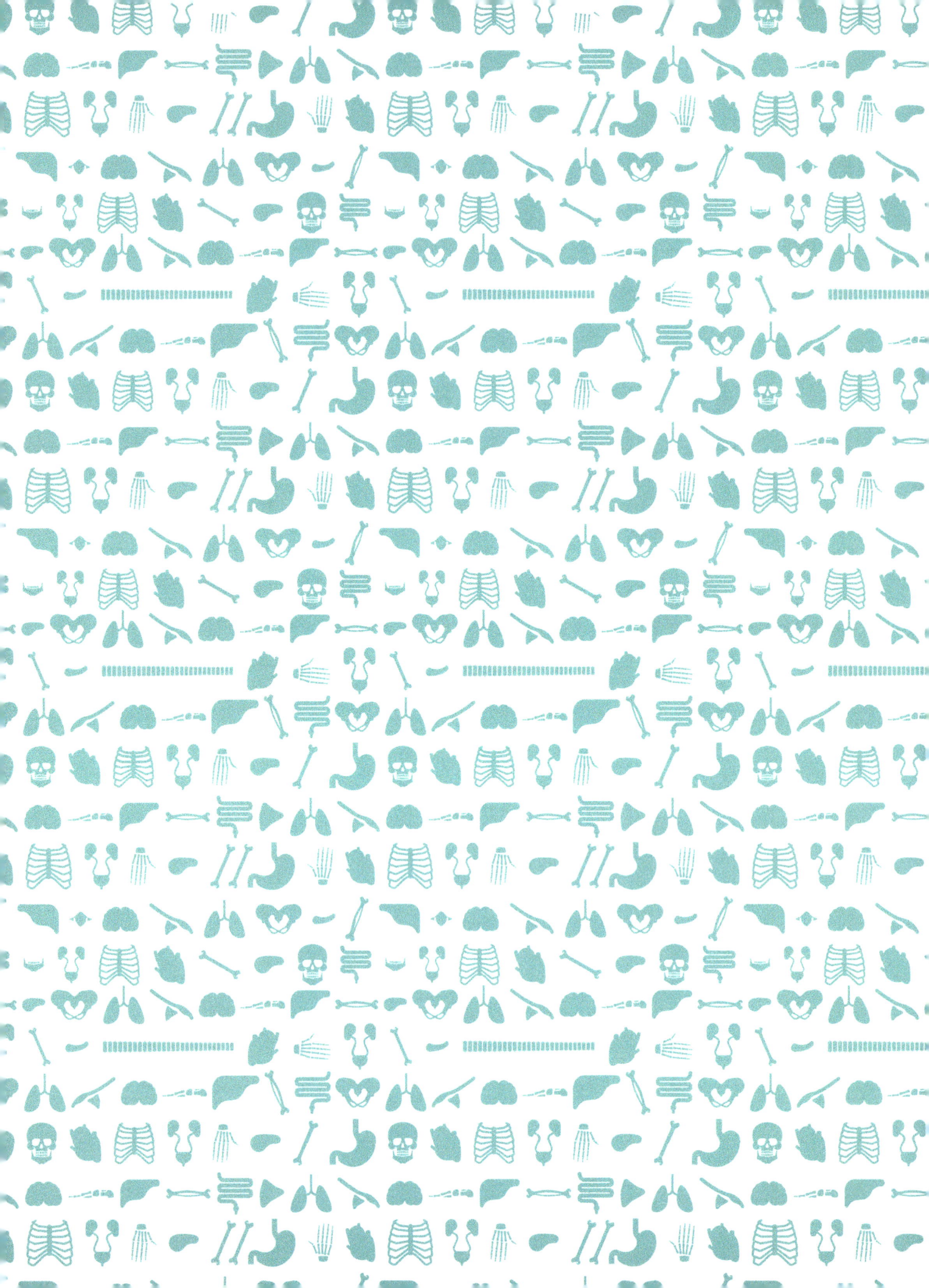

Female Urinary/Reproductive

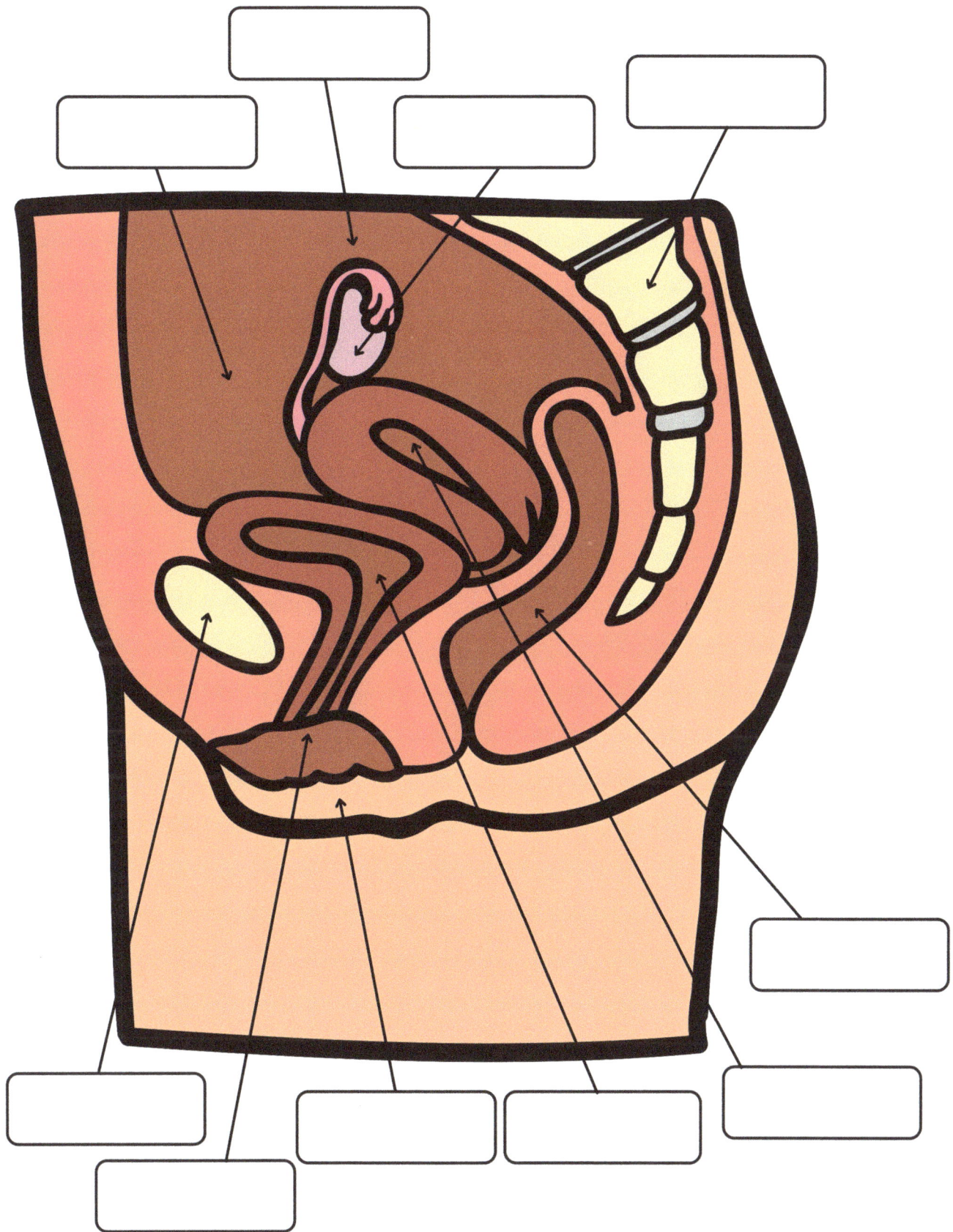

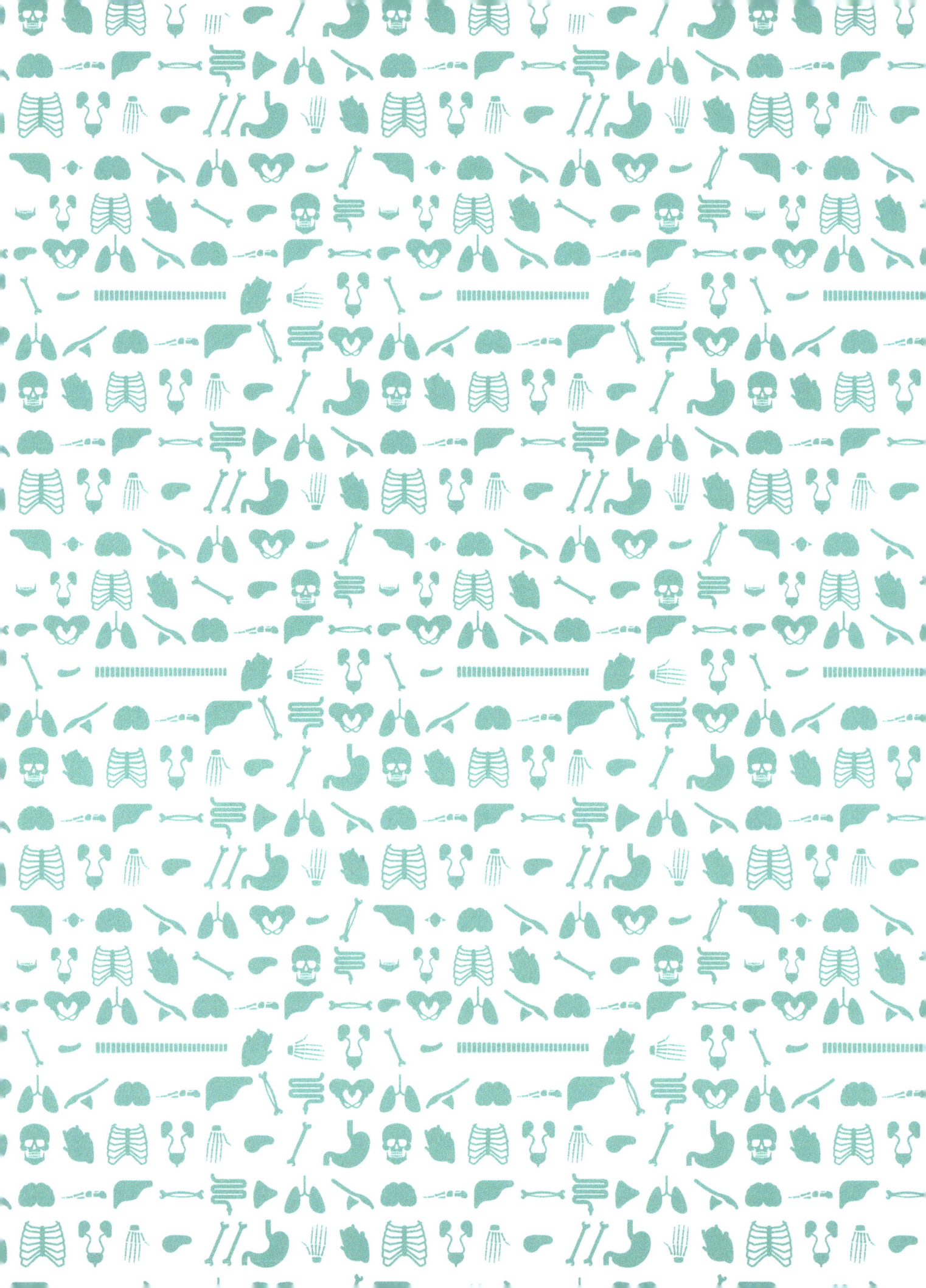

Male Urinary/Reproductive

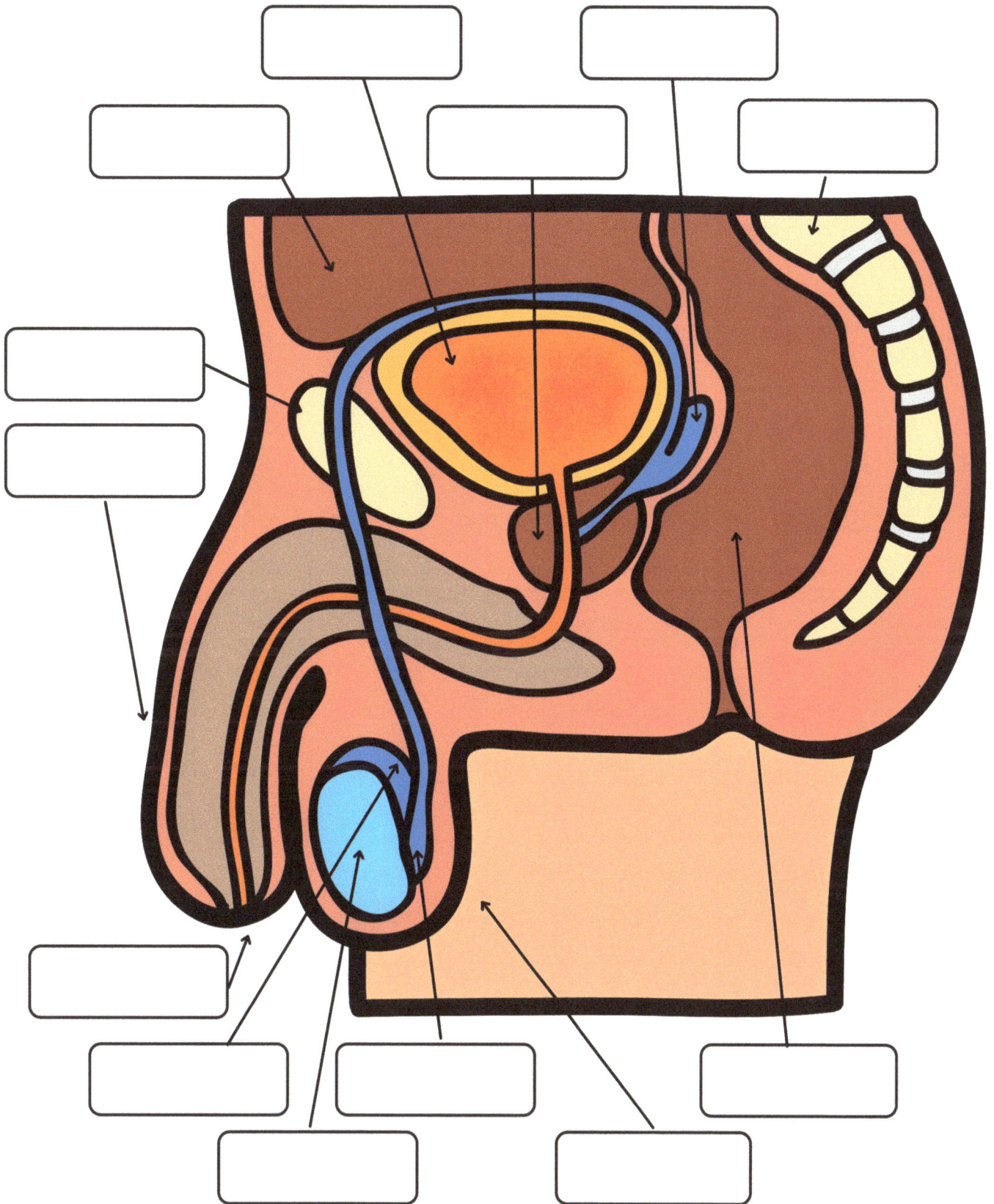

Human Fetus Development Spinner

Cut out both circles. Punch hole as indicated. Place indented circle over second circle and secure with brad. Twist top circle to show each stage of development in 4-week intervals.

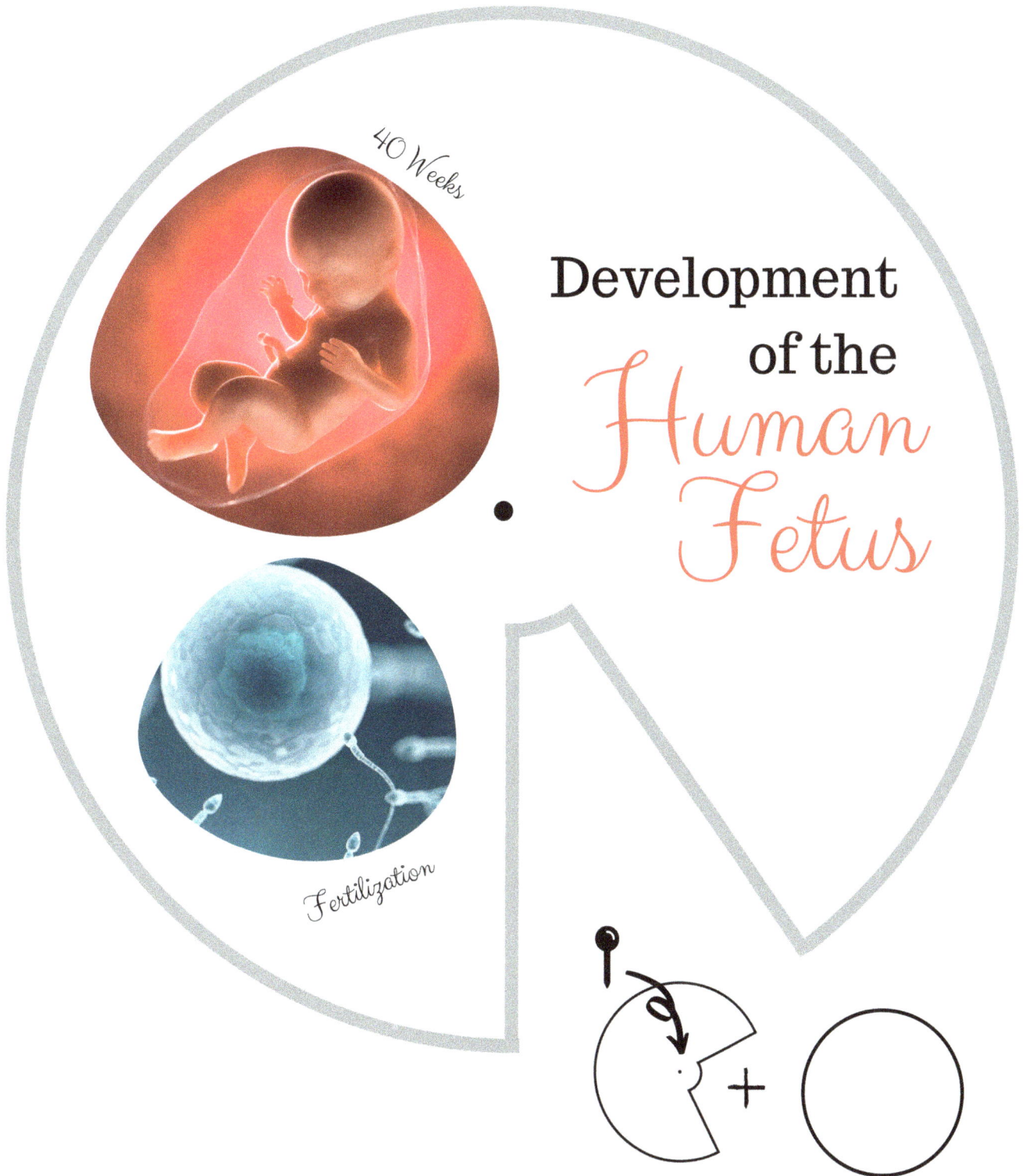

40 Weeks

Development of the *Human Fetus*

Fertilization

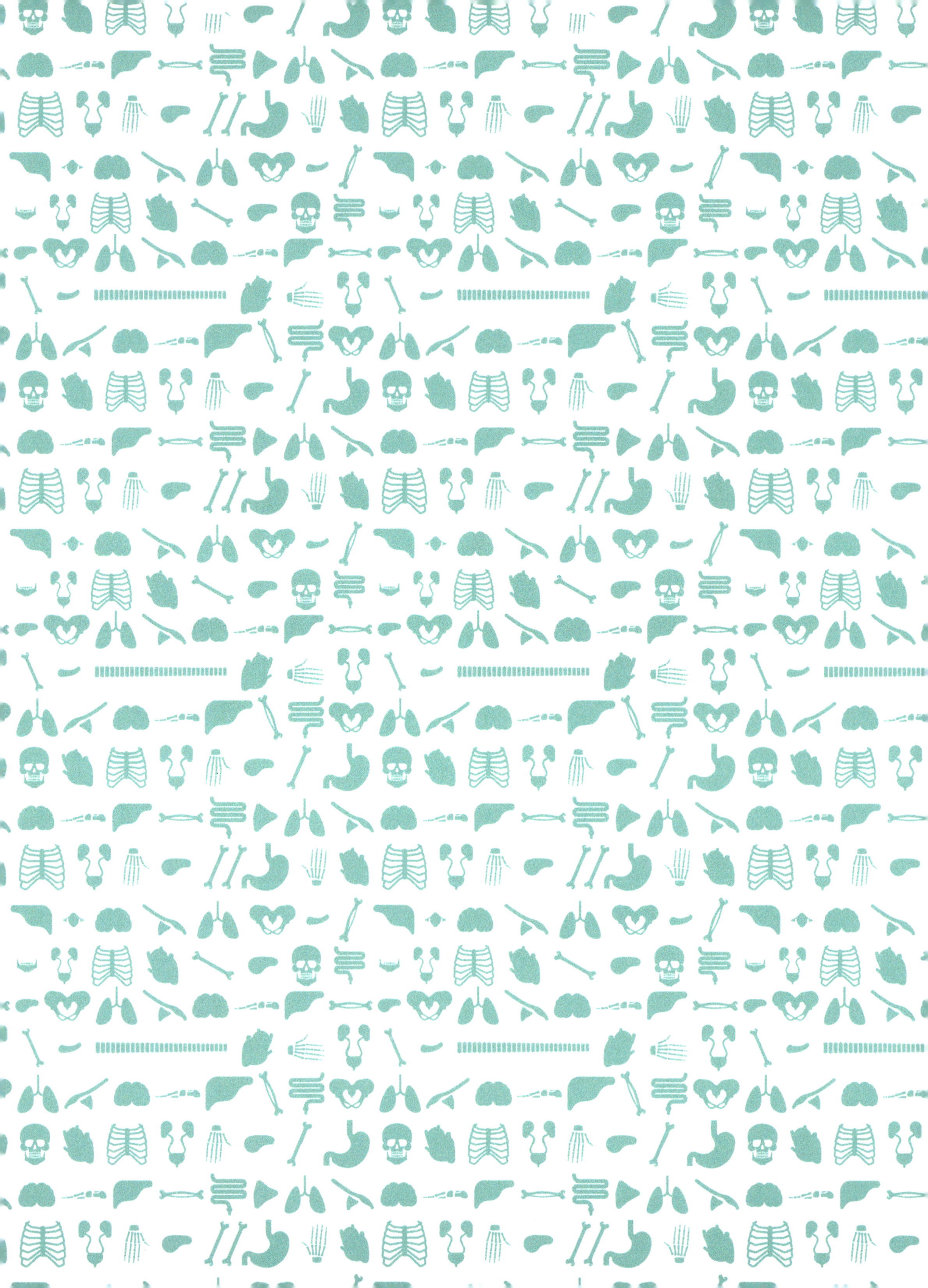

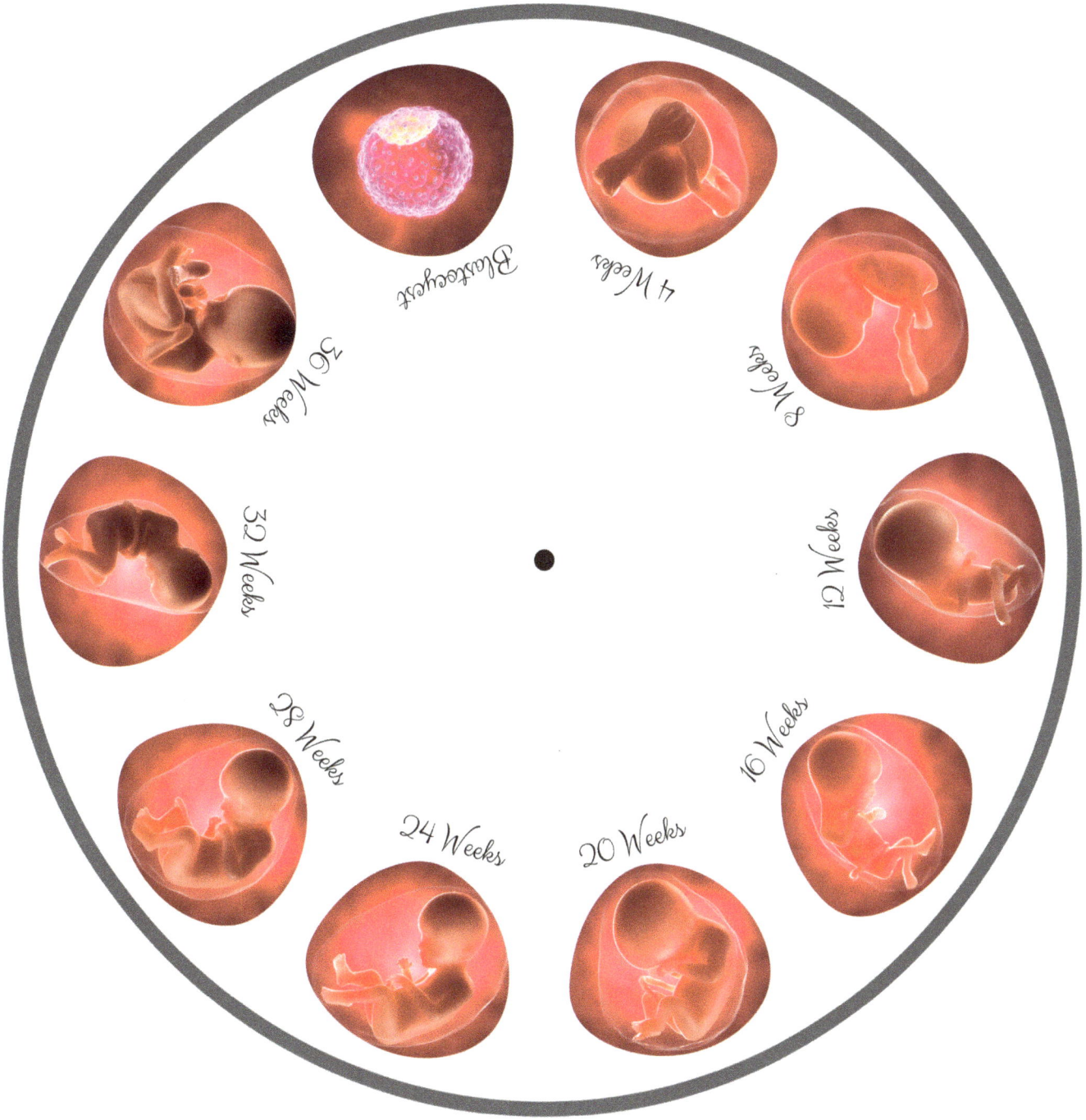

Blastocyst

4 Weeks

8 Weeks

12 Weeks

16 Weeks

20 Weeks

24 Weeks

28 Weeks

32 Weeks

36 Weeks

Stages of Digestion

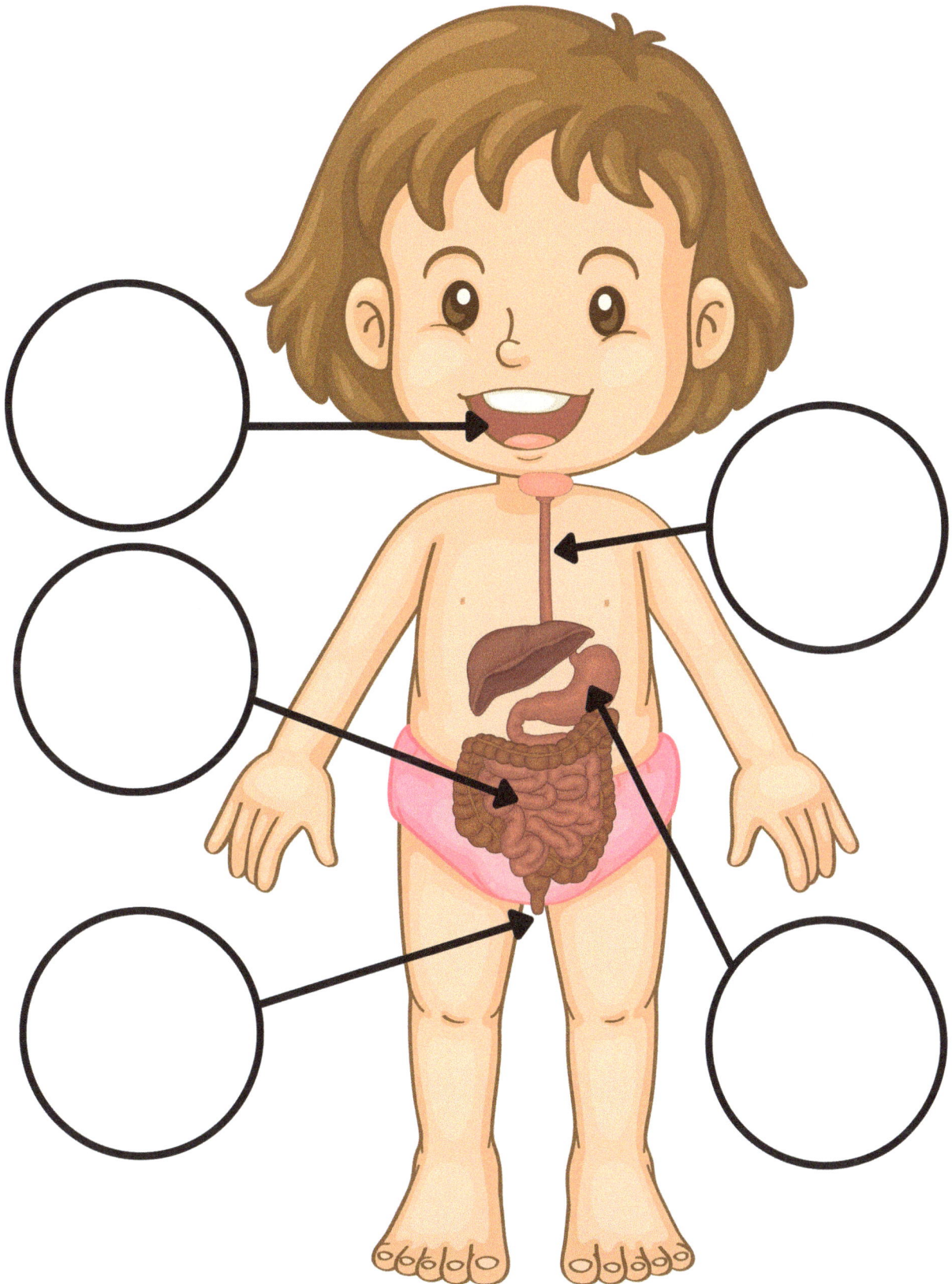

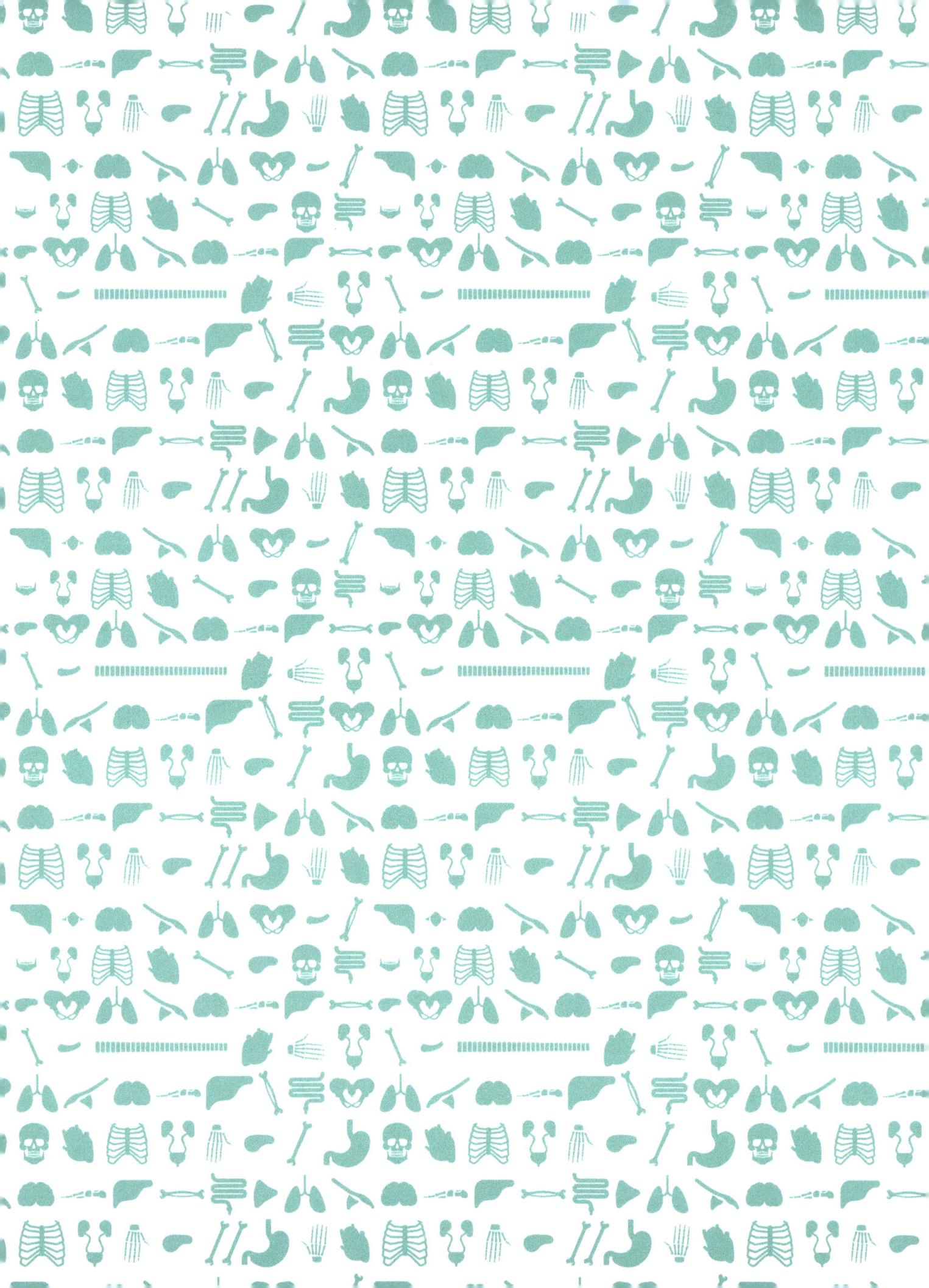

Stages of Digestion

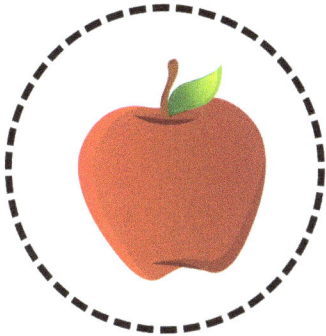

Mastication

Digestion starts in the mouth. The food is chewed by the teeth as part of the mechanical digestion process. It is then mixed with enzymes in the saliva, which starts breaking down the food.

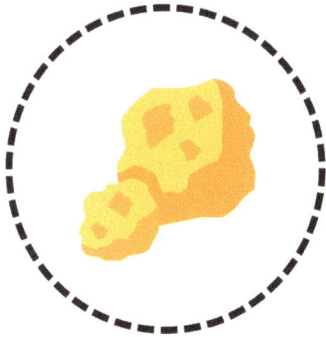

Ingestion

After the food is swallowed, it passes through the esophagus and then into the stomach. This process uses both gravity and peristalsis (muscular movement downward).

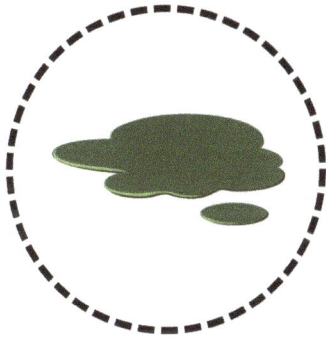

Digestion

In the stomach, the food particles are mixed with stomach acid, which is very powerful. This chemical digestion breaks down the food into simpler parts.

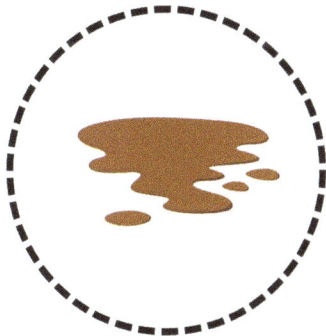

Absorption

The digested stomach contents travels through the small intestine where most of the nutrients are absorbed. The food moves through the many feet of intestines by peristalsis. As it passes through the large intestine, additional water is absorbed, and the resulting fecal matter becomes more solid.

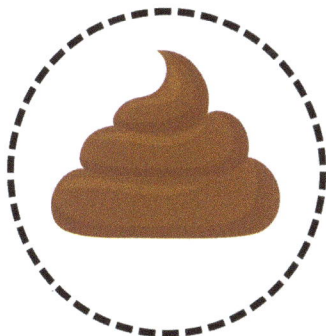

Defecation

After all usable nutrients and fluids are absorbed, the resulting fecal matter is stored in rectum to be expelled by defecation (pooping).

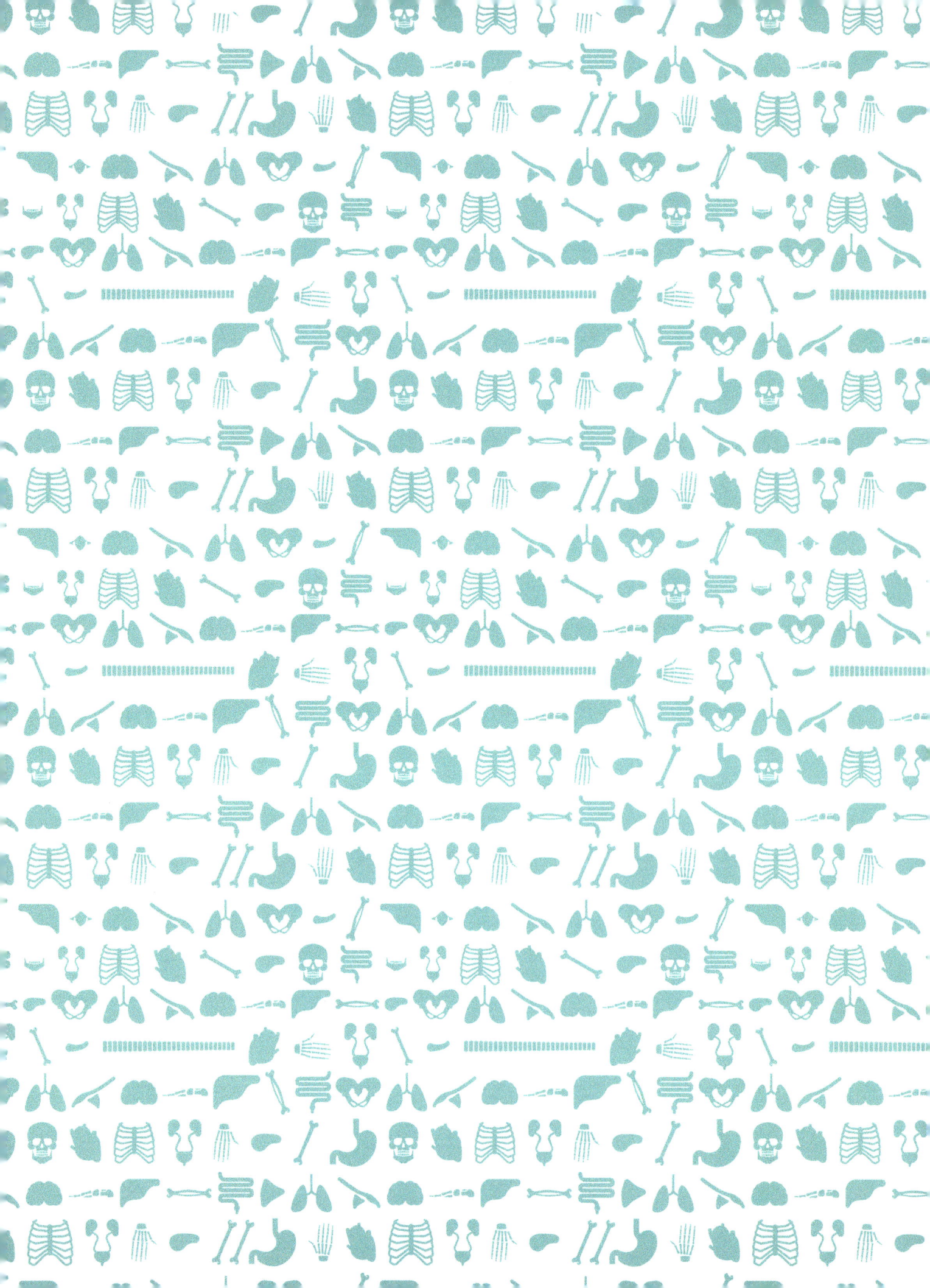

MAKING POOP SENSORY ACTIVITY

Instructions

Digestion is the process of turning ingested food into usable nutrients to fuel body processes. It starts in the mouth as food is masticated (chewed) and ends as poop (defecation).

Provide the child with a sealable bag of crackers - make sure they are easy to crush.

Materials
- Crackers
- Small Rocks
- Sealable Bag
- Vinegar
- Soy Sauce
- Nylon

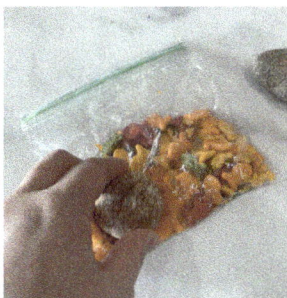

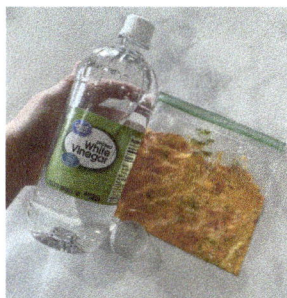

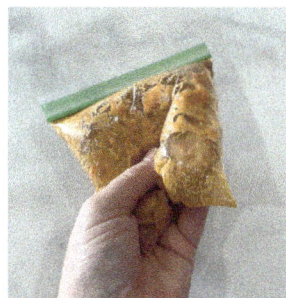

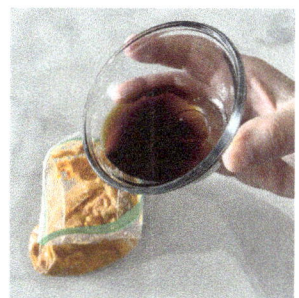

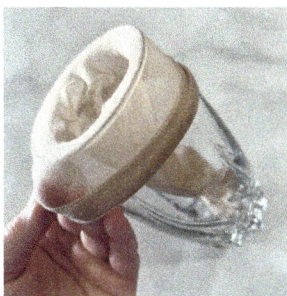

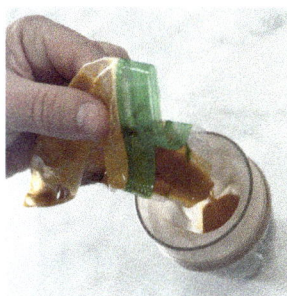

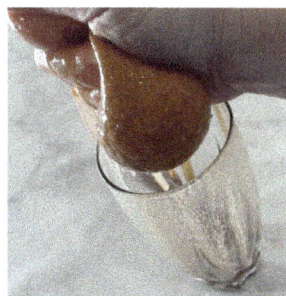

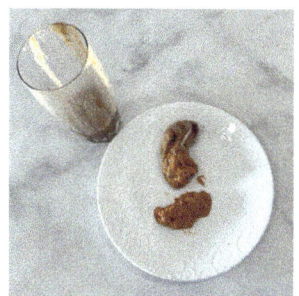

Using smooth stones (or wooden blocks, Legos) "chew" up the food by crunching them into soft pieces. Use 1-2 Tablespoons of vinegar - this represents the saliva and stomach acids as the food moves down the digestive track. Continue to mix thoroughly. Discuss how the small intestine continues to mix the food together in a process called segmentation and moves through the GI track by peristalsis. Add 2-3 Tablespoons of soy sauce. This represents bile, which is created in the liver and released by the gallbladder. The purpose of bile is to break down fats in the small intestine and assists in removing waste products from the body. Secure a nylon sock over a glass and pour the contents of the bag into the nylon sock. Squish the watery contents out of the nylon - discuss how the large intestine is a semi-permeable membrane and absorbs excess fluid back into the body. After all available fluid is squeezed out, look at what is left - how does it compare with real poop?

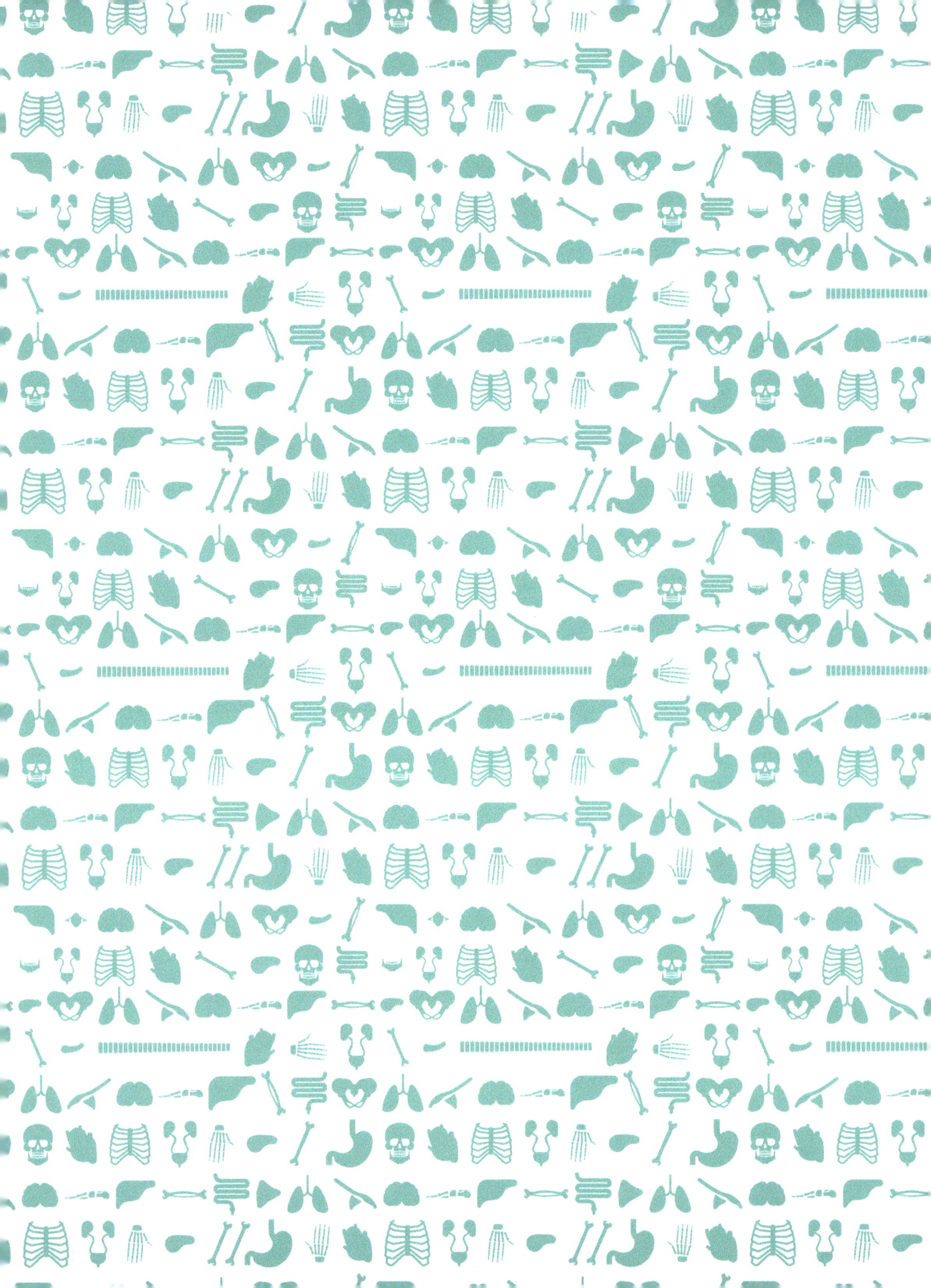

Healthy Plate Sorting

Cut out "Healthy Plate". Laminate for additional durability. Cut out food options and have child match the appropriate foods to appropriate categories. What foods do not belong? Discuss.

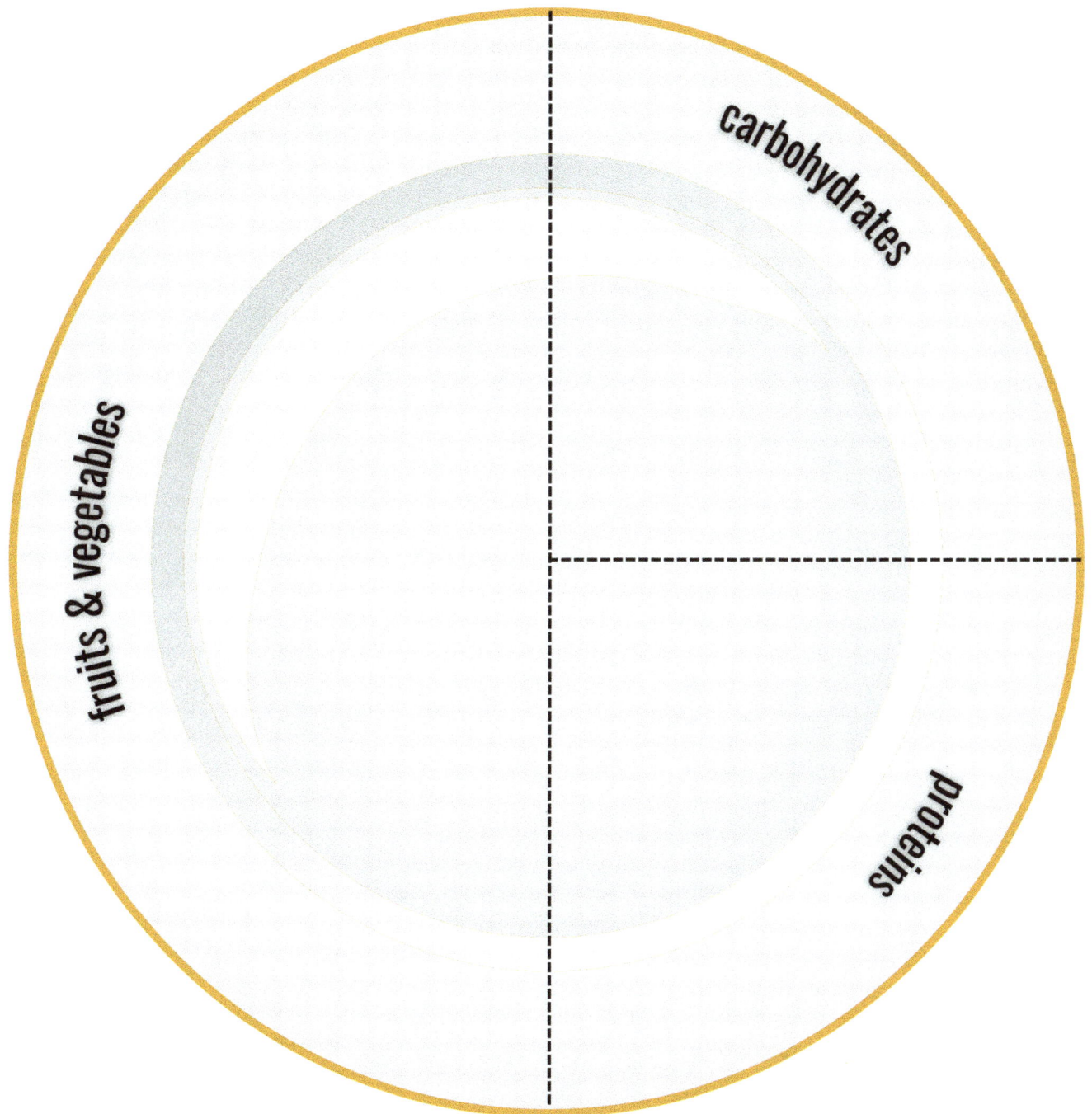

carbohydrates

fruits & vegetables

proteins

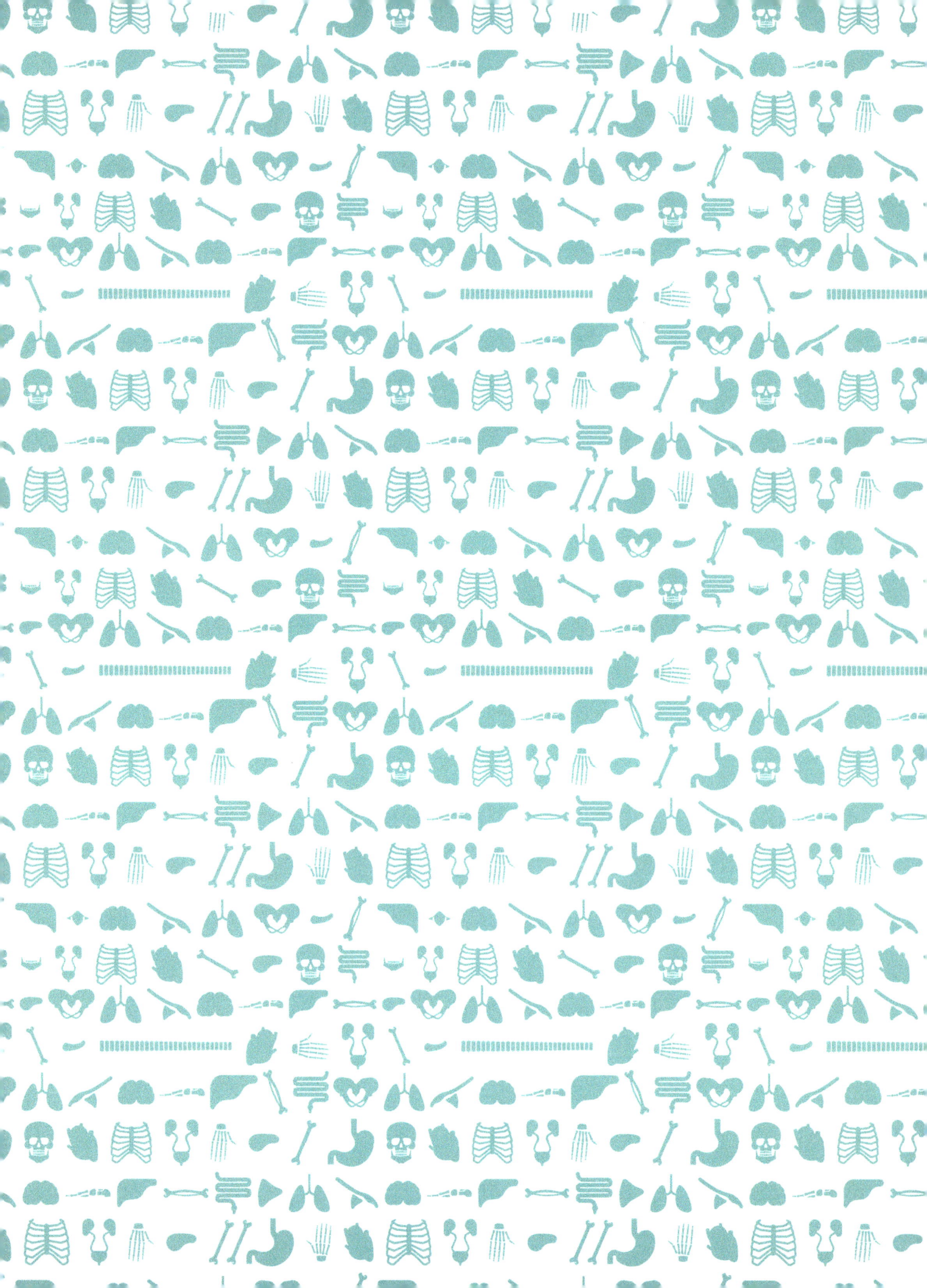

Healthy Plate Food Options

Fruits and Vegetables

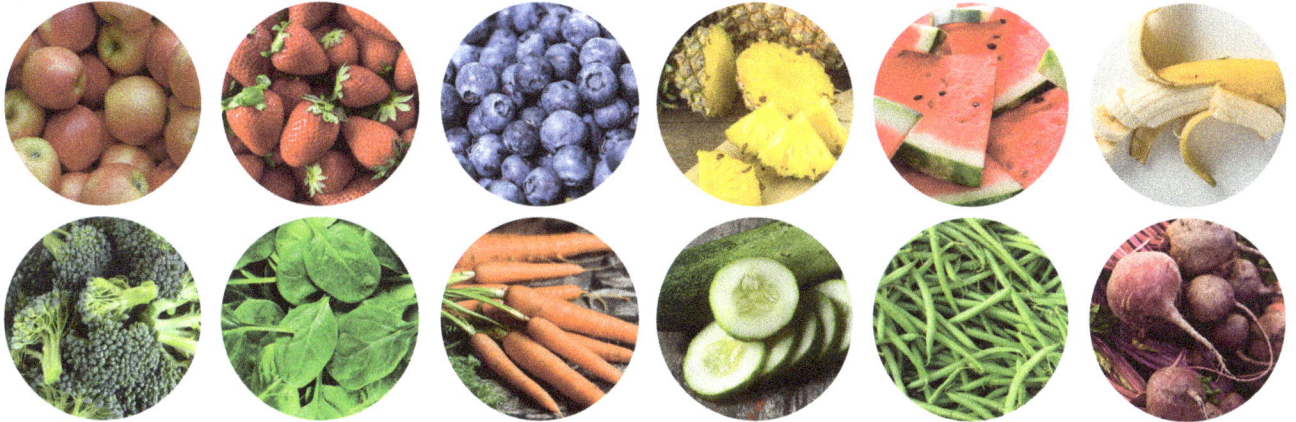

Carbohydrates

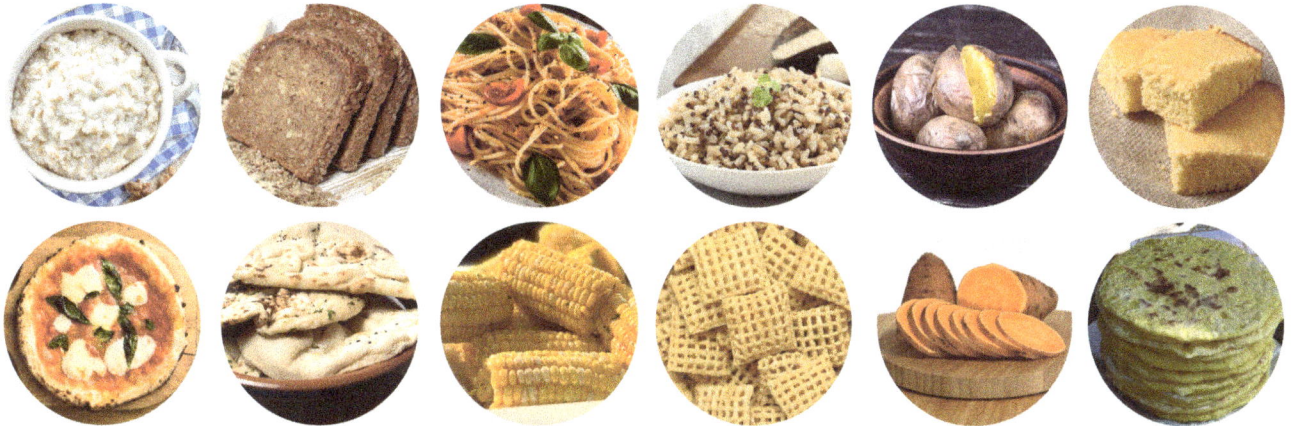

Proteins

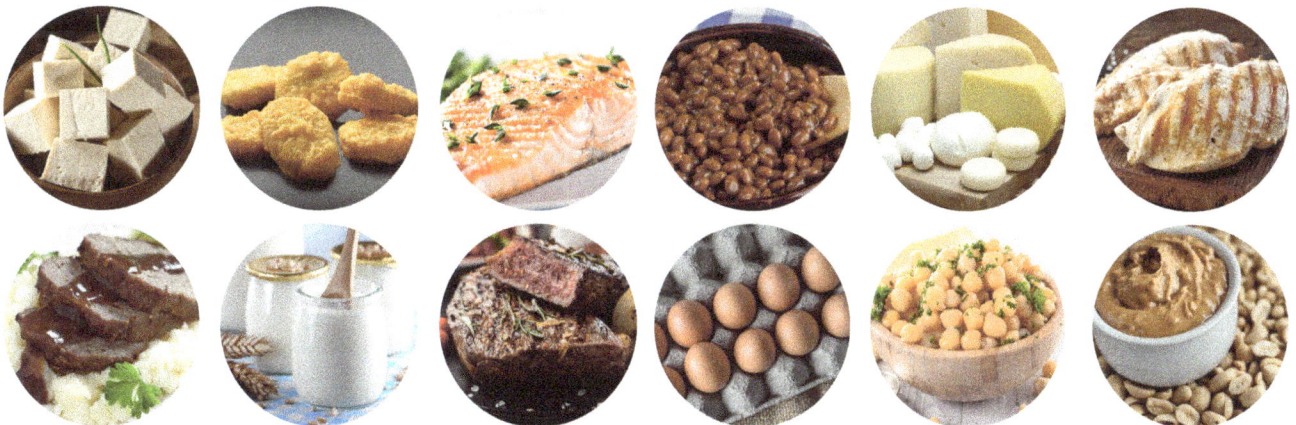

Other

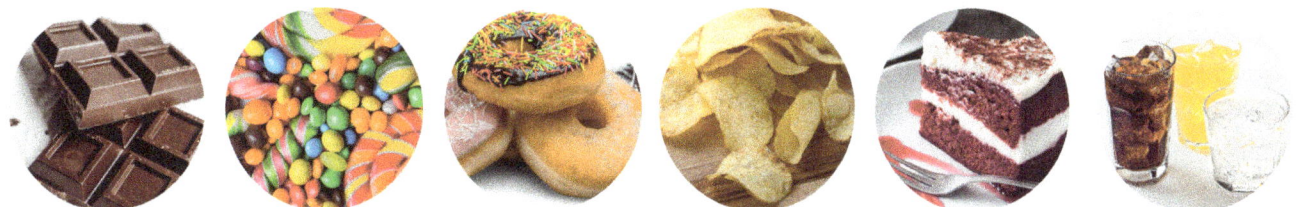

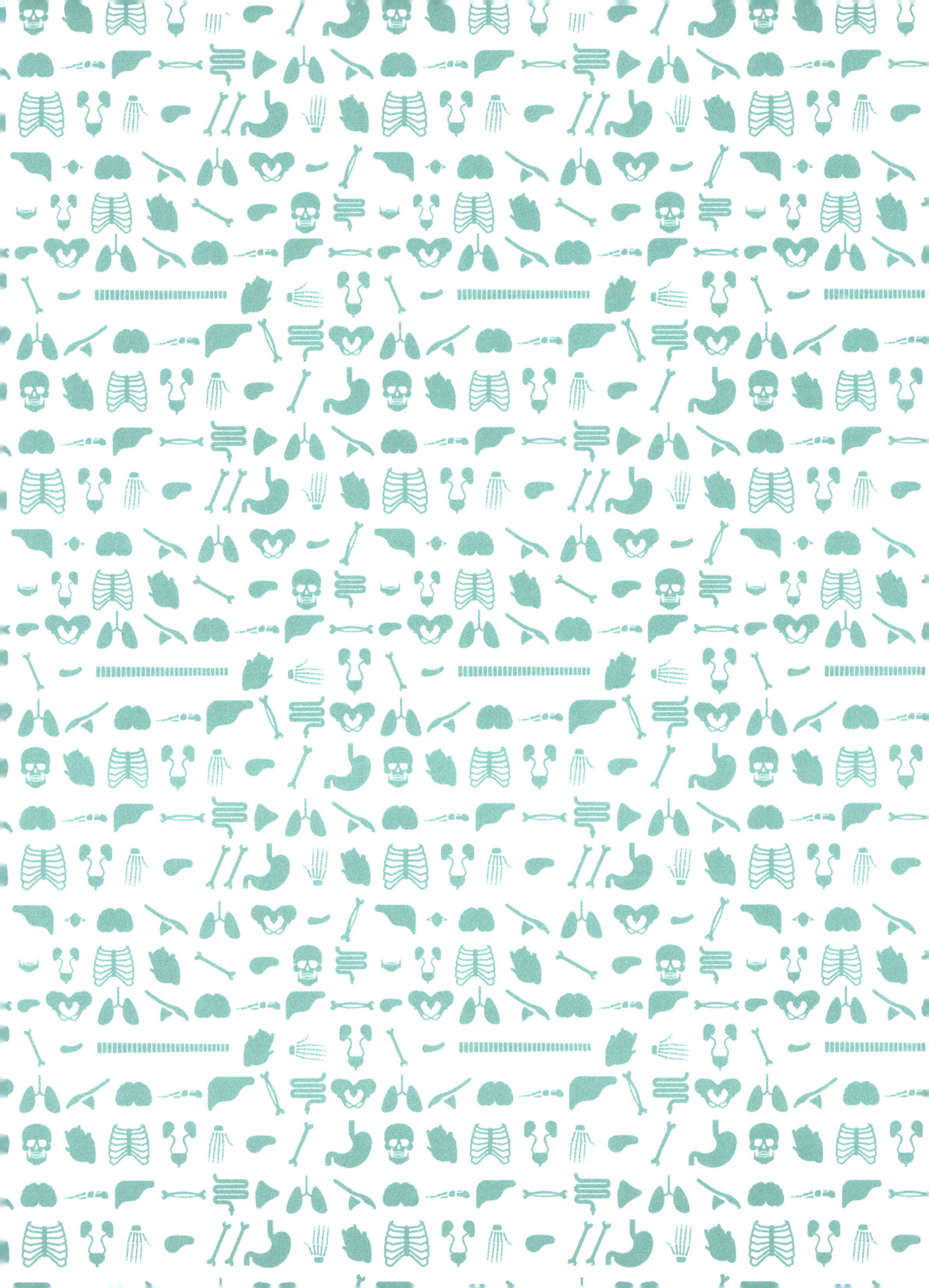

LAYERS OF THE SKIN

Instructions

The skin is the largest organ of the body, and protects the body from microbes, substances and helps regulate body temperature. It also allows the sensations of touch, heat, and cold. It is divided into three main layers, the epidermis, dermis and subcutaneous layers. The epidermis is further subdivided into five additional layers.

Materials

- Foam Sheet
- Plastic Sheet
- Construction Paper
- Felt
- Grip Liner
- 1" Foam
- Bubble Wrap
- Pipe Cleaners
- Grey, Red & Blue Yarn

Use the included template to cut out the different layers from different substances. It is important to note that the stratum basele (part of the epidermis) is the only layer that truly has a "color" due to the melanocytes - however for the sake of illustration, use whatever skin tone of foam sheet, construction paper, felt, etc. Layer the different layers in a stair-step pattern. Lay the yarn strands (nerves, veins & arteries) between the subcutaneous layer and using an awl or small knife, cut holes in the dermis and insert them into this layer. For the hair follicles, use a paper punch to cut through all the layers down to the dermis and thread the pipe cleaner "hairs" through. Label each layer using included tags.

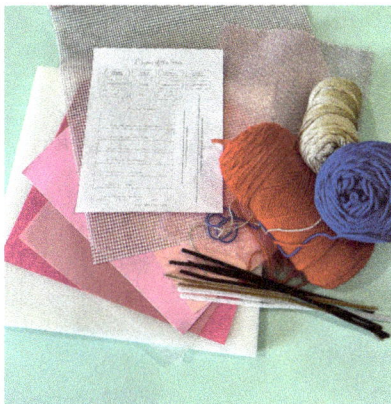

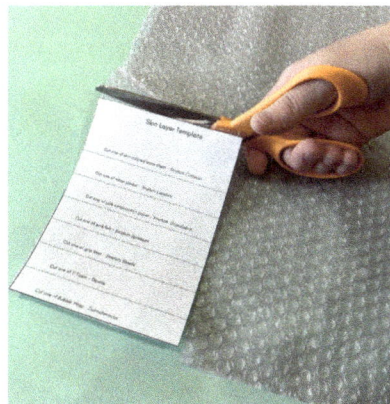

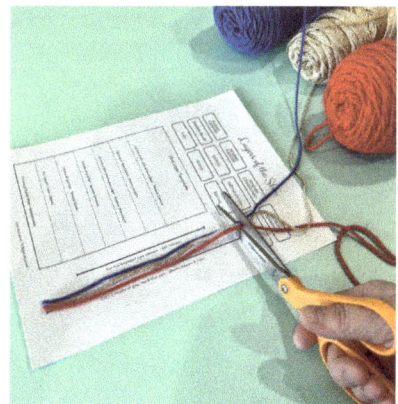

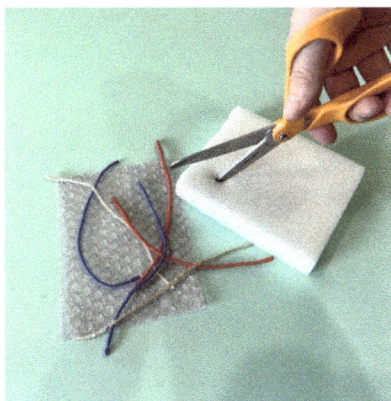

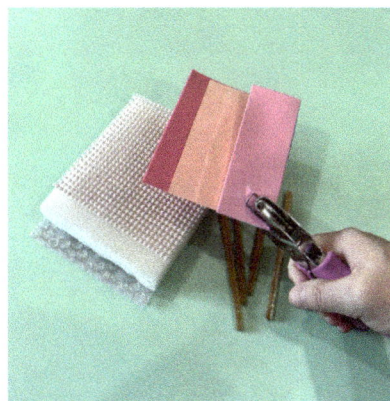

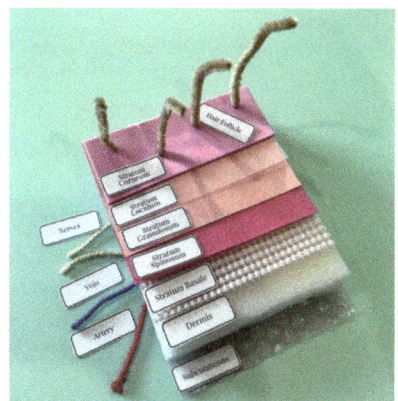

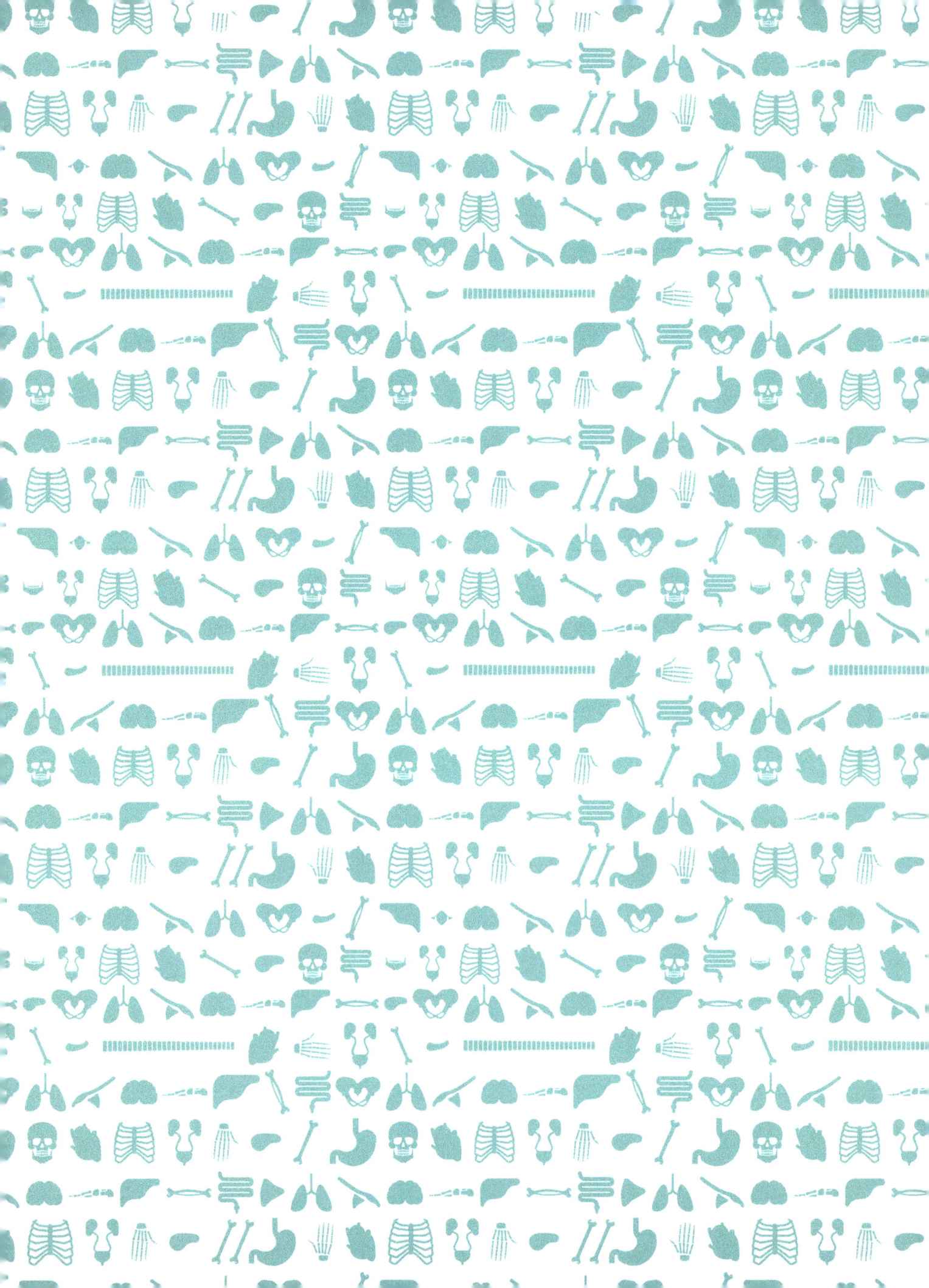

Layers of the Skin

Stratum Corneum	Stratum Lucidum	Stratum Granulosum	Stratum Spinosum
Stratum Basale	Dermis	Subcutaneous	Hair Follicle
Vein	Artery	Nerves	

Skin Layer Template

Cut one of skin colored foam sheet – *Stratum Corneum*

Cut one of clear plastic – *Stratum Lucidum*

Cut one of pink construction paper – *Stratum Granulosum*

Cut one of pink felt – *Stratum Spinosum*

Cut one of grip liner – *Stratum Basale*

Cut one of 1" Foam – *Dermis*

Cut one of Bubble Wrap – *Subcutaneous*

Cut 4-6 lengths of pipe cleaners – Hair Follicles

Cut 1-2 lengths of grey, red & blue yarn – Nerves, Arteries & Veins

BALLOON FINGERPRINTS

Instructions

The papillary ridges on the ends of the fingers and thumbs form unique fingerprints, an infallible means of personal identification, because the ridge arrangement on every finger of every human being is unique and does not alter with growth or age. Fingerprints are even more unique than DNA. Even identical twins don't have the same fingerprints.

Lay a deflated balloon on a flat surface. Press finger onto ink pad and cover surface with ink. Press carefully on balloon surface and carefully remove. Fingerprint should be visible. Allow to dry for 2-3 minutes. Blow up balloon and observe fingerprint. Repeat with a different finger.

Discuss: Compare the prints - how are they similar? How do they differ?

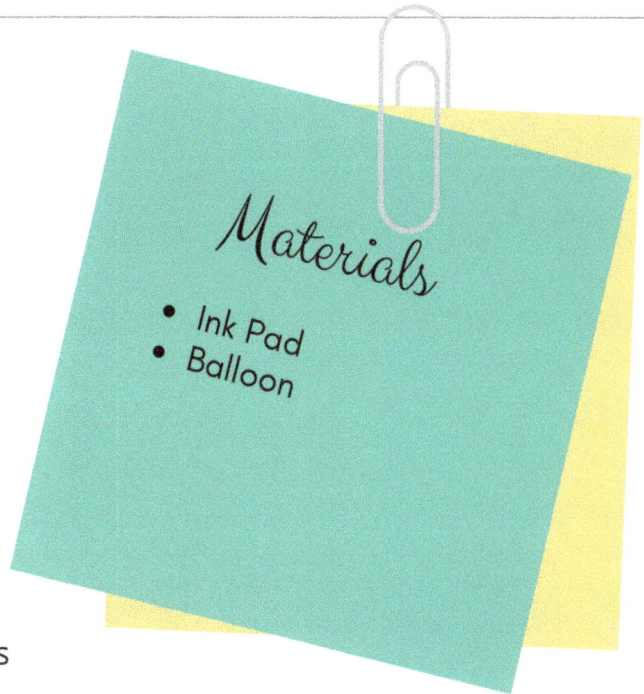

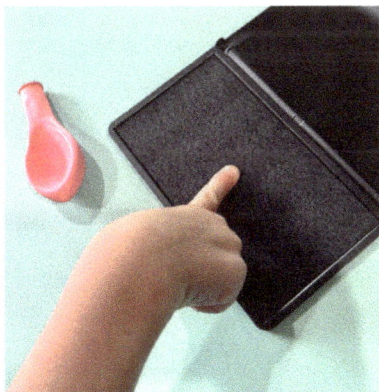

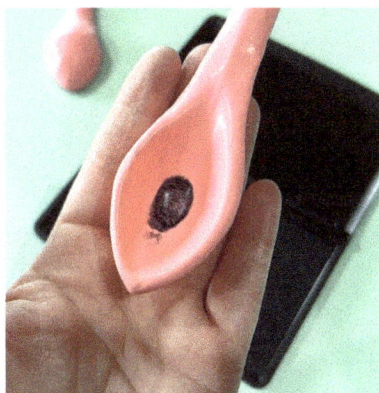

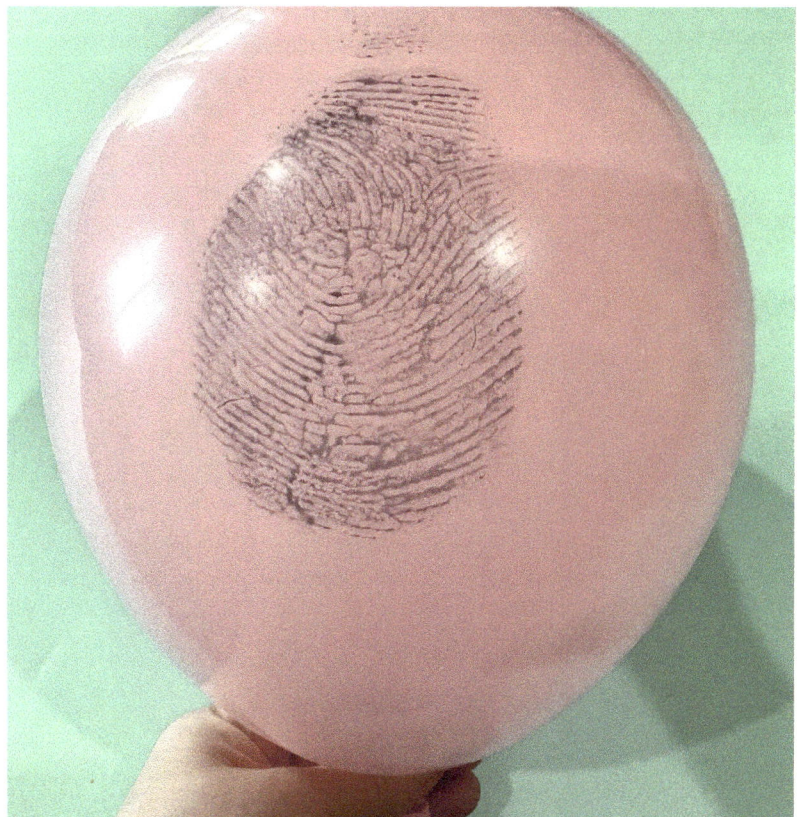

Materials
- Ink Pad
- Balloon

BRAIN HEMISPHERE HAT

Instructions

The human brain is the command center for the human nervous system. It receives signals from the body's sensory organs and outputs information to the muscles. It controls involuntary functions such as breathing and cardiac contractions. It also is the location of higher-level functions such as language, conscious thought and reasoning. This activity helps the child recognize the different sections of the brain and what each area is responsible for body and cognitive function. Cut out the included brain hemisphere hat template. Cut along each side of the wedges and pull each (now cut) dashed line over until it touches the opposite line and secure with tape or glue. Note: if using glue, hold together with clothes pins or paper clips while drying. Continue pleating until you form a half hemisphere. It should look now as a half-round shape. Attach both sides with tape to form a full brain. Attach the cerebellum and brain stem to back to complete hat. **Discuss:** What functions each lobe performs. Compare the right and left side, what functions are the same? Different?

Materials

- Brain Hemisphere Hat Template
- Scissors
- Tape

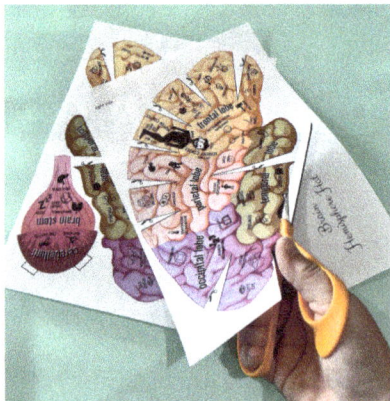

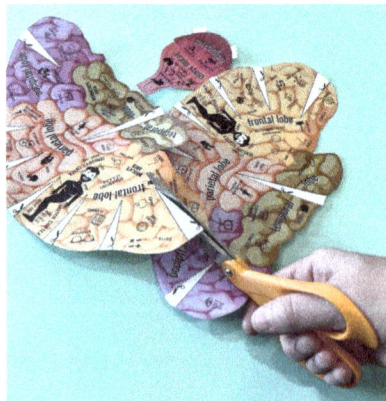

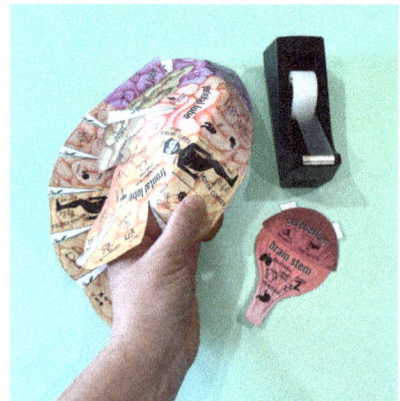

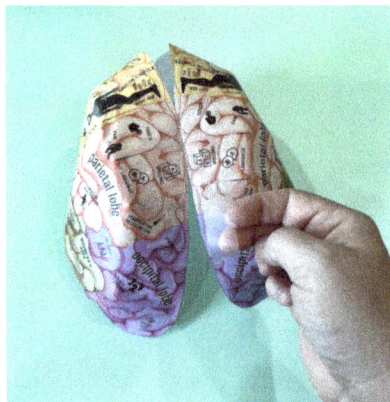

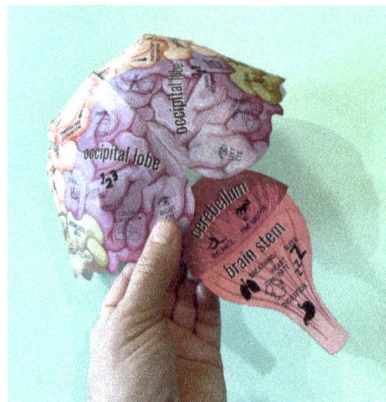

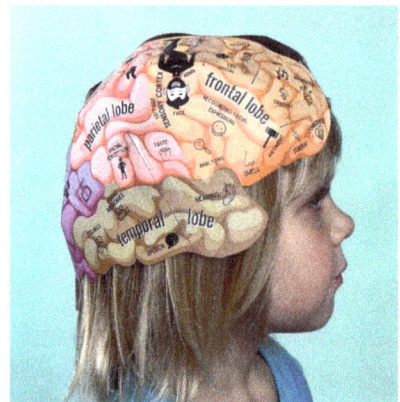

right side

frontal lobe

IDEAS

ART

SOCIAL

MUSIC

IMAGINATION

CREATIVITY

CONSCIENCE

EUREKA!

JUDGMENT

SMELL

ANALYZING

RECOGNIZING FACIAL EXPRESSIONS

MOTOR CORTEX

TOE
FOOT
LEG
TRUNK

LEFT SIDE

ARMS

SENSORY CORTEX

LEFT SIDE

FACE

TOUCH

PAIN

parietal lobe

TASTE

SPATIAL PERCEPTION

SPELLING

LANGUAGE

TEMPERATURE RECOGNITION

HEARING

temporal lobe

VISUAL MEMORIES

FEELINGS

SPEECH

occipital lobe

DIMENSIONS

READING

NUMBER RECOGNITION

COLOR PERCEPTION

LEFT EYE

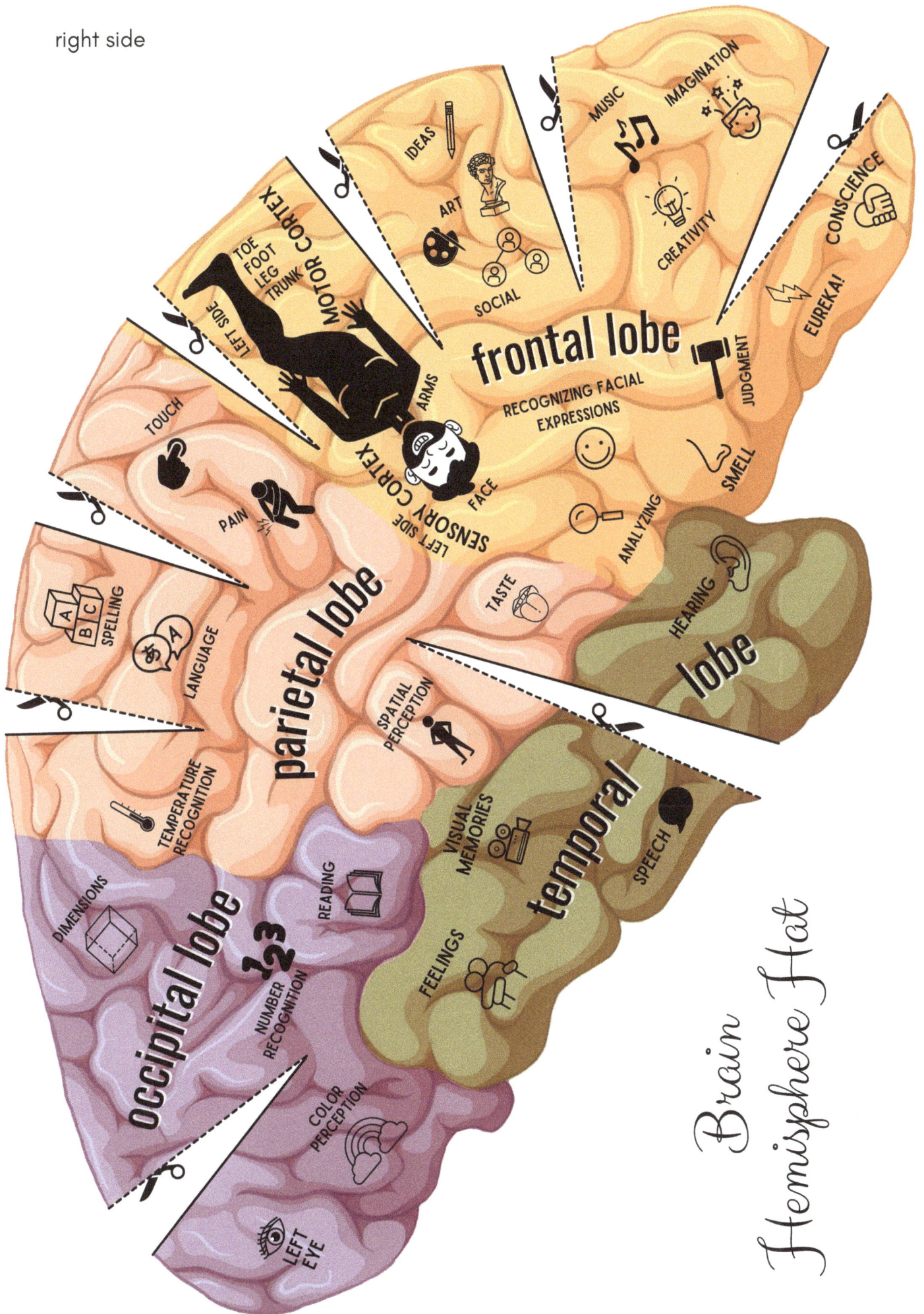

Brain Hemisphere Hat

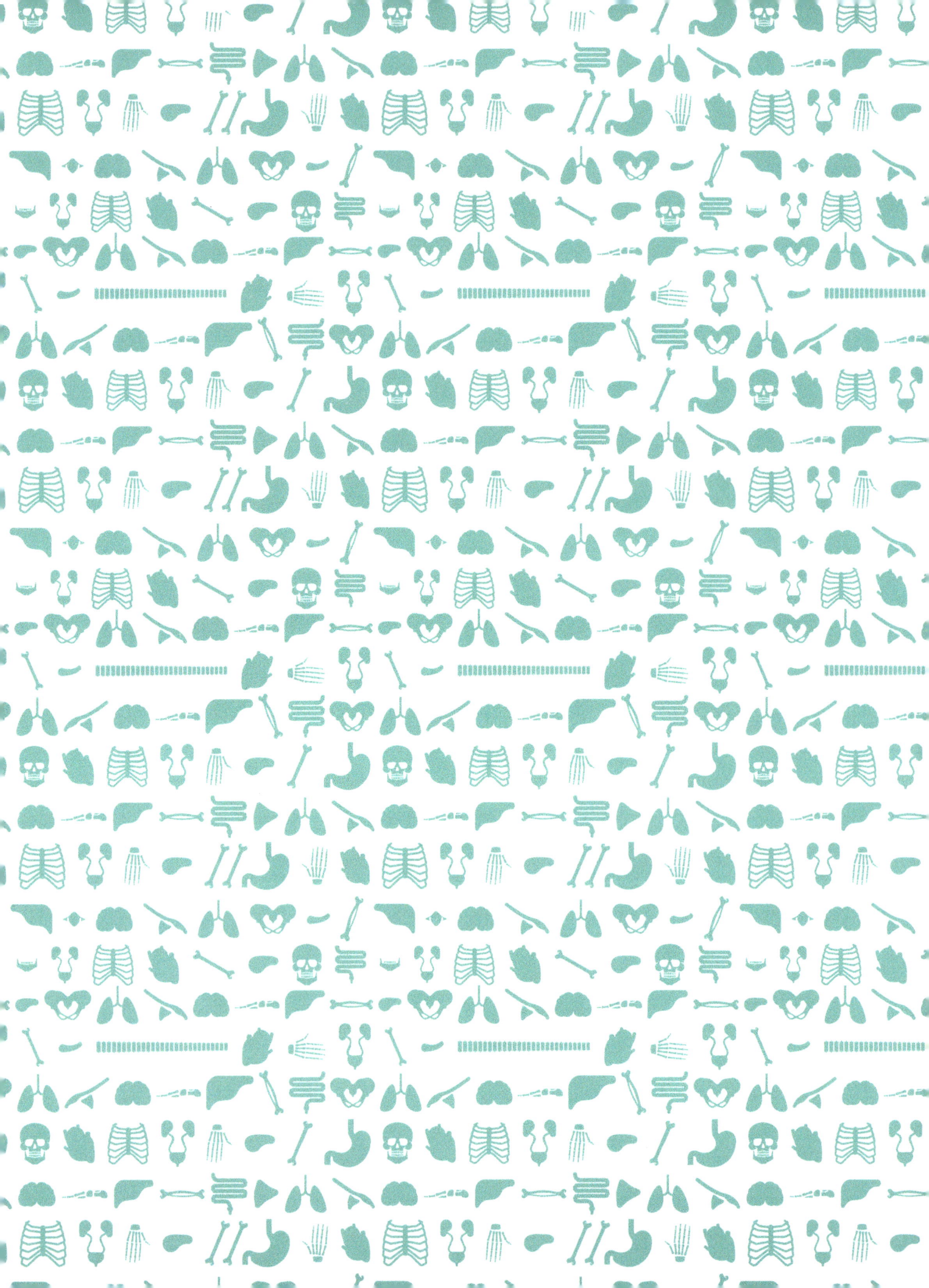

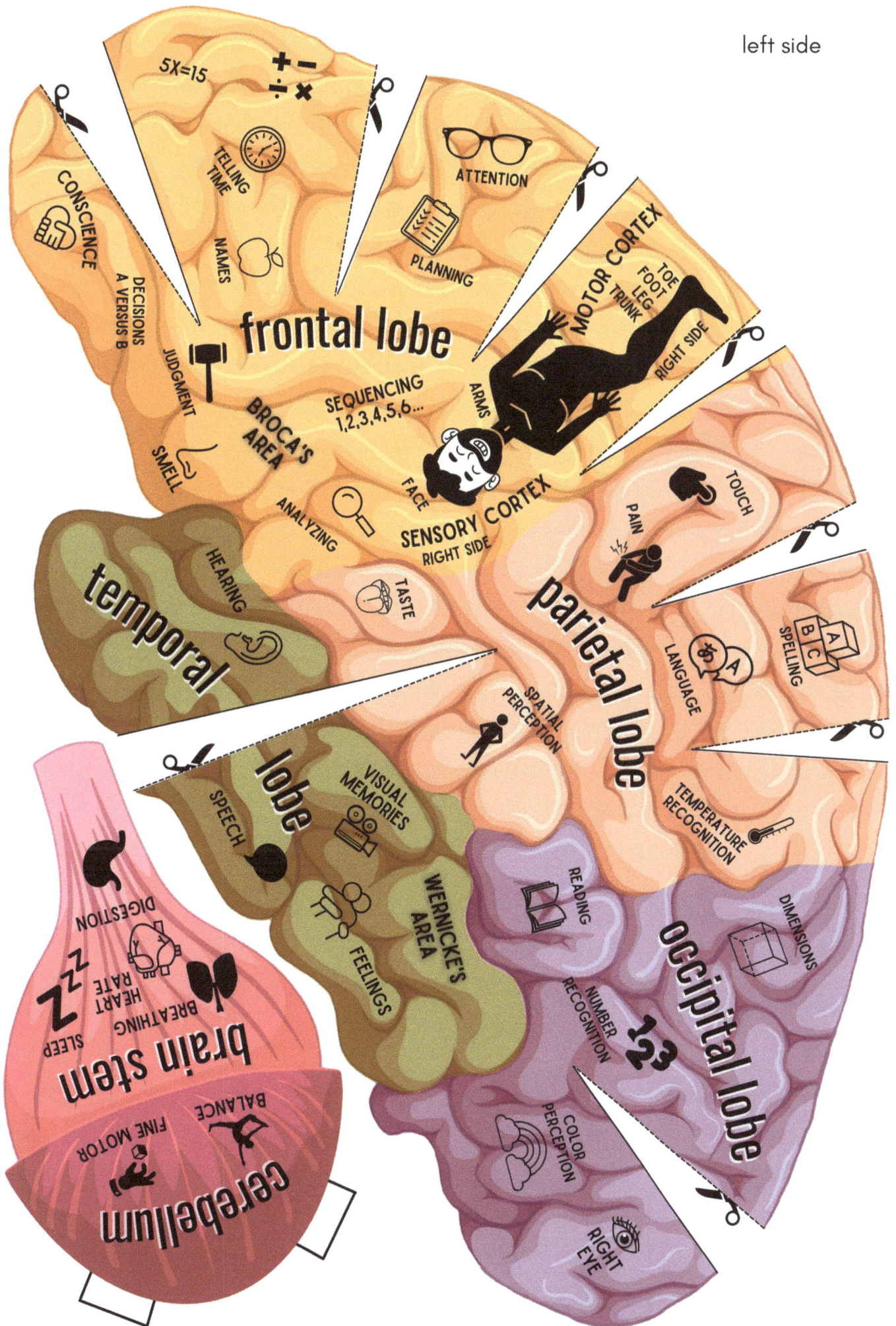

left side

frontal lobe

- CONSCIENCE
- DECISIONS A VERSUS B
- JUDGMENT
- SMELL
- 5X=15
- TELLING TIME
- NAMES
- BROCA'S AREA
- SEQUENCING 1,2,3,4,5,6...
- ANALYZING
- FACE
- ATTENTION
- PLANNING

MOTOR CORTEX
- TOE
- FOOT
- LEG
- TRUNK
- ARMS
- RIGHT SIDE

SENSORY CORTEX
RIGHT SIDE

temporal
- HEARING

lobe
- SPEECH
- VISUAL MEMORIES
- WERNICKE'S AREA
- FEELINGS

parietal lobe
- TASTE
- PAIN
- TOUCH
- SPATIAL PERCEPTION
- LANGUAGE
- SPELLING
- TEMPERATURE RECOGNITION

occipital lobe
- READING
- DIMENSIONS
- NUMBER RECOGNITION
- 123
- COLOR PERCEPTION
- RIGHT EYE

brain stem
- DIGESTION
- HEART RATE
- BREATHING
- SLEEP
- ZZZ

cerebellum
- FINE MOTOR
- BALANCE

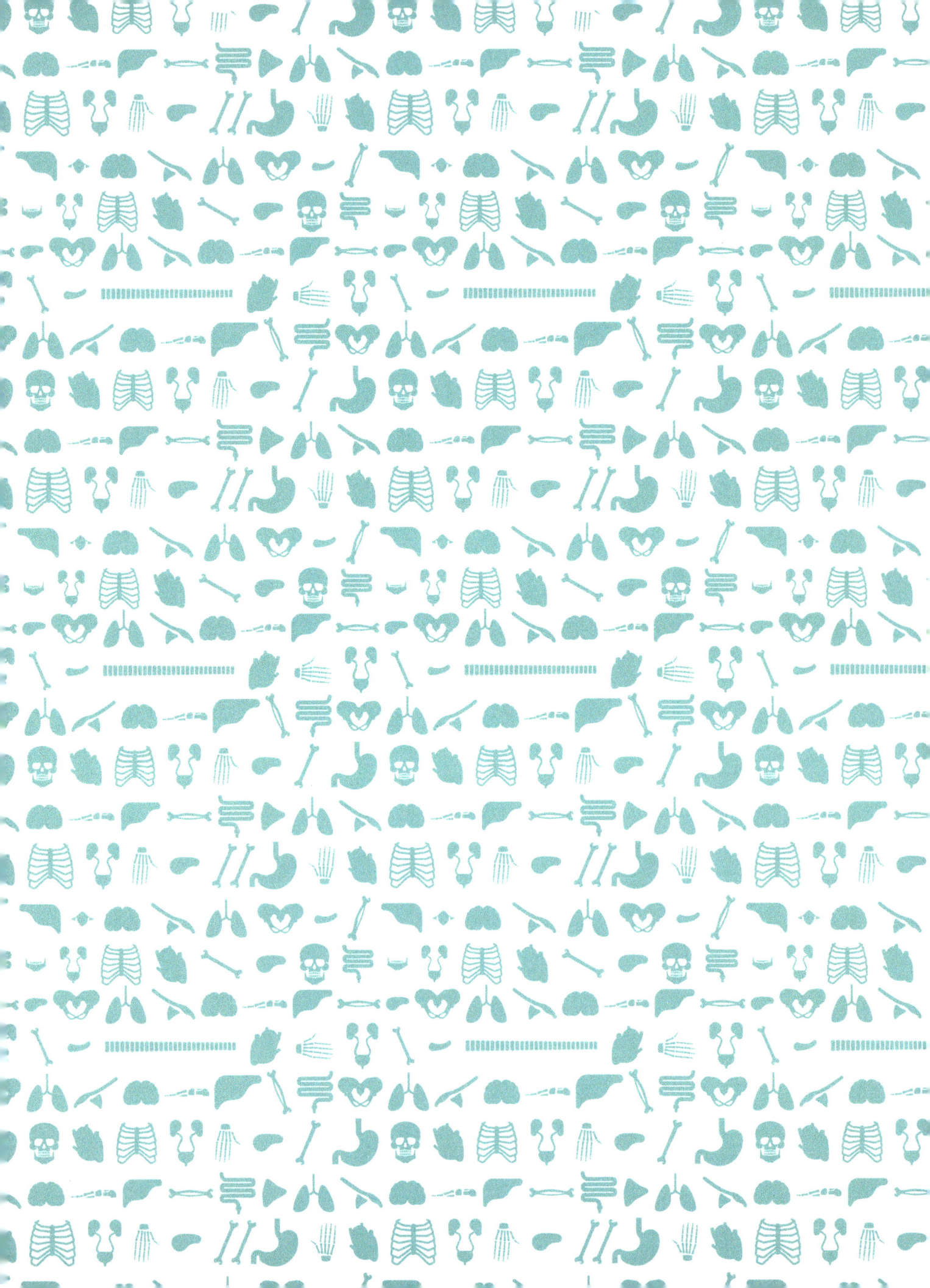

Lobes of the Brain

Frontal Lobe
- Problem solving
- Emotional traits
- Reasoning (Judgement)
- Speaking
- Voluntary motor activity

Temporal Lobe
- Understanding language
- Behavior
- Memory
- Hearing

Brain Stem
- Breathing
- Body temperature
- Digestion
- Alertness/sleep
- Swallowing

Cerebellum
- Balance
- Coordination and control of voluntary movement
- Fine muscle control

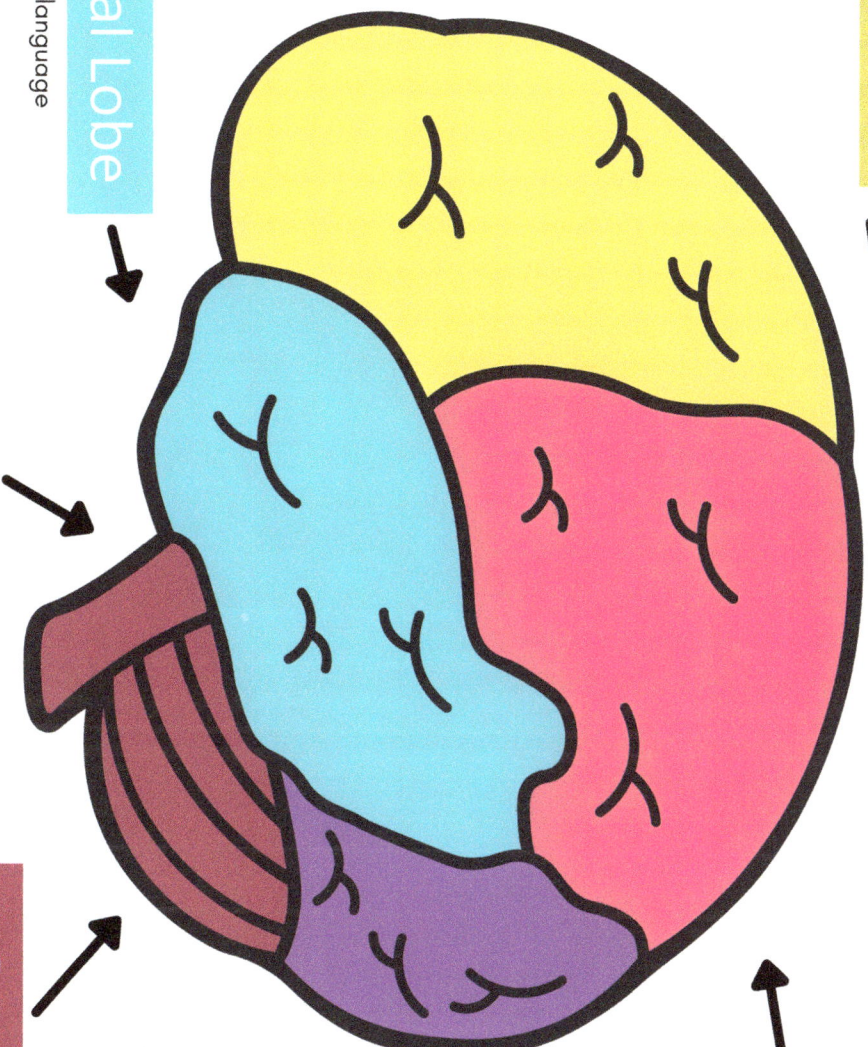

Occipital Lobe
- Vision
- Color perception

Parietal Lobe
- Knowing right from left
- Sensation
- Reading
- Body orientation

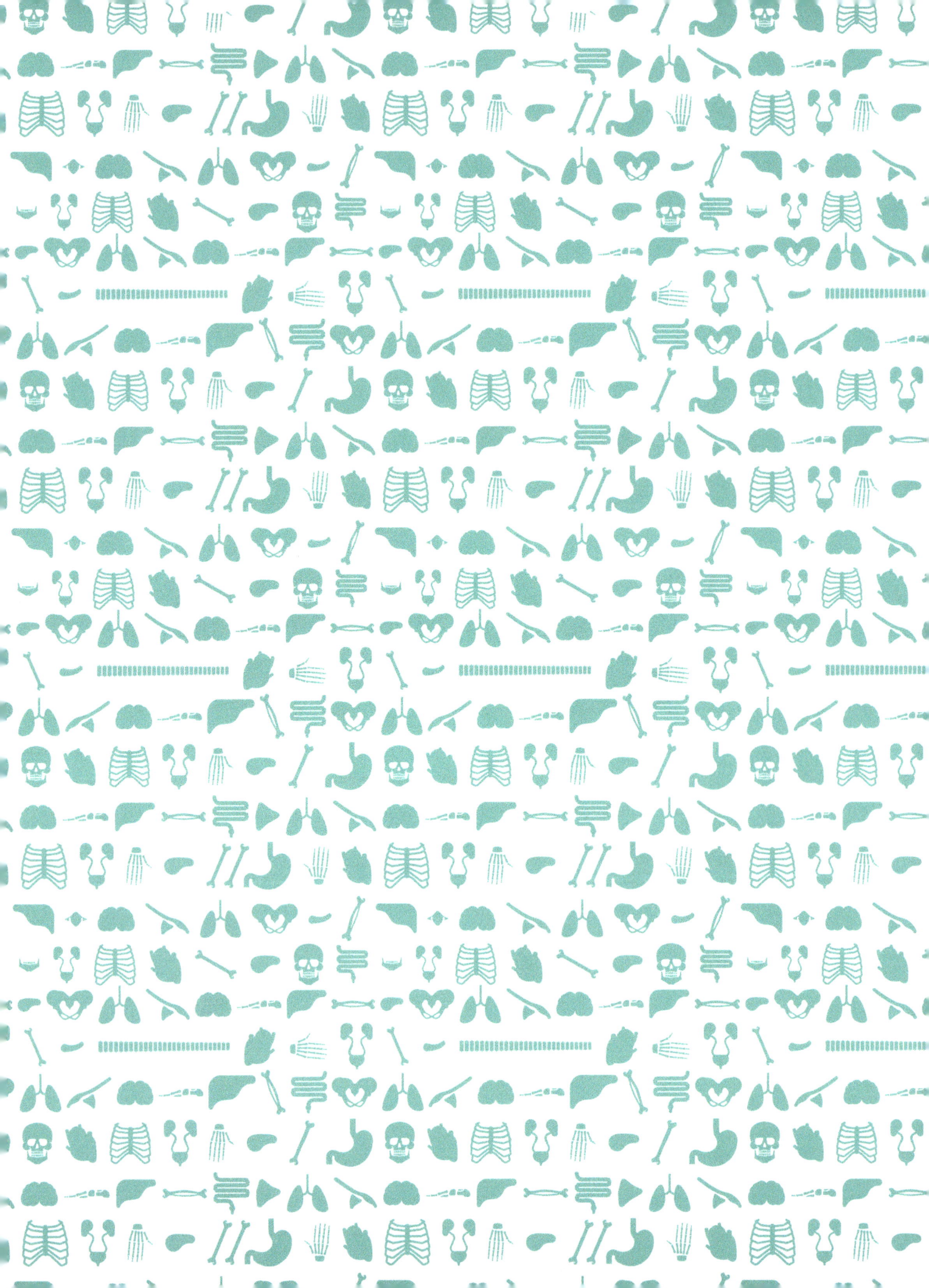

PLAYDOUGH NEURON ANATOMY

Instructions

Neurons are the fundamental units of the brain and nervous system, the cells responsible for receiving sensory input from the external world, for sending motor commands to our muscles, and for transforming and relaying the electrical signals at every step in between. They also have a very unique shape, which helps their function. Use the included template to help shape the cell parts. It is helpful to have at least 3-4 different types of playdough or clay to easily identify the different features of this cell. Have the child form the different parts of the neuron and then use the included labels to label each part of the neuron.

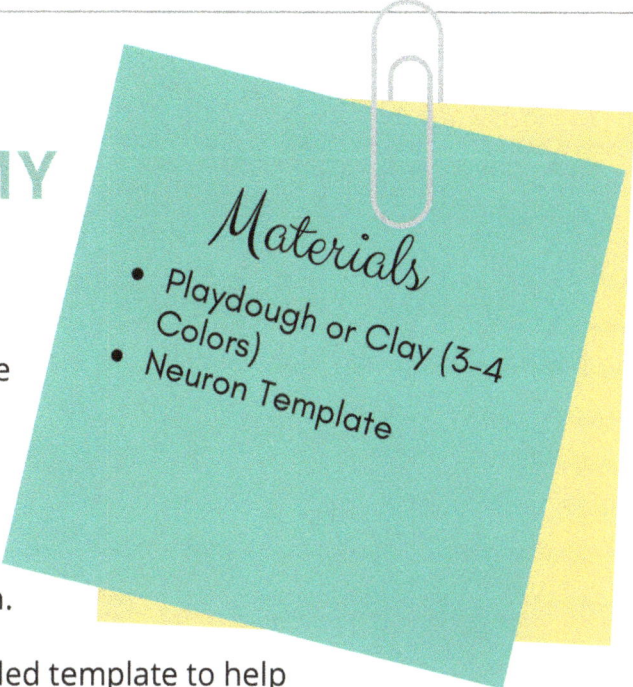

Materials
- Playdough or Clay (3-4 Colors)
- Neuron Template

Discuss: What is the main part of the cell? How does the structure of the cell help it send electrical signals? What purpose does the myelin sheath perform?

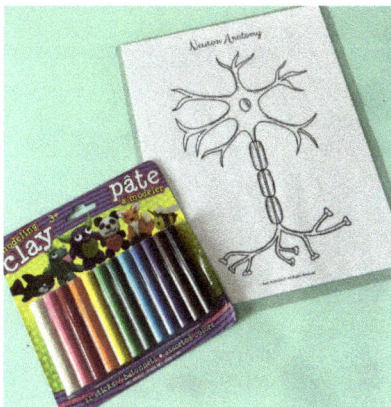

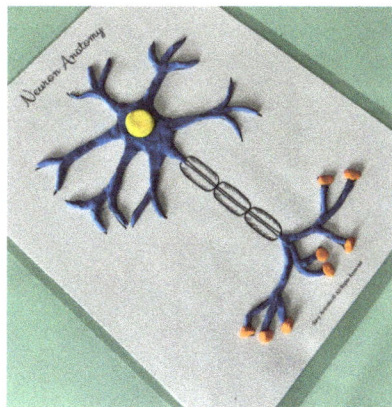

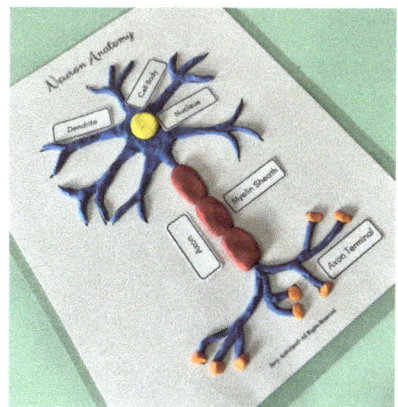

Dendrite	Cell Body	Nucleus
Axon	Myelin Sheath	Axon Terminal

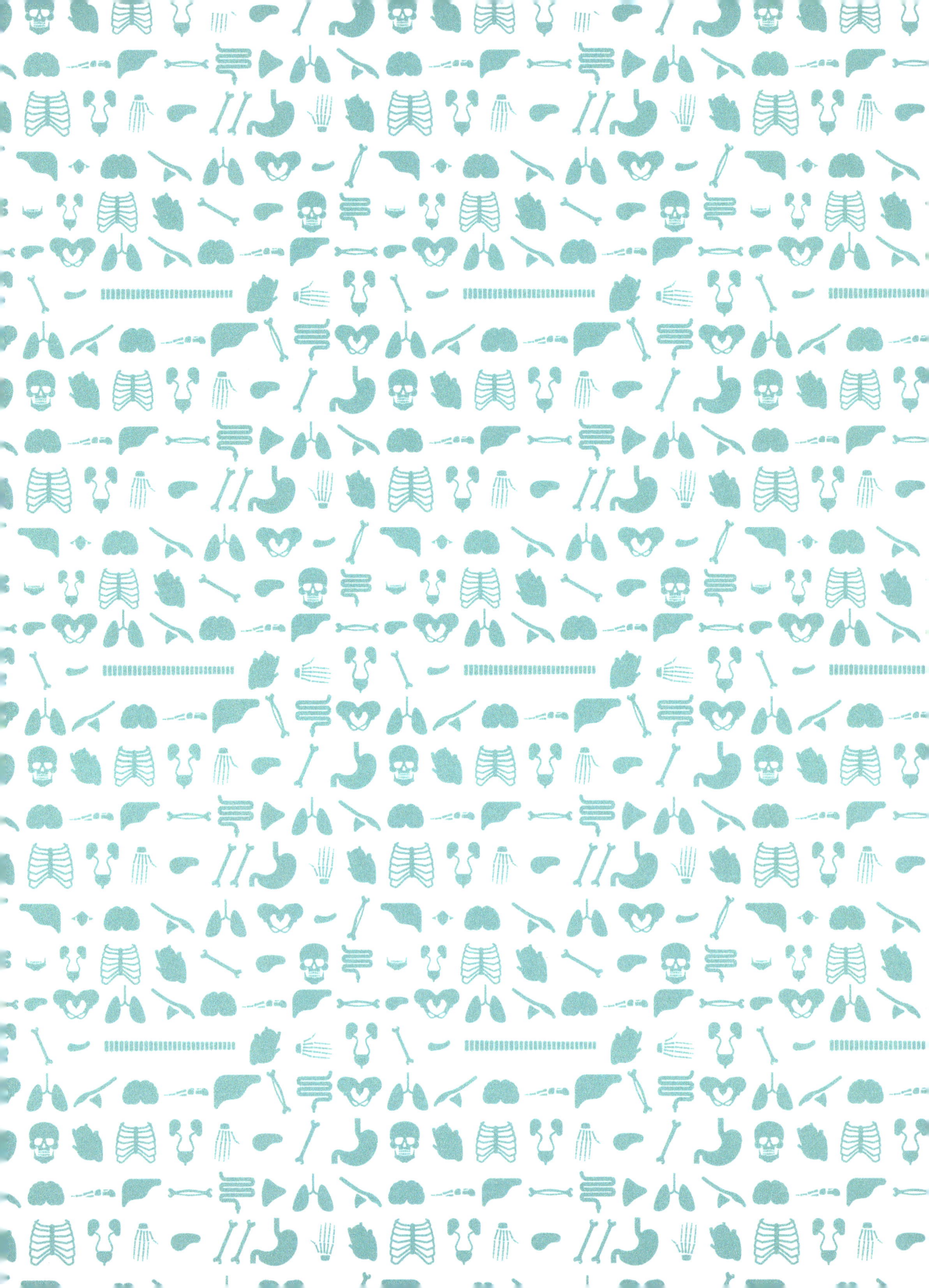

Neuron Anatomy

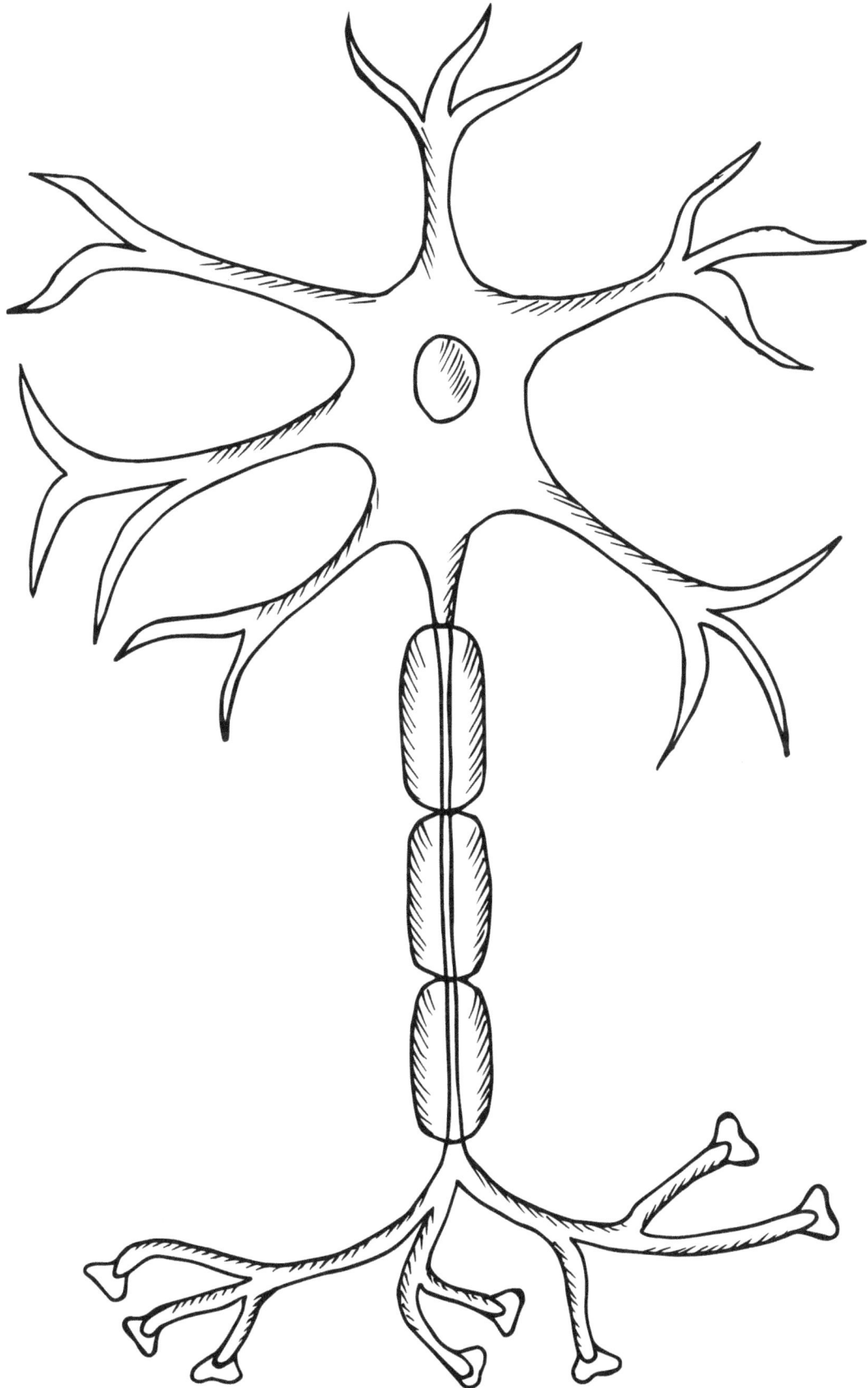

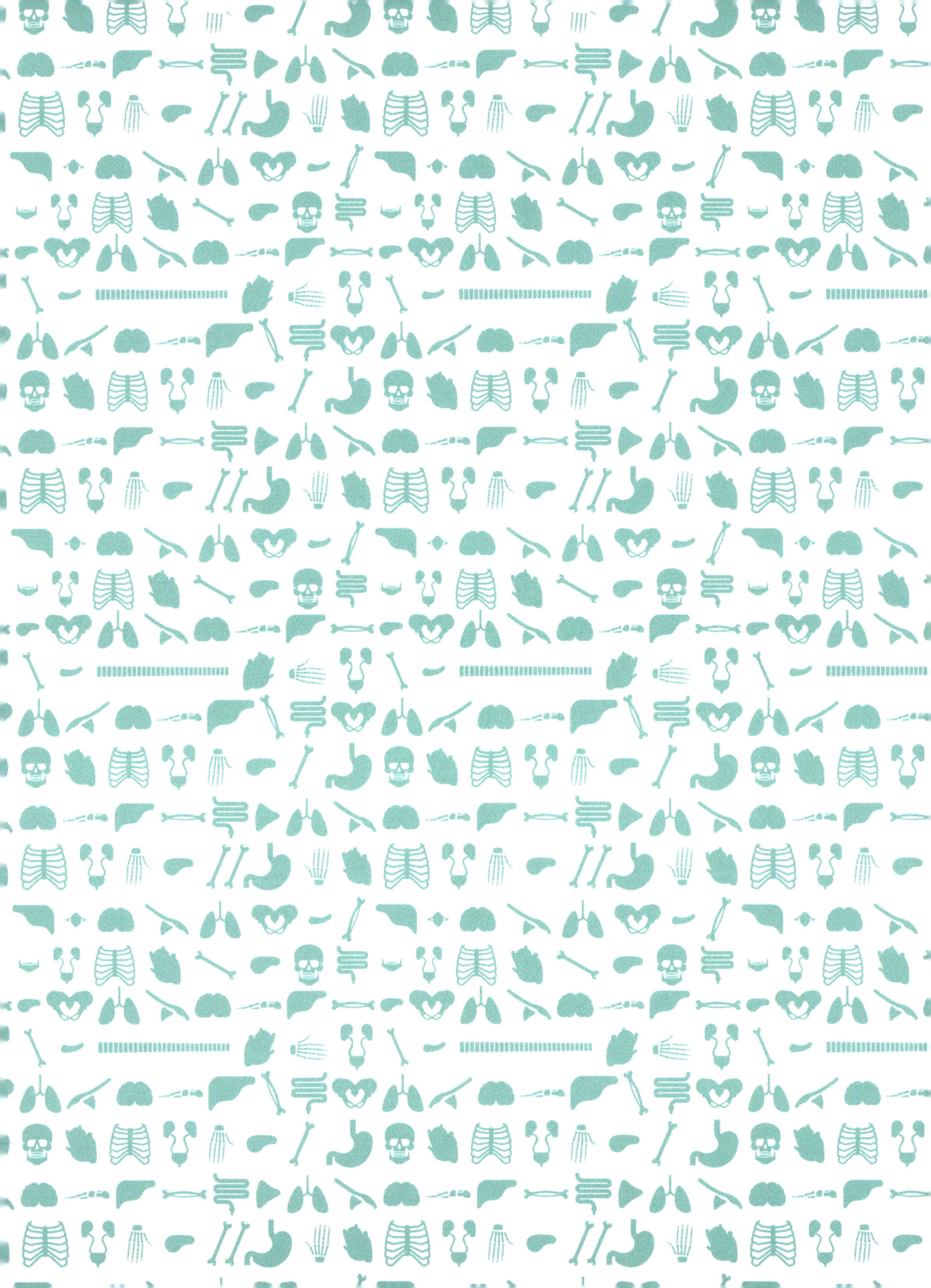

Emotion Matching

Emotions are mental states brought on by neurophysiological changes, associated with thoughts, feelings, behavioral responses, and a degree of pleasure or displeasure.

Cut out each emotion card. Have child match identify the emotions in the faces of the photos of the children and match them with the appropriate emotion.

Discuss when they felt these emotions - what happened? How did it make them feel? What are ways to help deal with this emotion? Repeat for the other four cards.

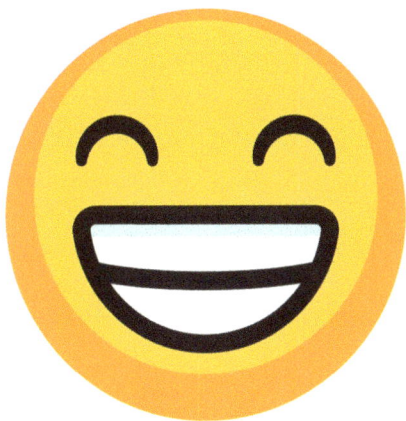

HAPPY

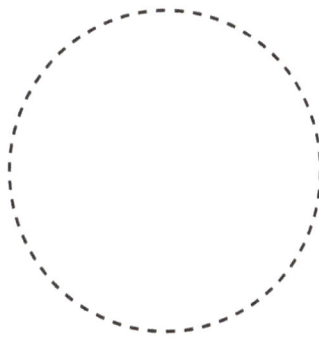
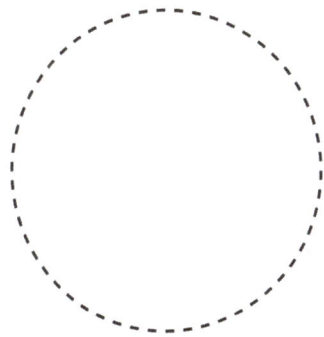
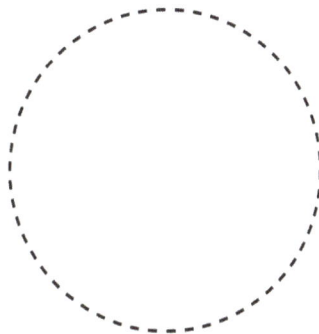
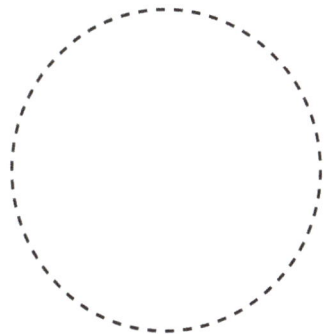

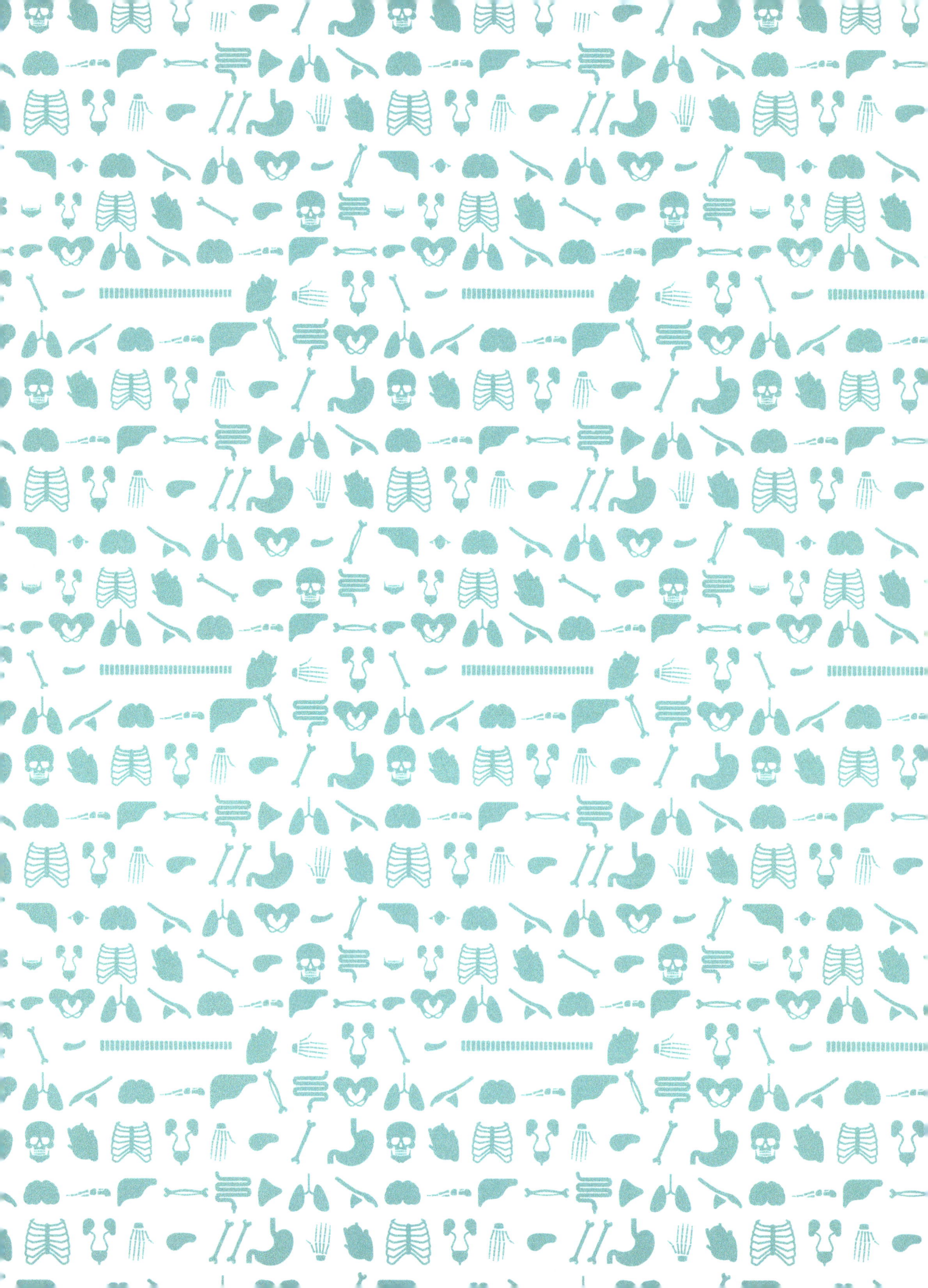

Emotion Matching

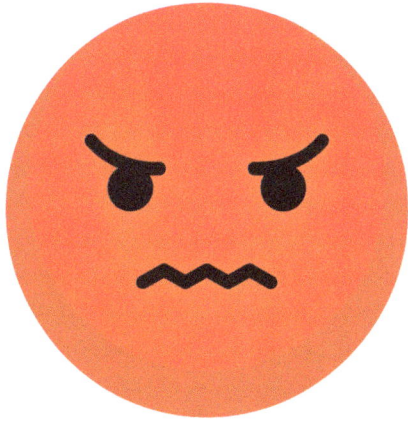

ANGER

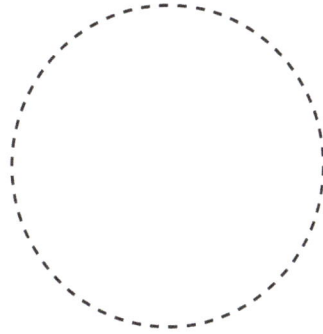
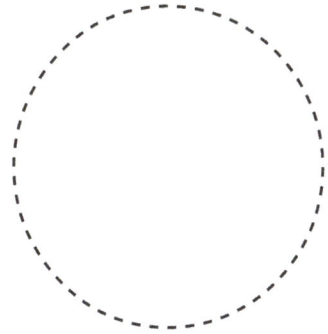
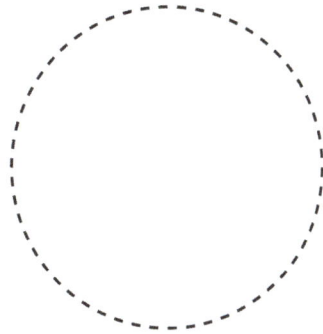
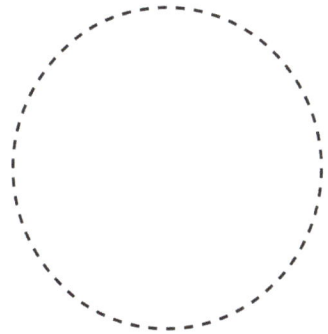

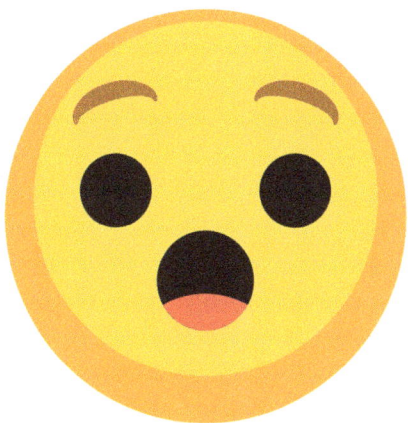

FEAR

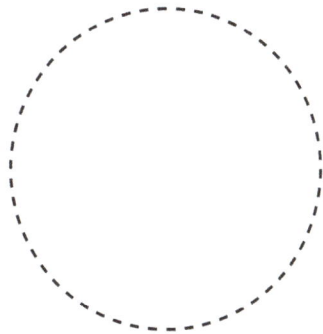
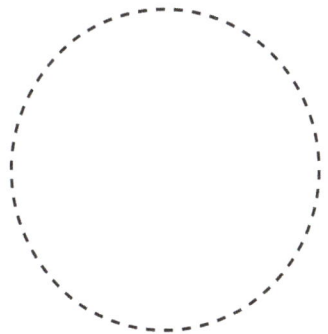
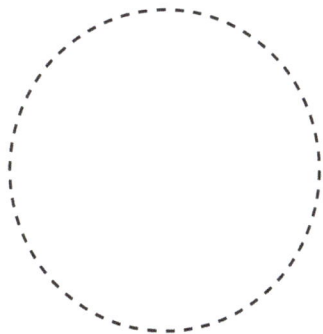
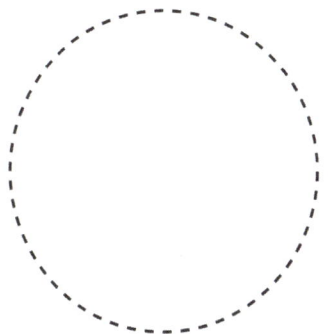

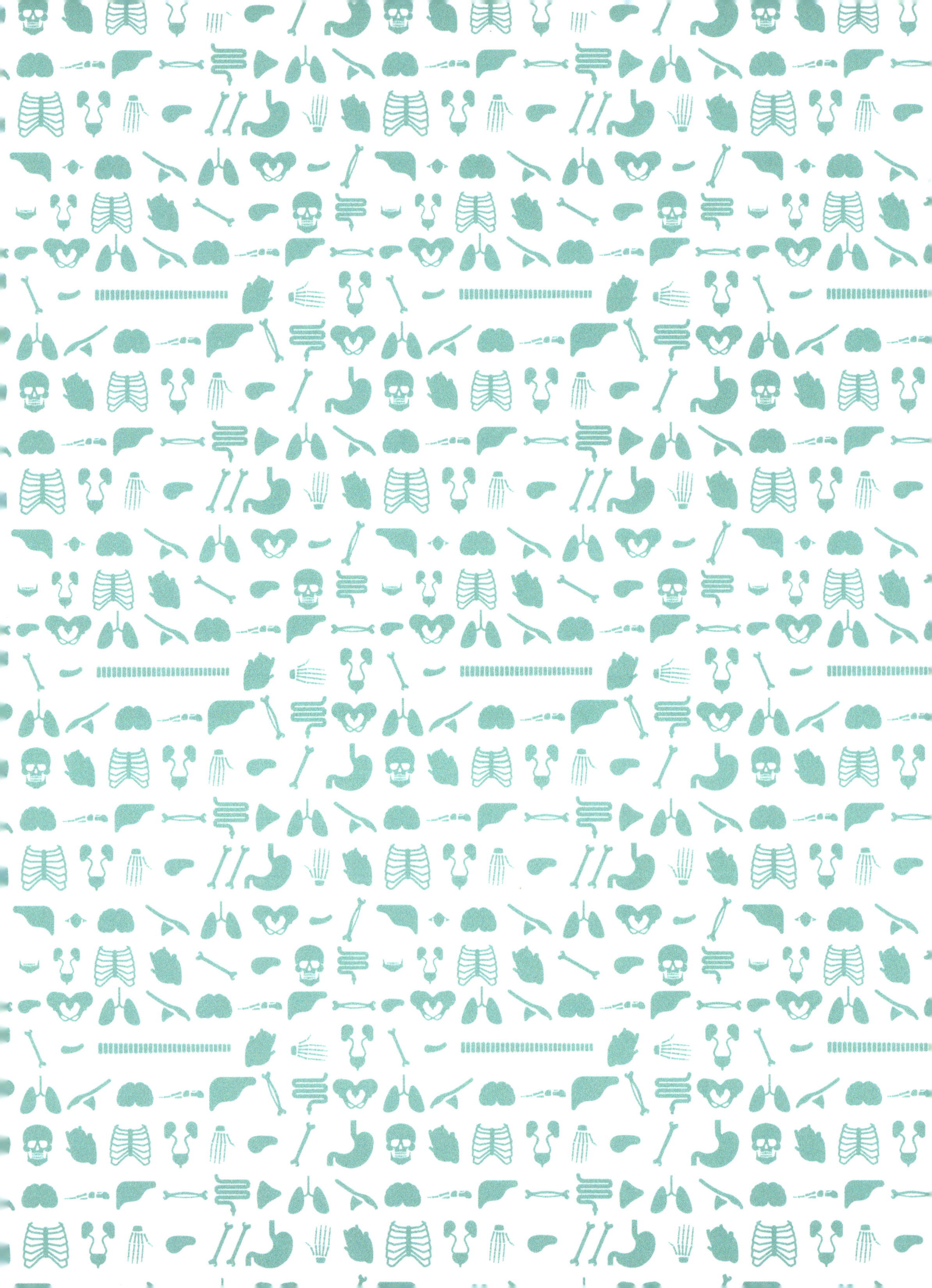

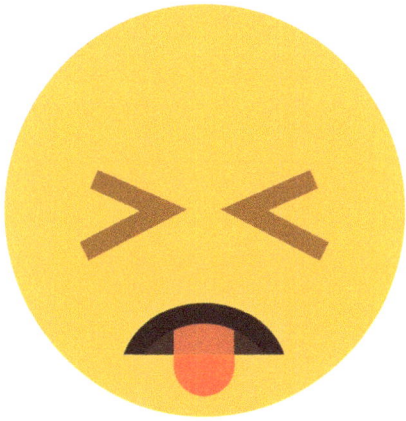

DISGUST

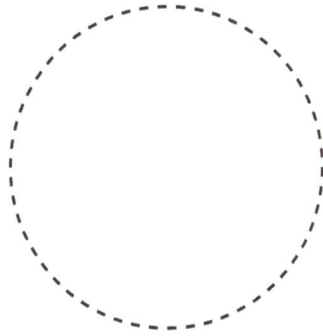
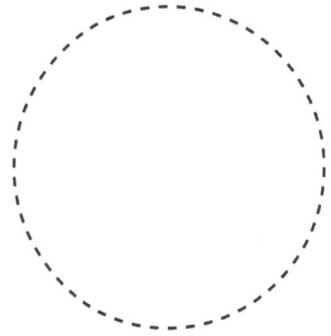
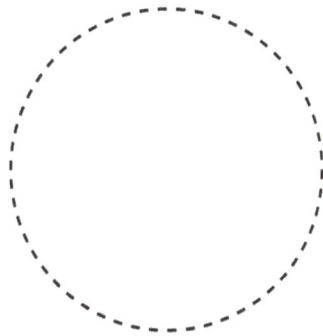
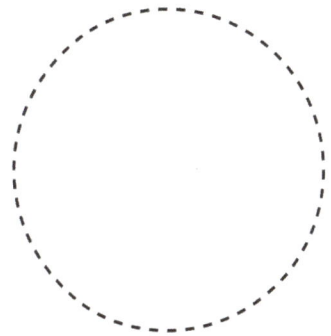

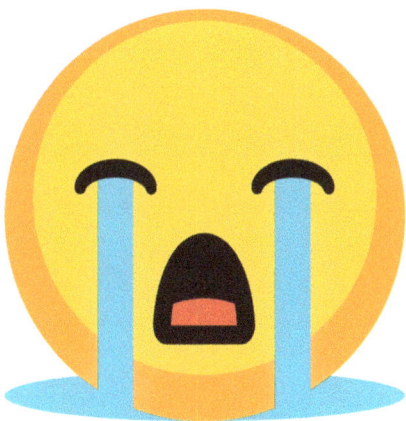

SAD

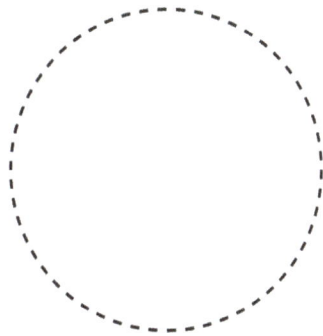
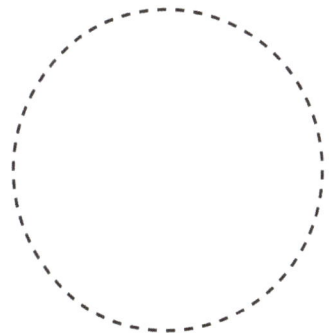
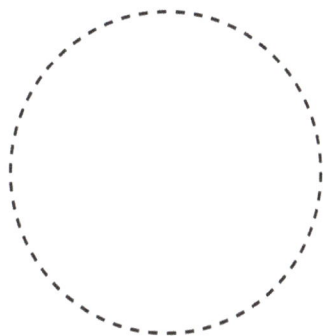
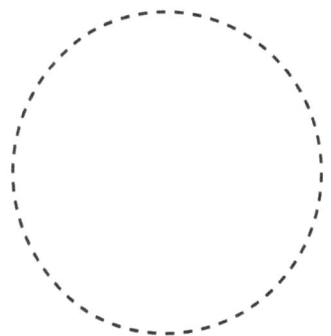

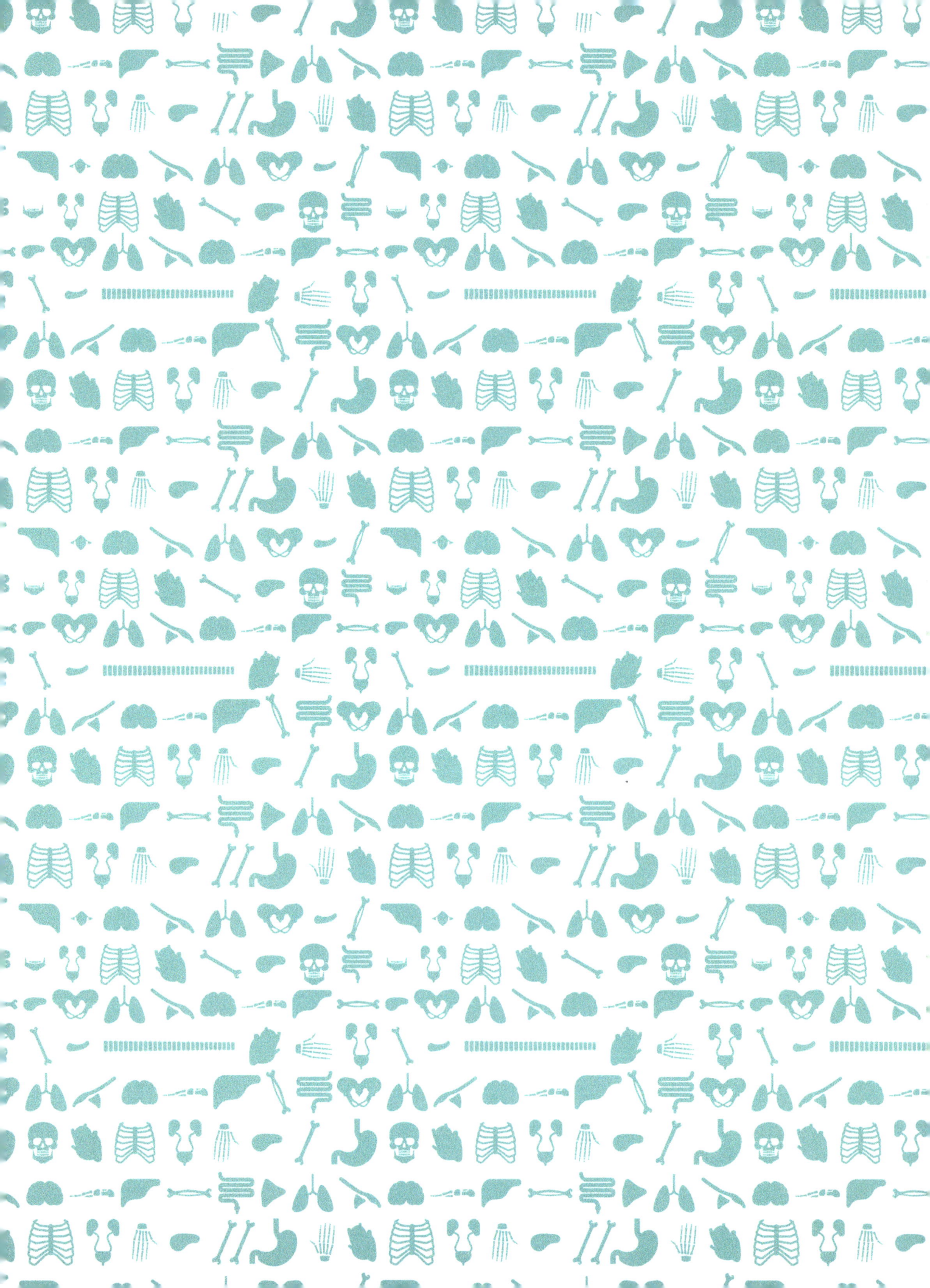

Emotion Matching

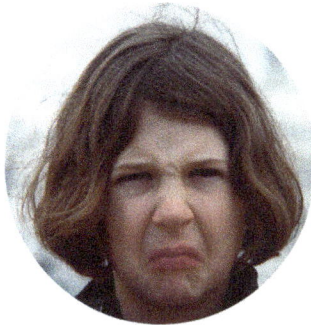

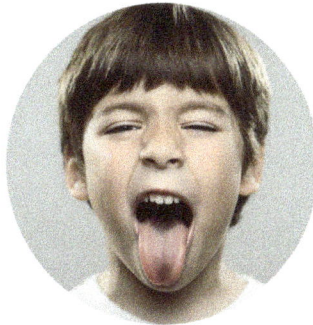

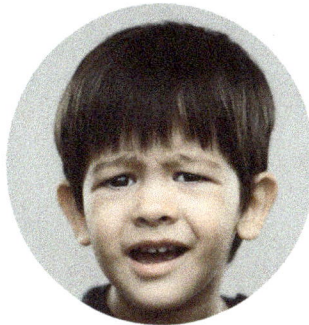

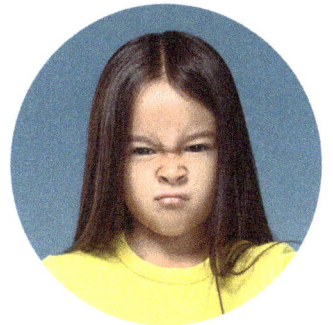

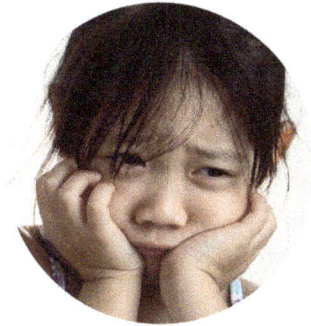

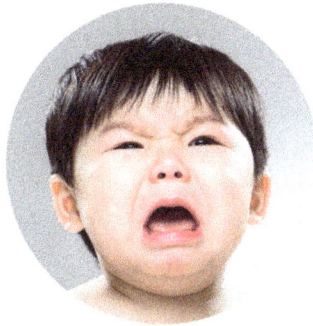

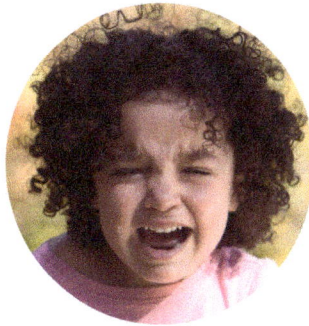

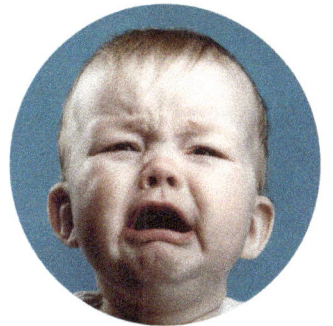

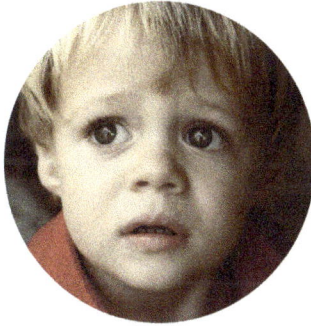

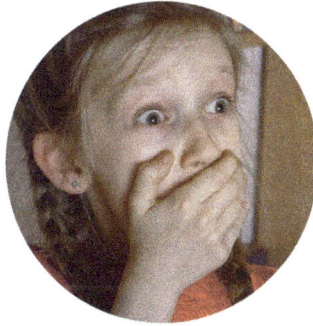

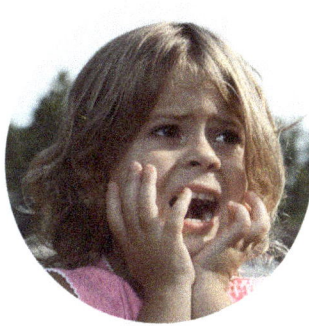

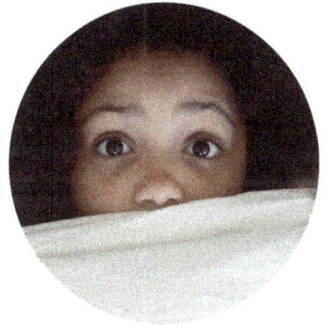

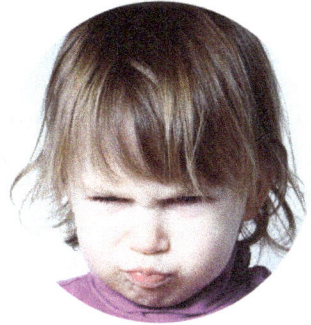

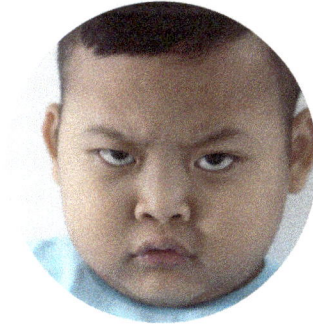

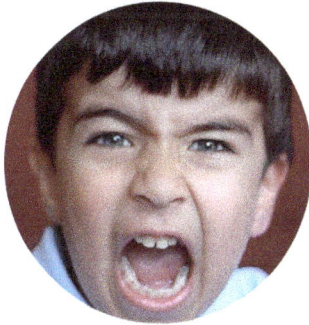

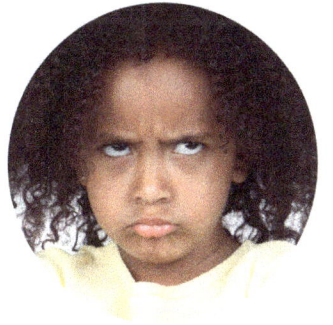

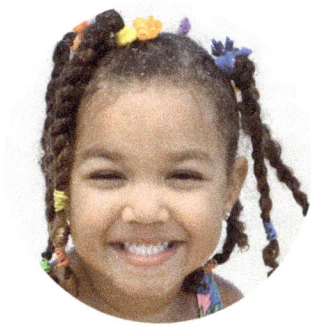

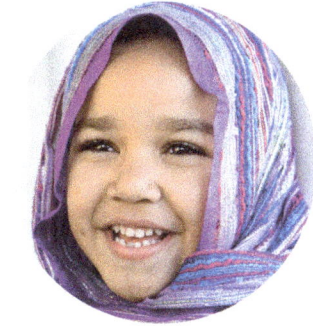

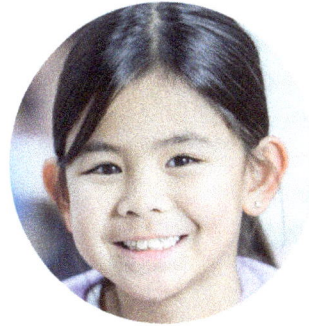

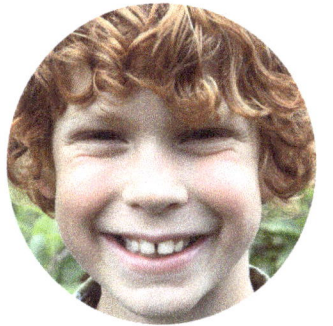

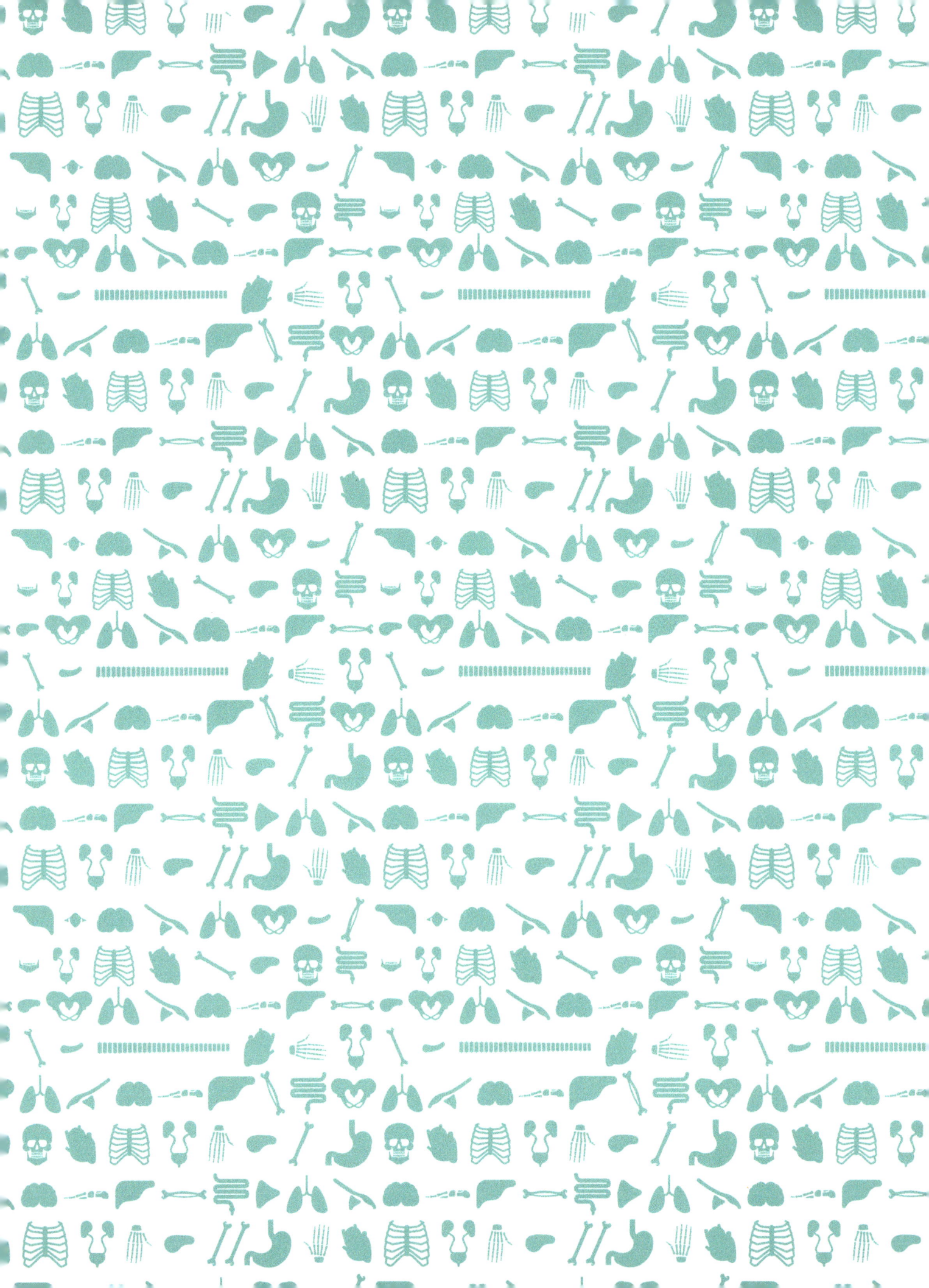

Endocrine System Matching

Hypothalamus

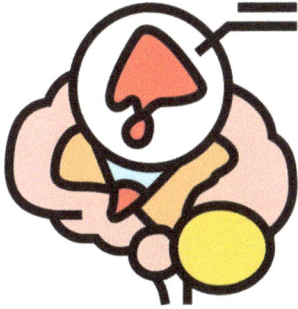

About the size of an almond, this organ is located above the brainstem at the base of your brain. Known as the "gatekeeper" of the endocrine system, it directly controls the pituitary gland.

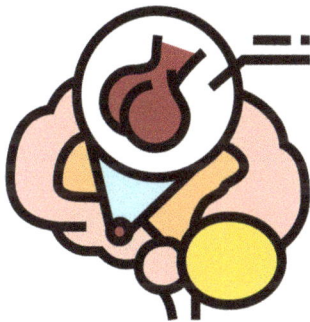

Pituitary Gland

Located at the base of the brain and is about the size of a pea. Known as the "master gland" of the body. Produces hormones that indirectly or directly affect body growth, fluid balance, metabolism and reproduction.

Pineal Gland

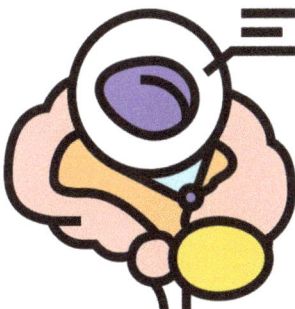

Located deep in the brain where the two halves of the brain join. Produces melatonin which affects the sleep/wake cycle.

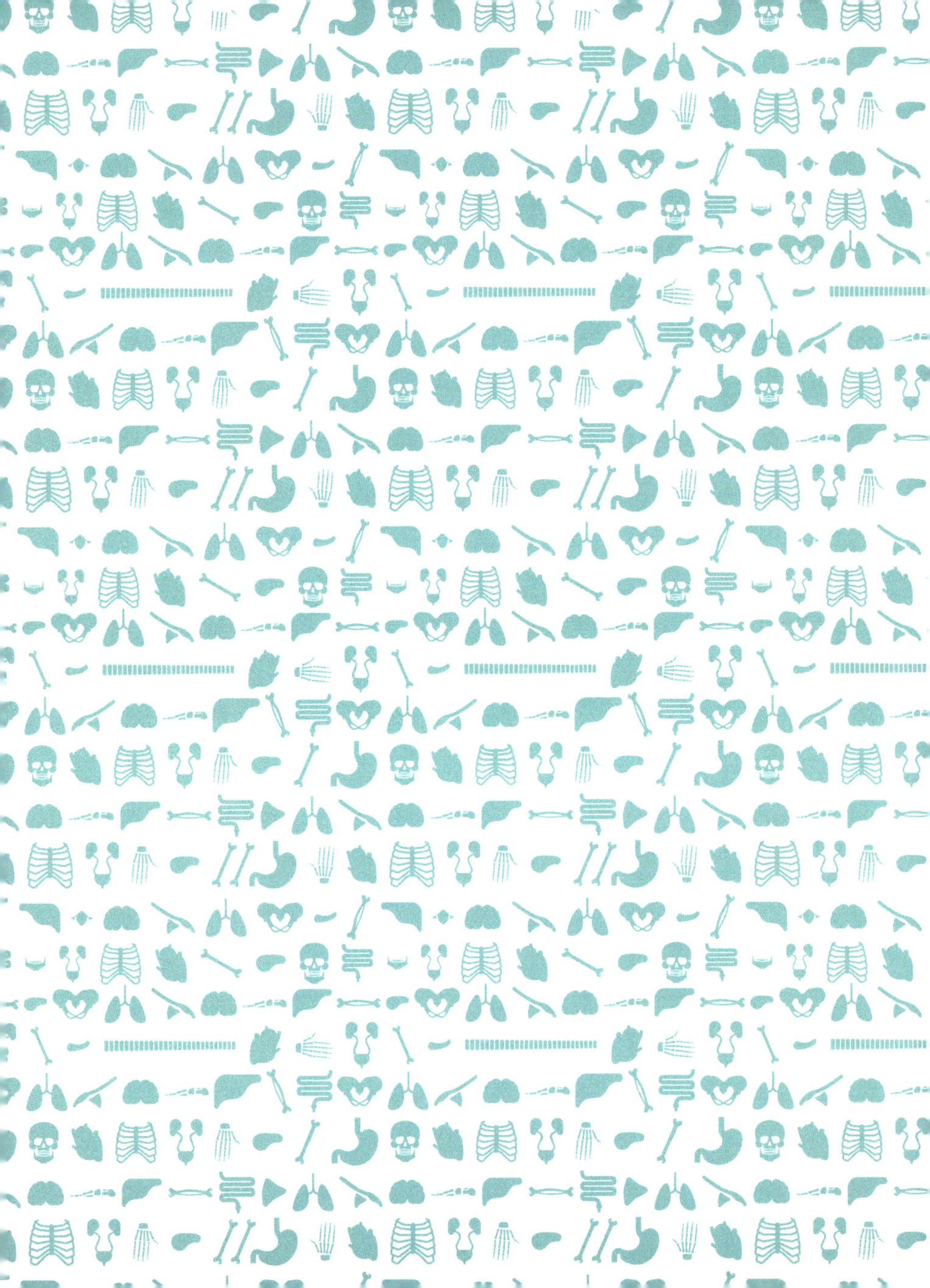

Endocrine System Matching

Pancreas

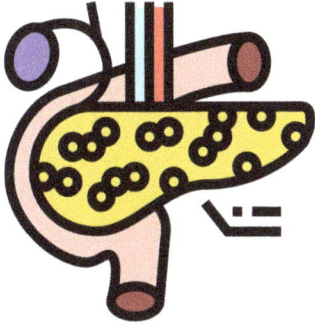

Located behind the stomach and in front of the spine. Consists of islet cells that create and release important hormones like insulin, which acts to lower blood sugar, and glucagon, which acts to raise blood sugar.

Adrenal Glands

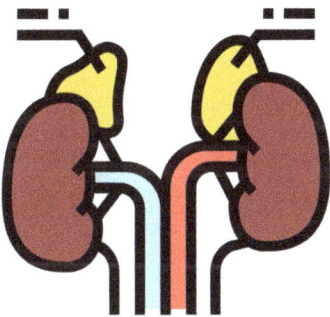

Located on top of the kidneys, these glands produce hormones that regulate metabolism, immune system, blood pressure, stress response, etc.

Thyroid

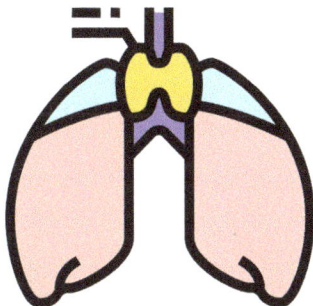

Located in the front of the neck, wrapped around the trachea, this gland makes hormones that are secreted into the blood and carried to all body tissues. These hormones play a vital role in metabolism and heat regulation.

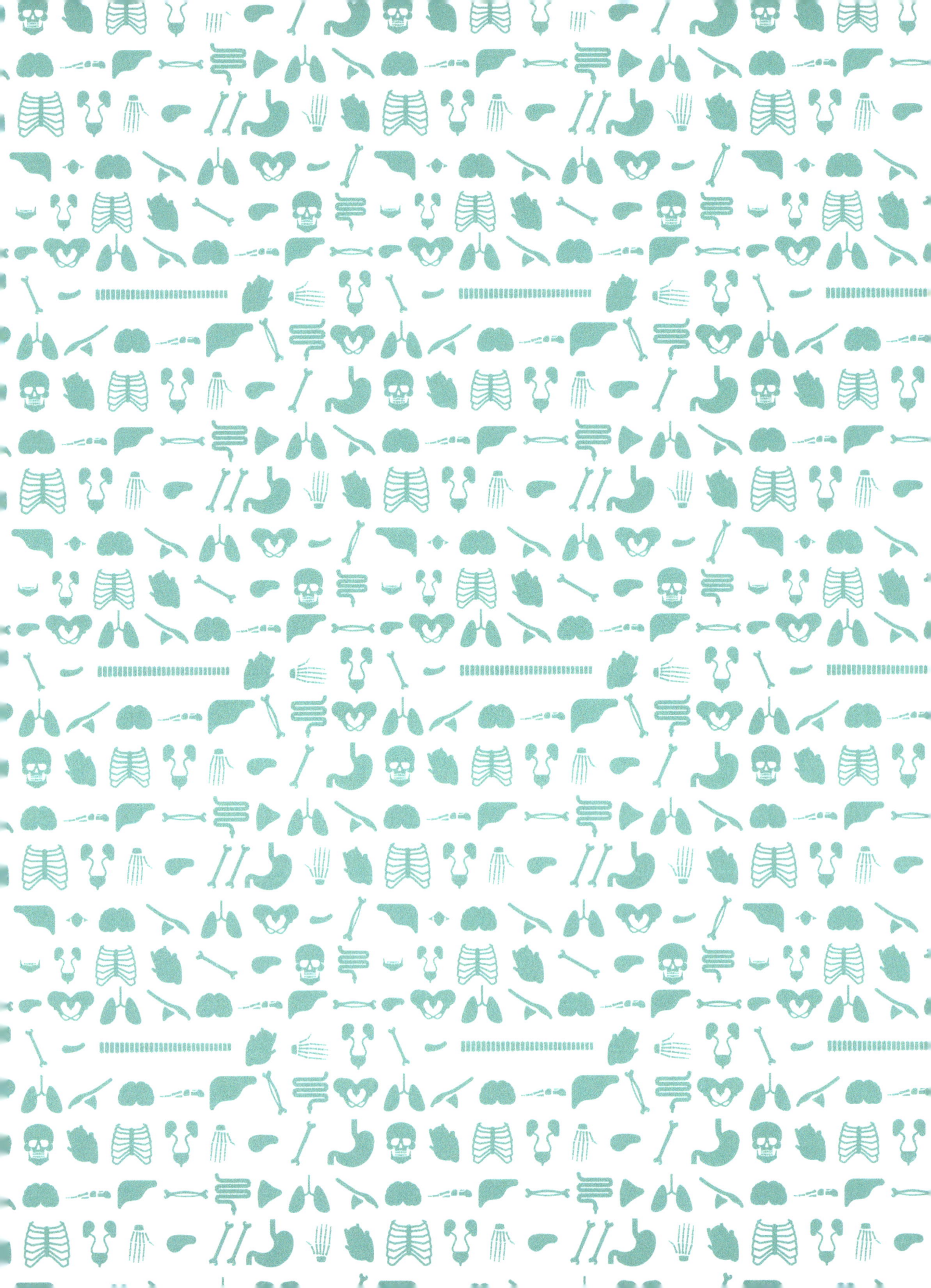

Endocrine System Matching

Parthyroid Glands

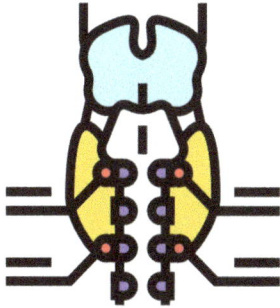

Located next to the thyroid gland, each of these four glands is about the size of a pea. These glands regulate calcium levels in the blood, which maintains healthy muscles and nerves.

Ovaries

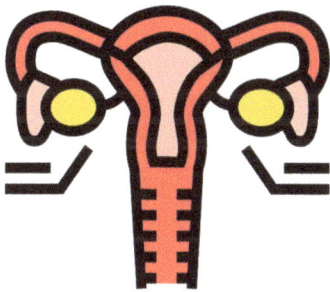

Located on either side of the uterus, these organs secrete estrogen and progesterone which are hormones vital to normal reproductive development and fertility in females.

Testes

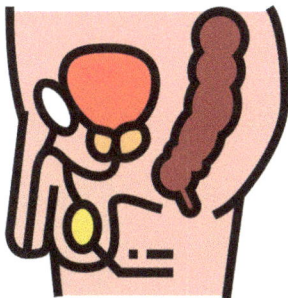

Located in the scrotum, these organs secrete testosterone, a hormone that is vital to normal reproductive development and fertility in males.

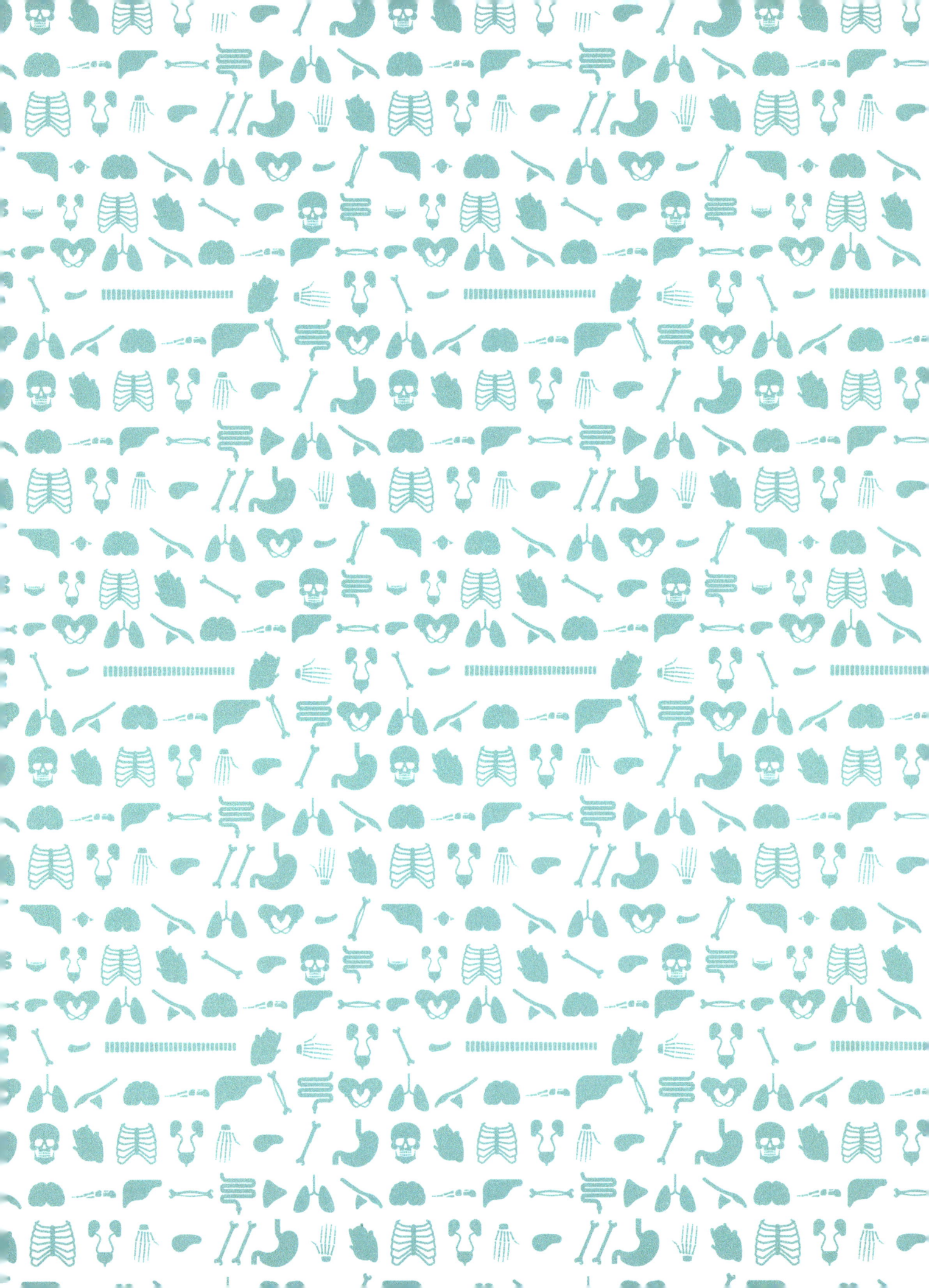

The Five Major Senses

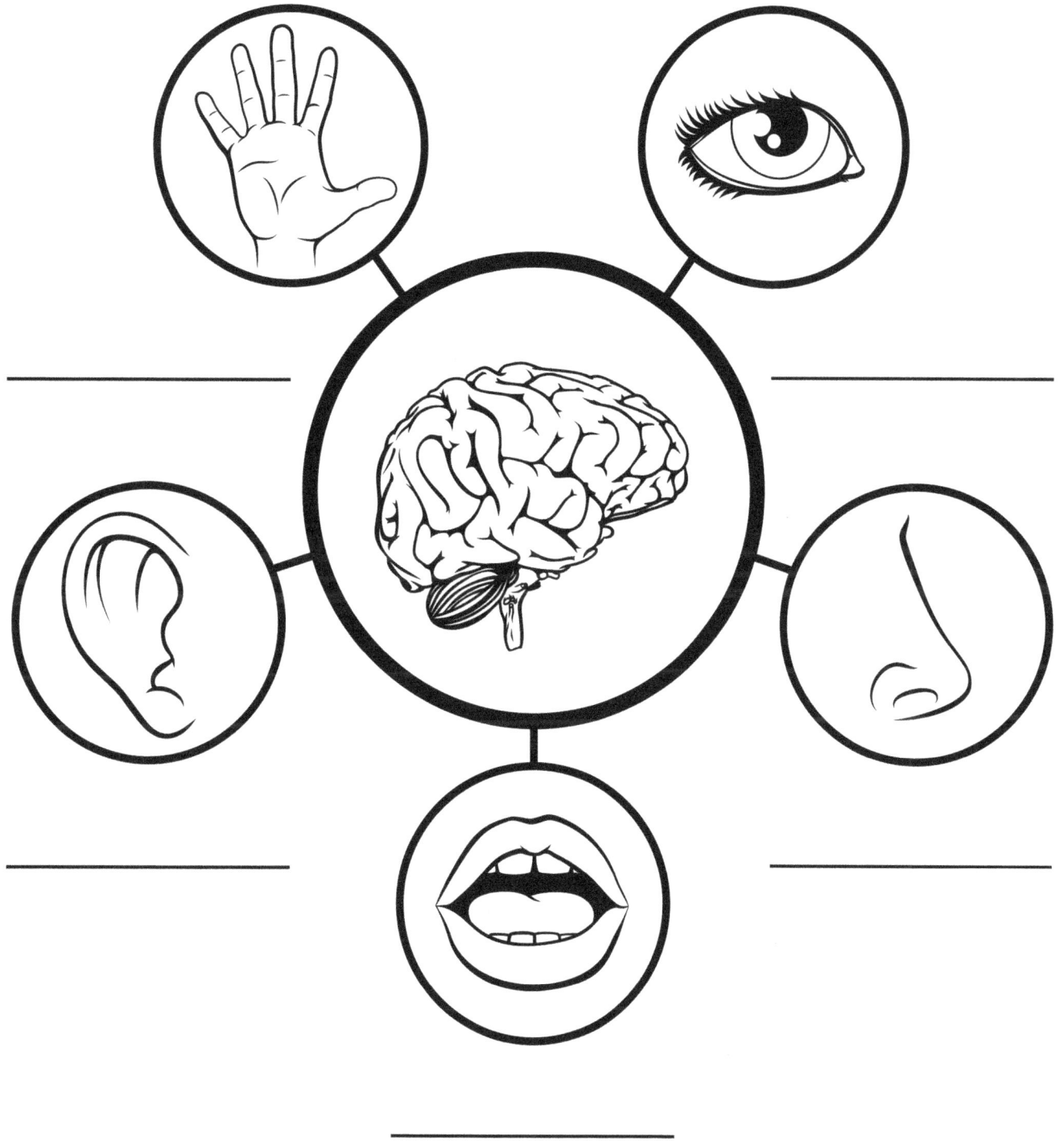

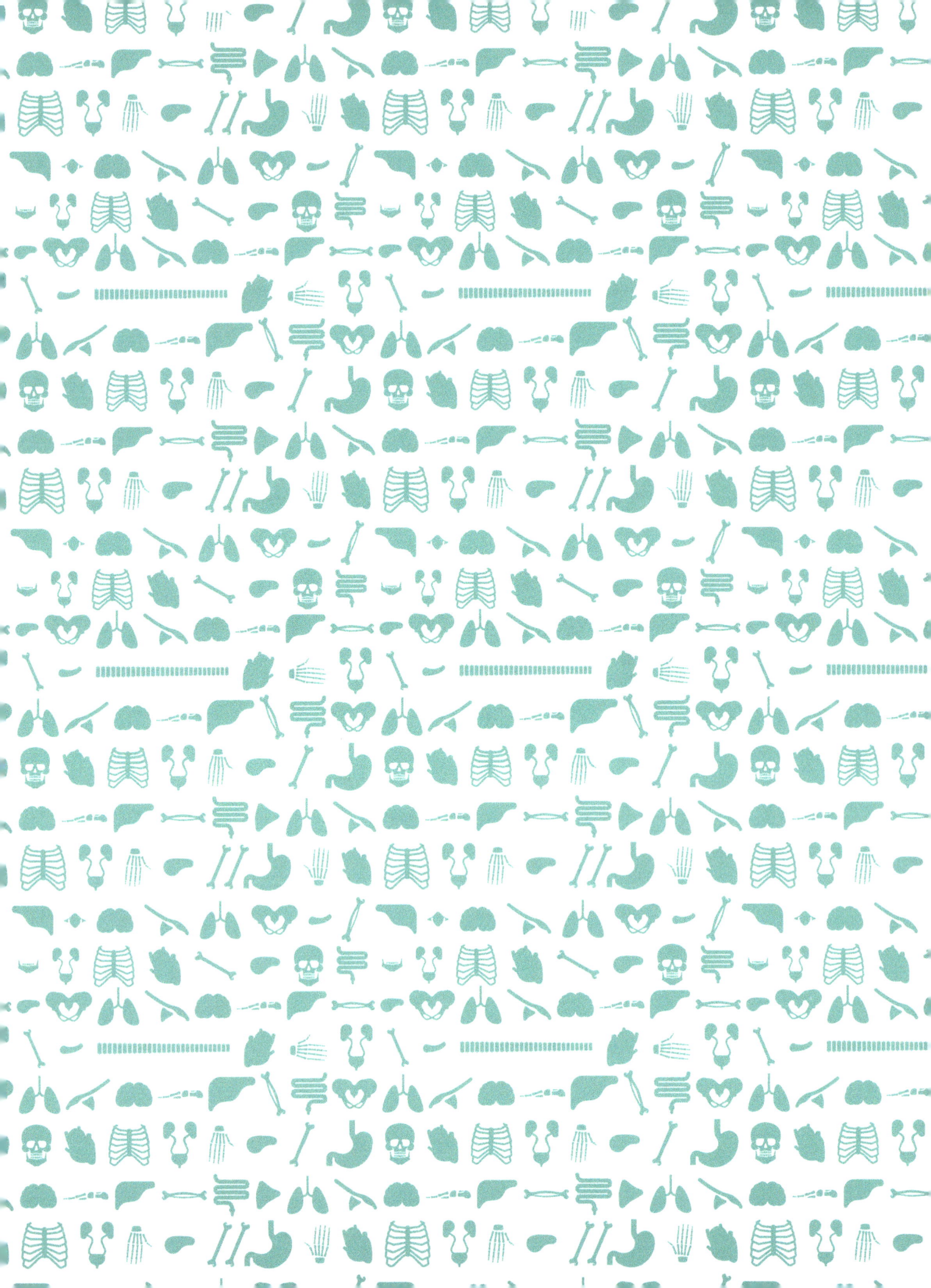

SENSORY: SIGHT

Instructions

The Snellen Chart is the most common method used to test a person's sense of sight. This standardized chart is placed 20 feet away and the client identifies the letters as far down as possible, demonstrating their ability to see at a certain accuracy. In addition, color blindness is assessed using a test known as the Ishihara Test, using numbers out of dots that are a different color than the dots surrounding them. A person with color blindness cannot differentiate between the colors.

Materials
- Snellen Chart Template
- Ishihara Test Template

Place the included Snellen-inspired sign several feet away from the child. Have them hold their hand over one eye and identify the letters they can see. Repeat with the opposite eye. Show them the Ishihara-inspired color pattern circles. Ask them to identify the letter, number or object.

This should NOT be considered a medical test, only for educational purposes.

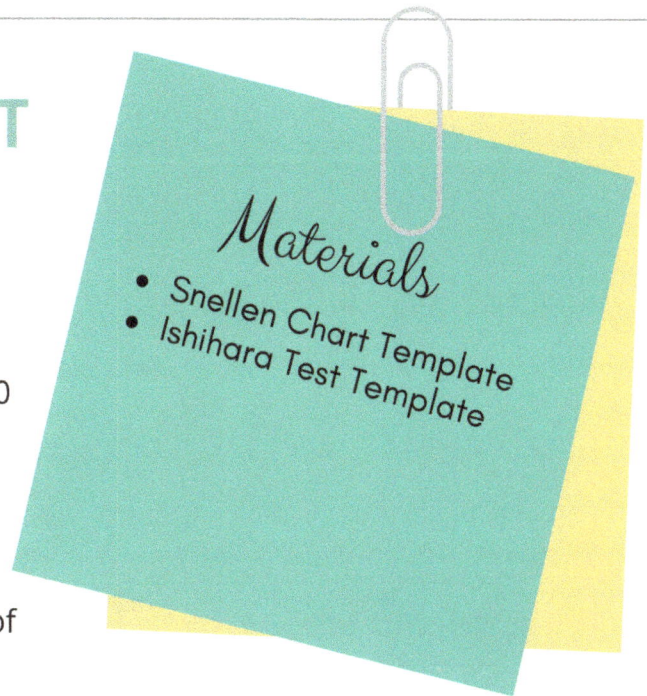

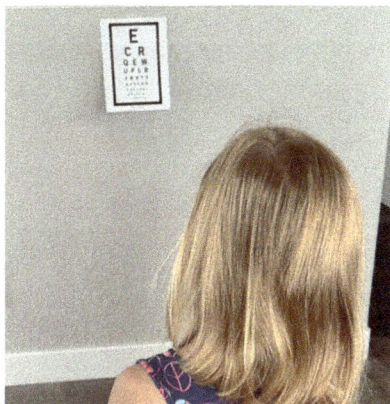

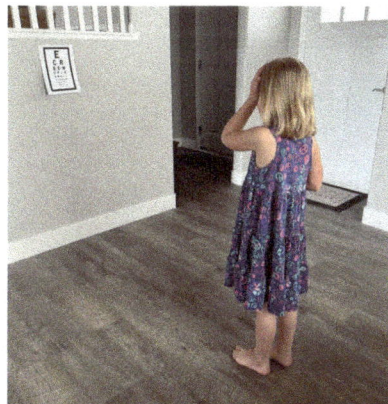

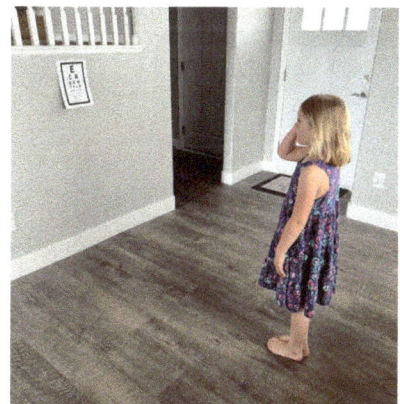

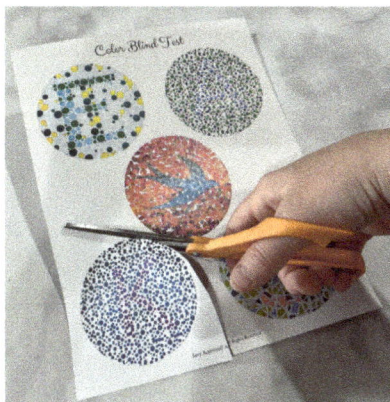

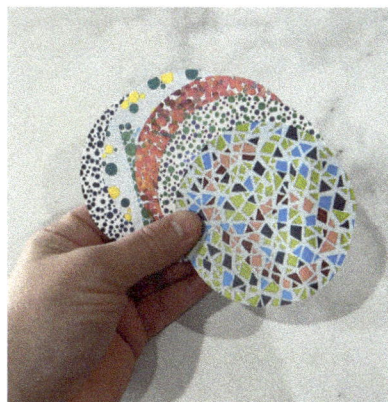

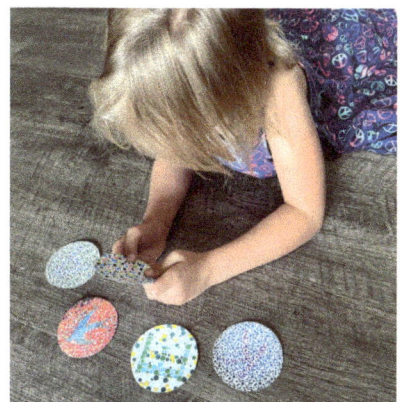

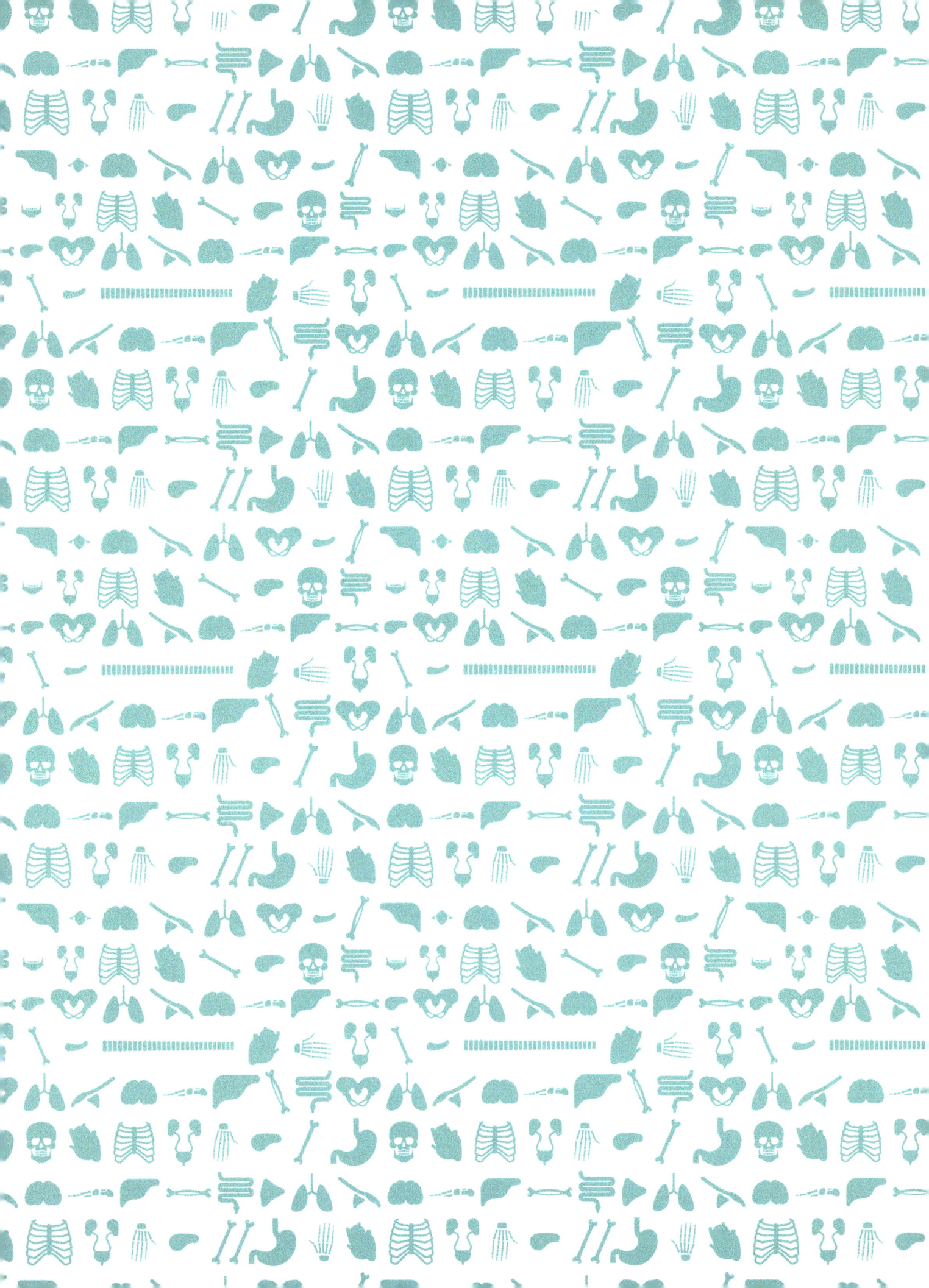

E

C R

Q E W

U P L B

A M N T Y

G F V X O N

T R V C Q S J

E W X C G Y A K

S O L B M H F R A

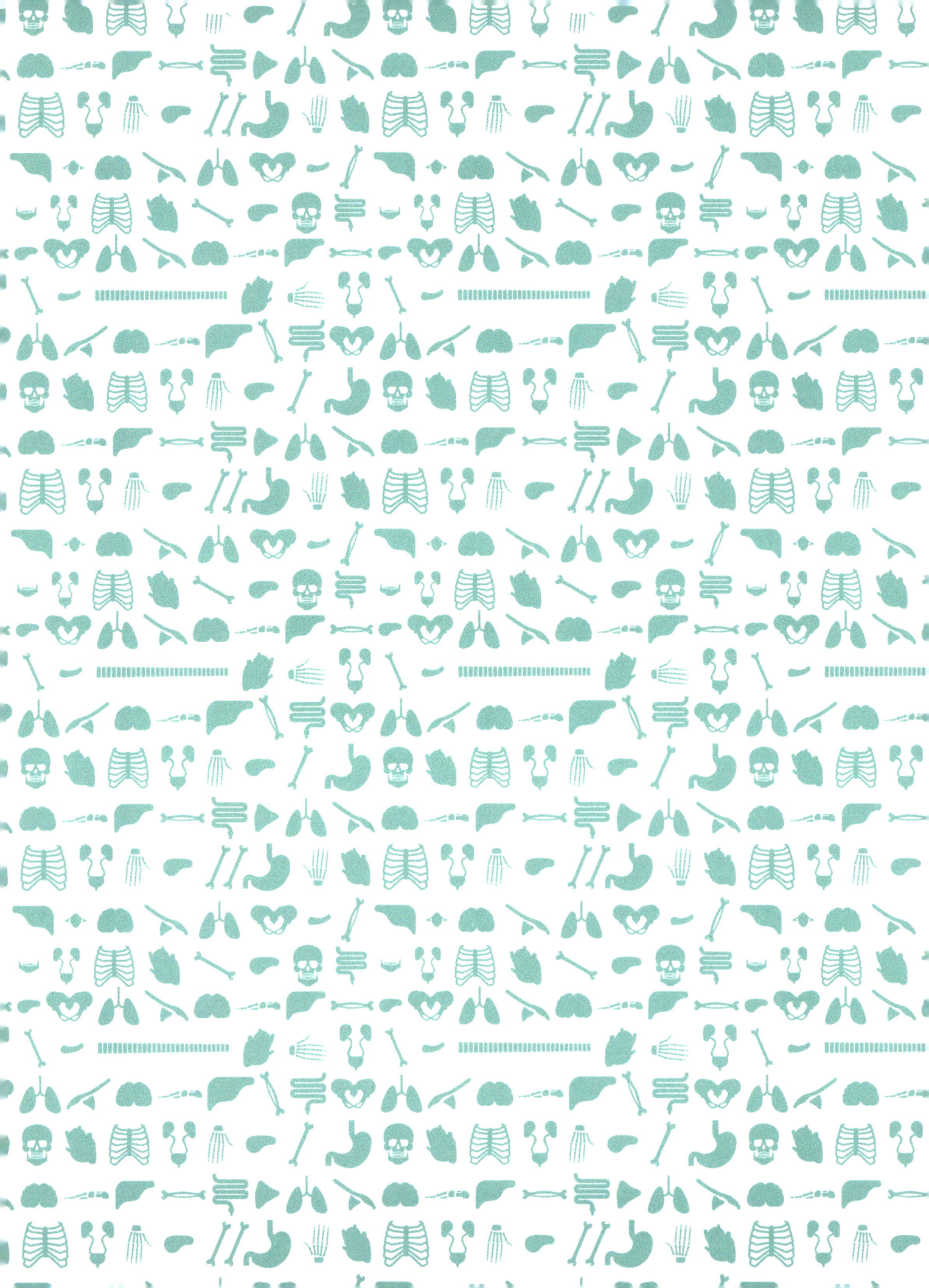

Ishihara Test

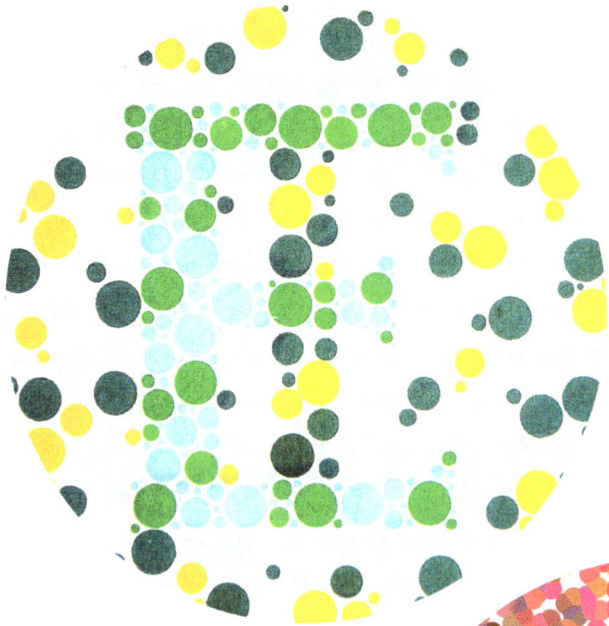

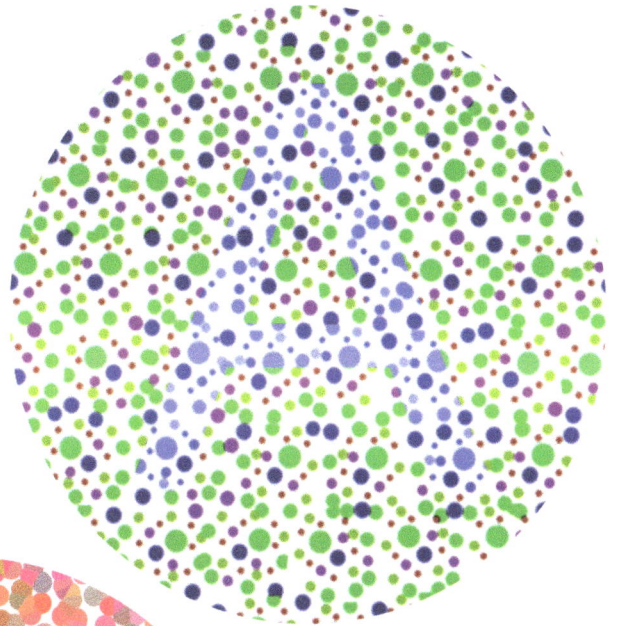

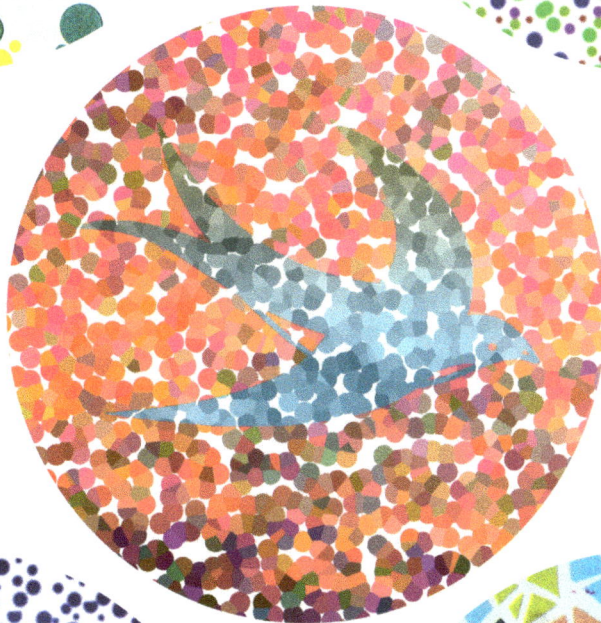

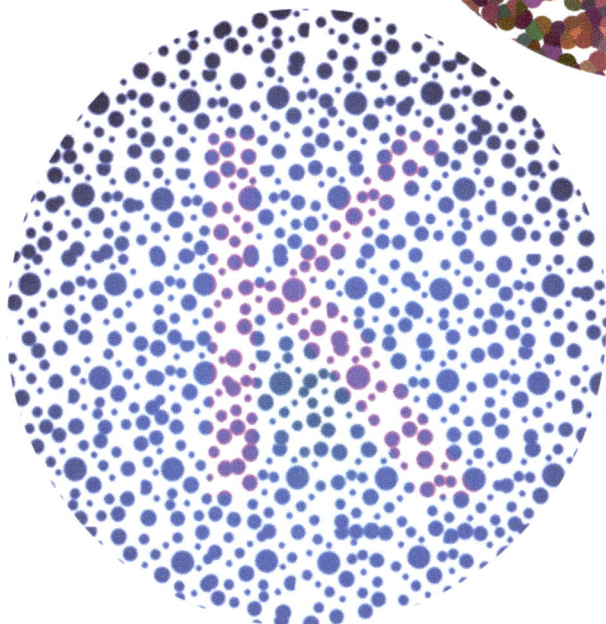

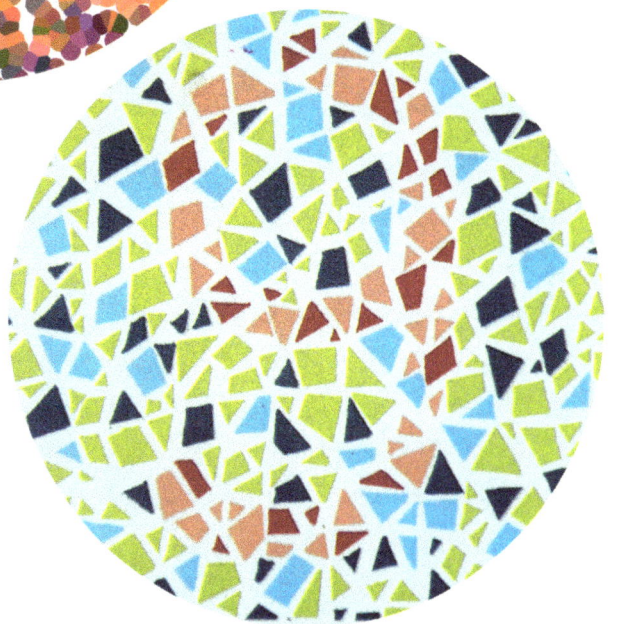

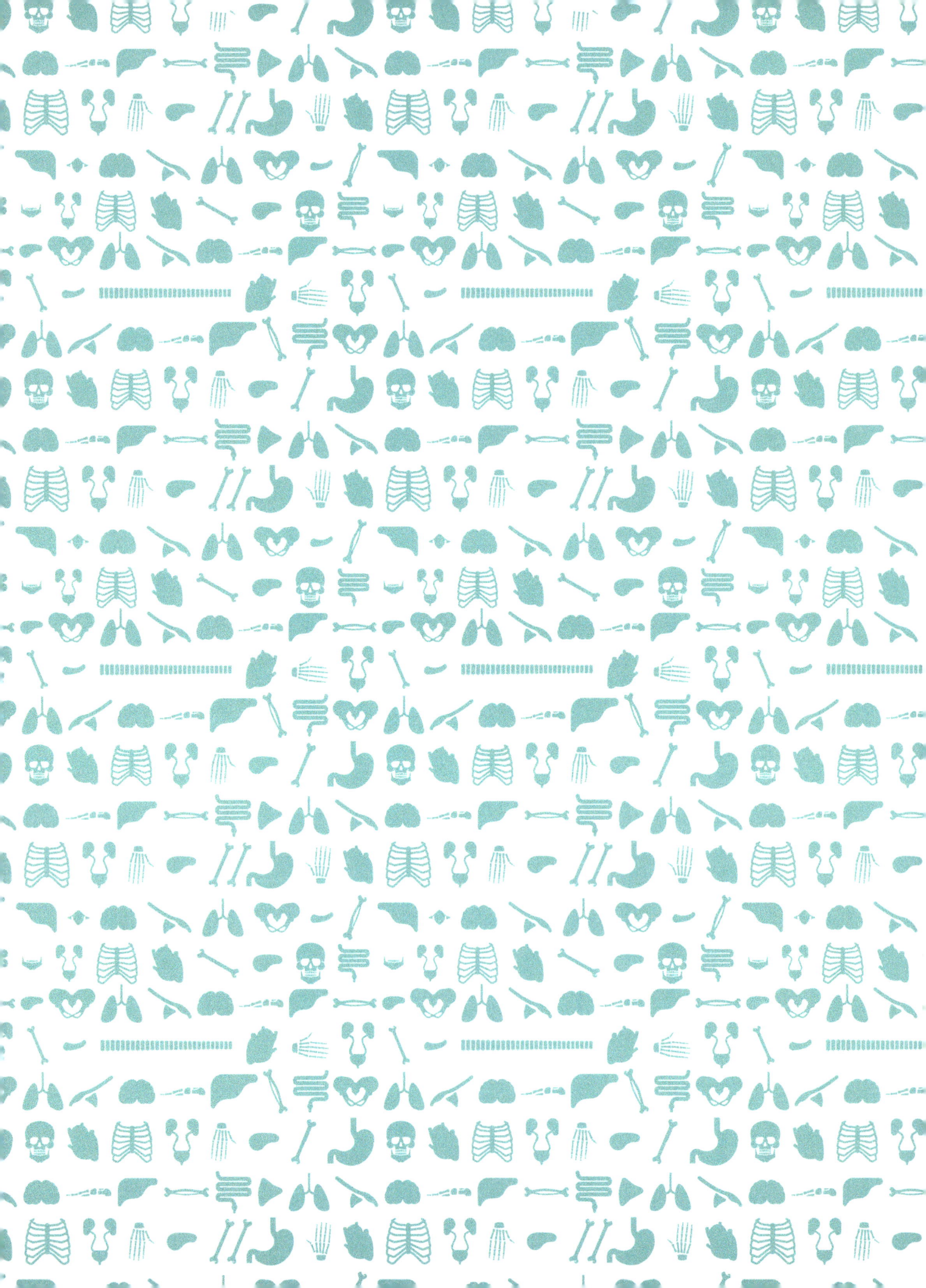

SENSORY: TASTE

Instructions

Taste buds are located primarily on the tongue. The adult human tongue contains between 2,000 and 8,000 taste buds, each of which are made up of 50 to 150 taste receptor cells, which are responsible for reporting the sense of taste to the brain. Taste buds can detect five major tastes, include bitter, sweet, salty, sour and savory. While traditionally it was believed that certain areas of the tongue ONLY detected certain tastes, recent evidence indicates that all areas of the tongue can detect all flavors, just some areas may detect certain flavors easier. Provide the child with five examples of the five different flavors. Examples of these include coffee, sugar, salt, lemon juice and brown gravy, but these can be substituted due to preference or dietary needs. Have the child taste each item individually and using the crayons indicate where on the tongue they most "tasted" that particular flavor. Have them wash their mouth out between tastes with water and repeat with other flavors. Once completed, look at the colored tongue map and see where they "tasted" certain flavors more.

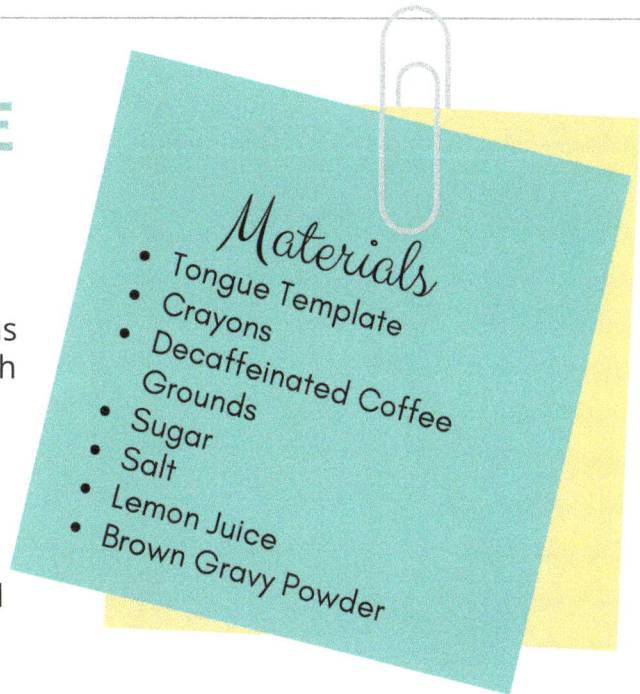

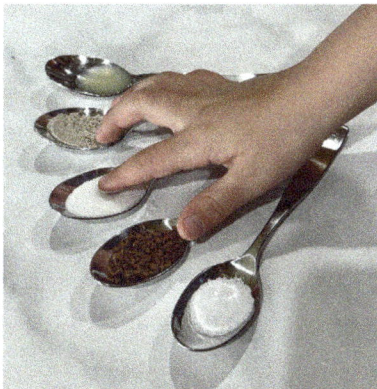

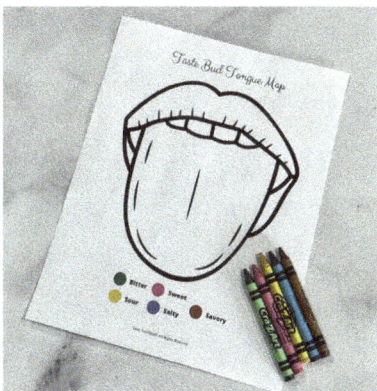

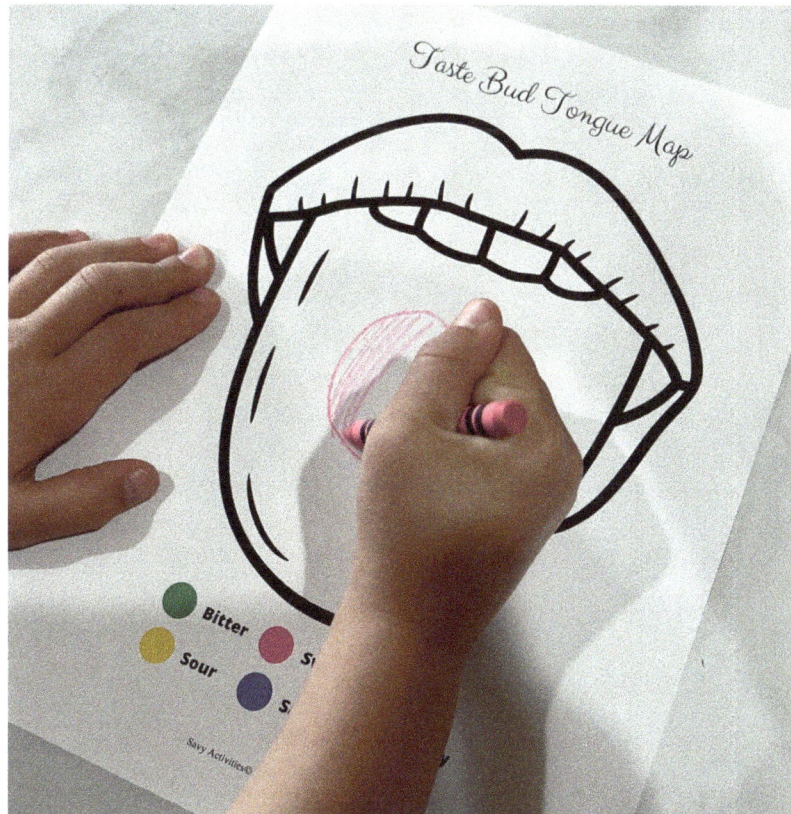

Materials

- Tongue Template
- Crayons
- Decaffeinated Coffee Grounds
- Sugar
- Salt
- Lemon Juice
- Brown Gravy Powder

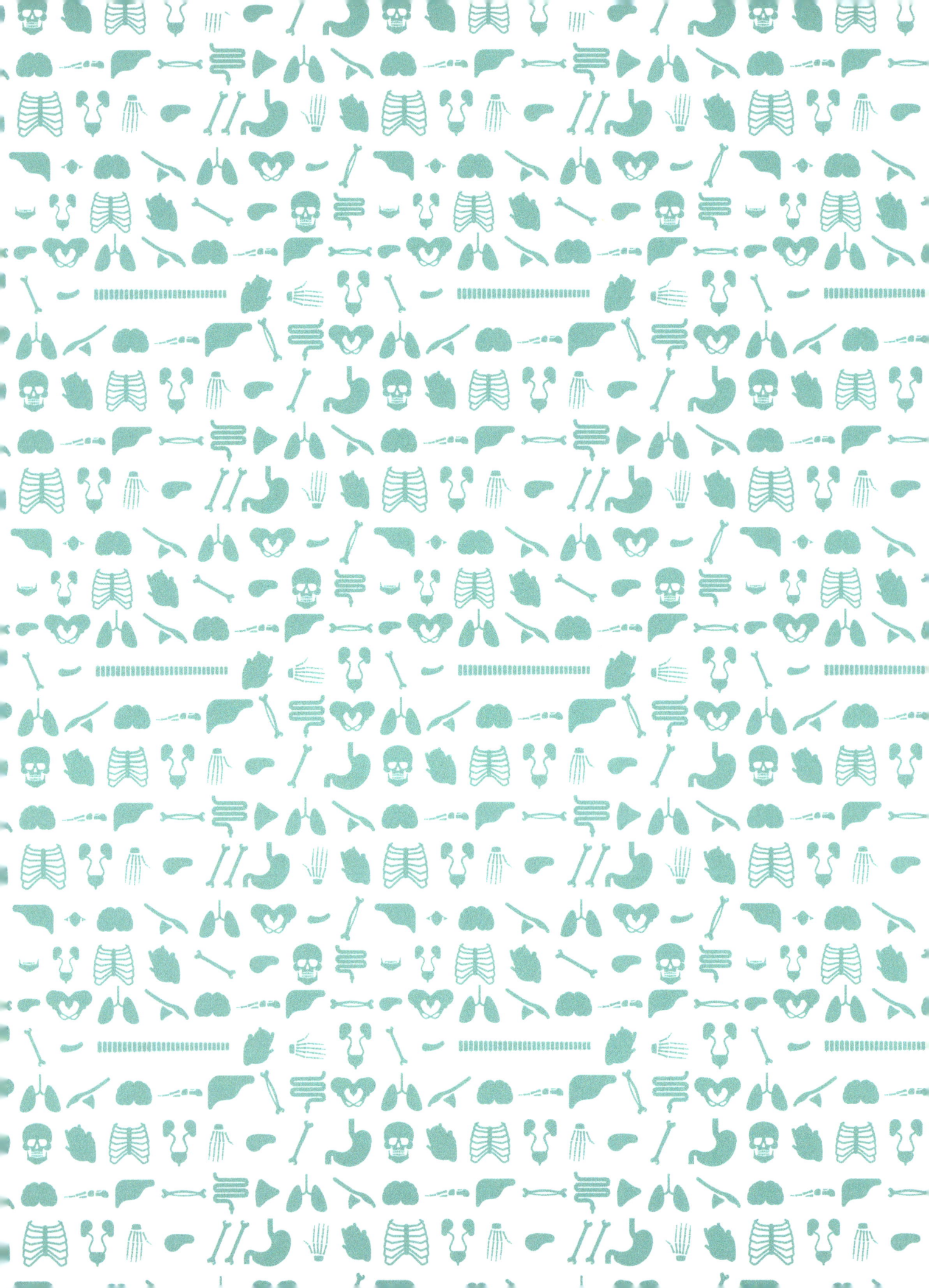

Taste Bud Tongue Map

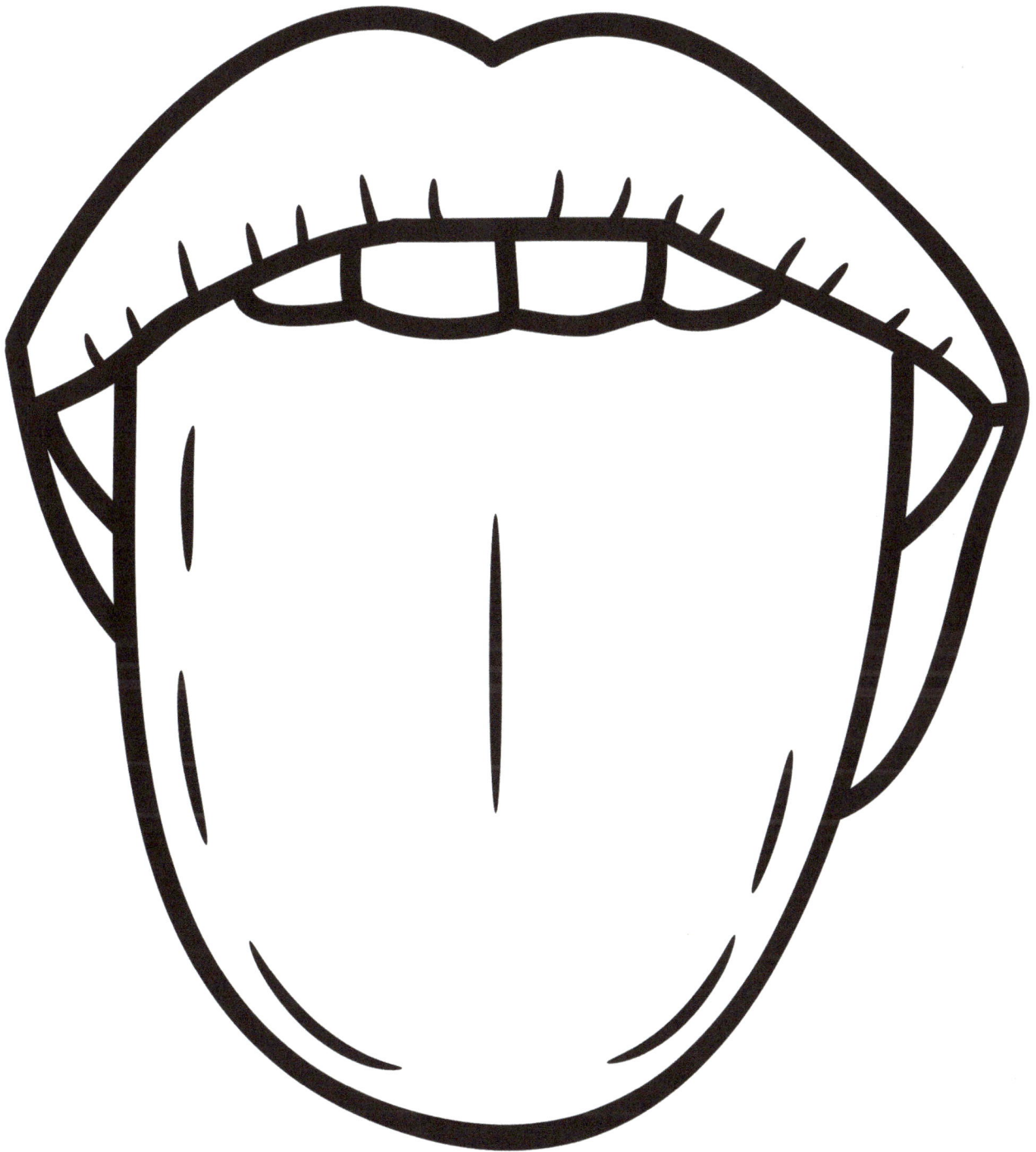

🟢 **Bitter**   🩷 **Sweet**

🟡 **Sour**   🔵 **Salty**   🟤 **Savory**

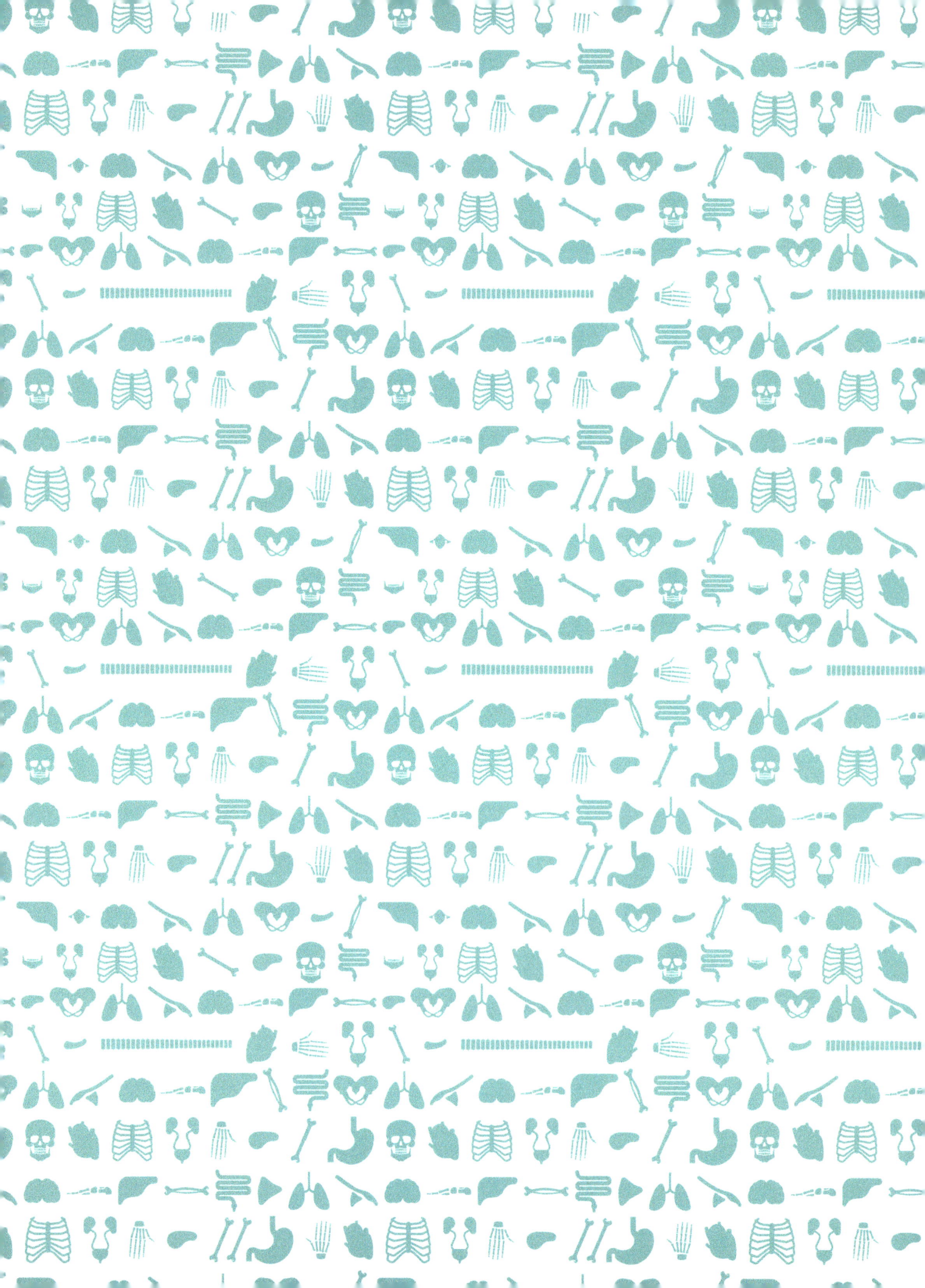

SENSORY: SMELL

Instructions

The sense of smell is a chemical sense and is identified in specialized sensory cells, called olfactory sensory neurons, which are found in a small patch of tissue high inside the nose. These cells connect directly to
the brain through the nervous system.

Materials

- 8-10 Small Containers
- Cotton Balls
- 4-5 Scented Oils
- Colored Stickers

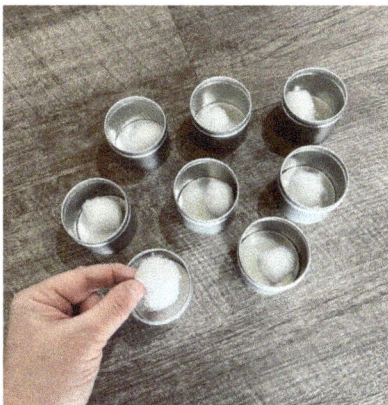

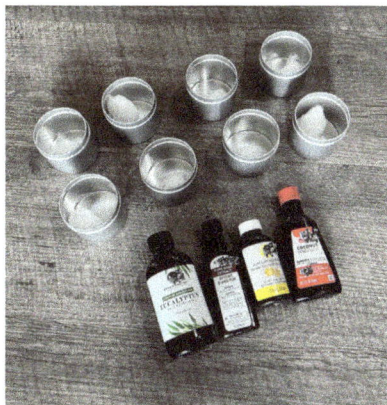

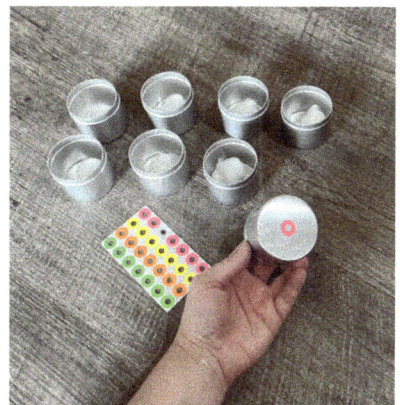

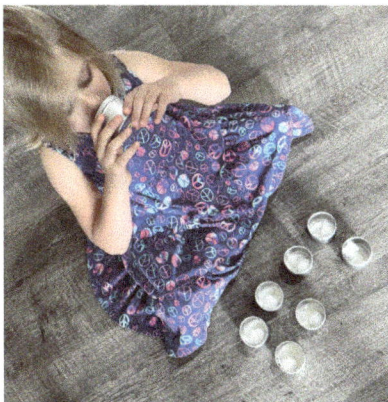

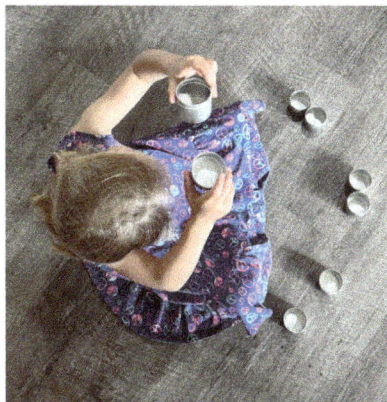

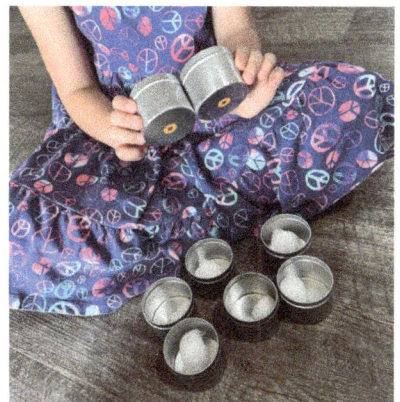

Provide the child with 8-10 small containers. Place a cotton ball inside each and add a few drops of an essential oil or cooking flavoring on two of the containers. Make sure it's saturated enough to be easily detected. Place stickers on the bottom of the containers to indicate which pairs contain the same scent. Repeat with 3-4 additional pairs of scents.

Have the child smell each container identify which scents are the same, based ONLY on the smell. Have them double check their guesses based on the colored stickers on the bottom of the containers. What scents were easiest to guess? Hardest?

SENSORY: HEARING

Instructions

Hearing is a mechanical sense. It turns physical movement into the electrical signals that make up the language of the brain, translating these vibrations into the experience of sound.

Activity #1 - Blindfold a child and place a sound source (ticking clock, electronic music, etc.) nearby the child. Can they identify where the sound is coming from?

Activity #1.2 - Place an ear plug in one of the child's ear - be careful to not injure the delicate ear canal. Again, place the blindfold and see if they can identify where the sound is coming from? Move around the child and have them continue to guess. Is it harder or easier to identify the sound with one ear plugged? Humans use two important cues to help determine where a sound is coming from: (1) which ear the sound hits first (known as interaural time differences), and (2) how loud the sound is when it reaches each ear (known as interaural intensity differences). It is much harder to identify location of sound without the use of both ears.

Activity #2 - This activity works best with multiple persons. Whisper a sentence into the ear of one person. Have them repeat the sentence to the next person, and so on until it reaches the last person. Have them repeat out loud what they heard; how close was it to the original? Discuss how easy it is to misinterpret auditory communication. Has this ever happened to them in real life? What happened?

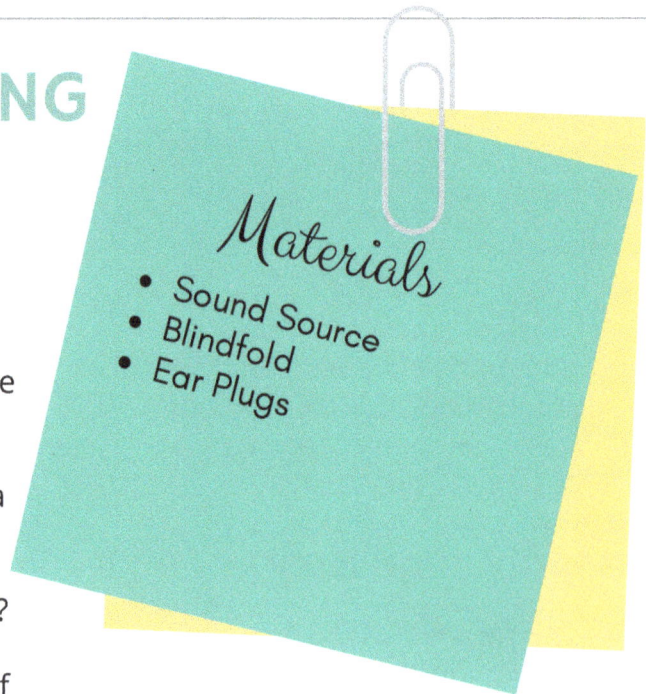

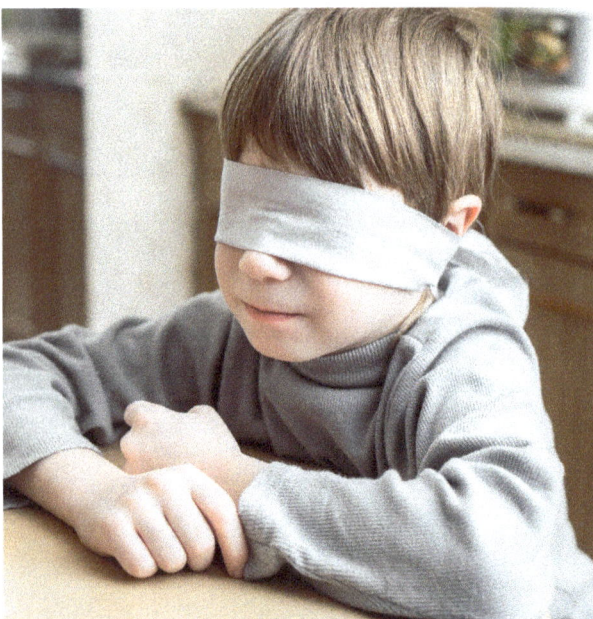

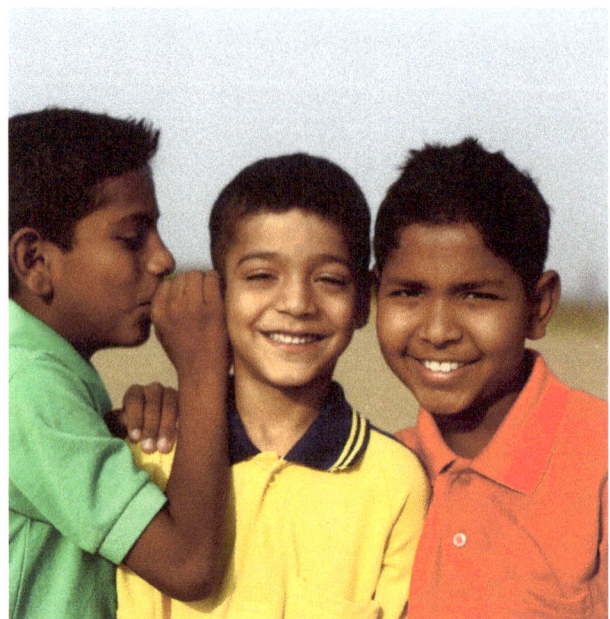

SENSORY: TOUCH

Instructions

The sense of touch consists of several distinct sensations communicated to the brain through specialized neurons in the skin. Pressure, temperature, light touch, vibration, pain and other sensations are all part of the touch sense and are all attributed to different receptors in the skin.

Fill a soft bag with 10-15 small objects. Consider items that have different sizes, shapes, textures, etc. They should be safe items that a child cannot hurt themselves on if manipulated. Have the child place their hand into the bag and locate one of the objects. Have them try to guess what the object is based solely on their sense of touch. What do they think it is? Have them remove ONLY that object from the bag. Are they correct? Repeat with the remaining objects. Keep track if desired on what they correctly identified. What items were harder to recognize? What were easiest? Why?

Materials
- Soft Bag
- 10-15 Objects (Varying size, shape, texture, etc.)

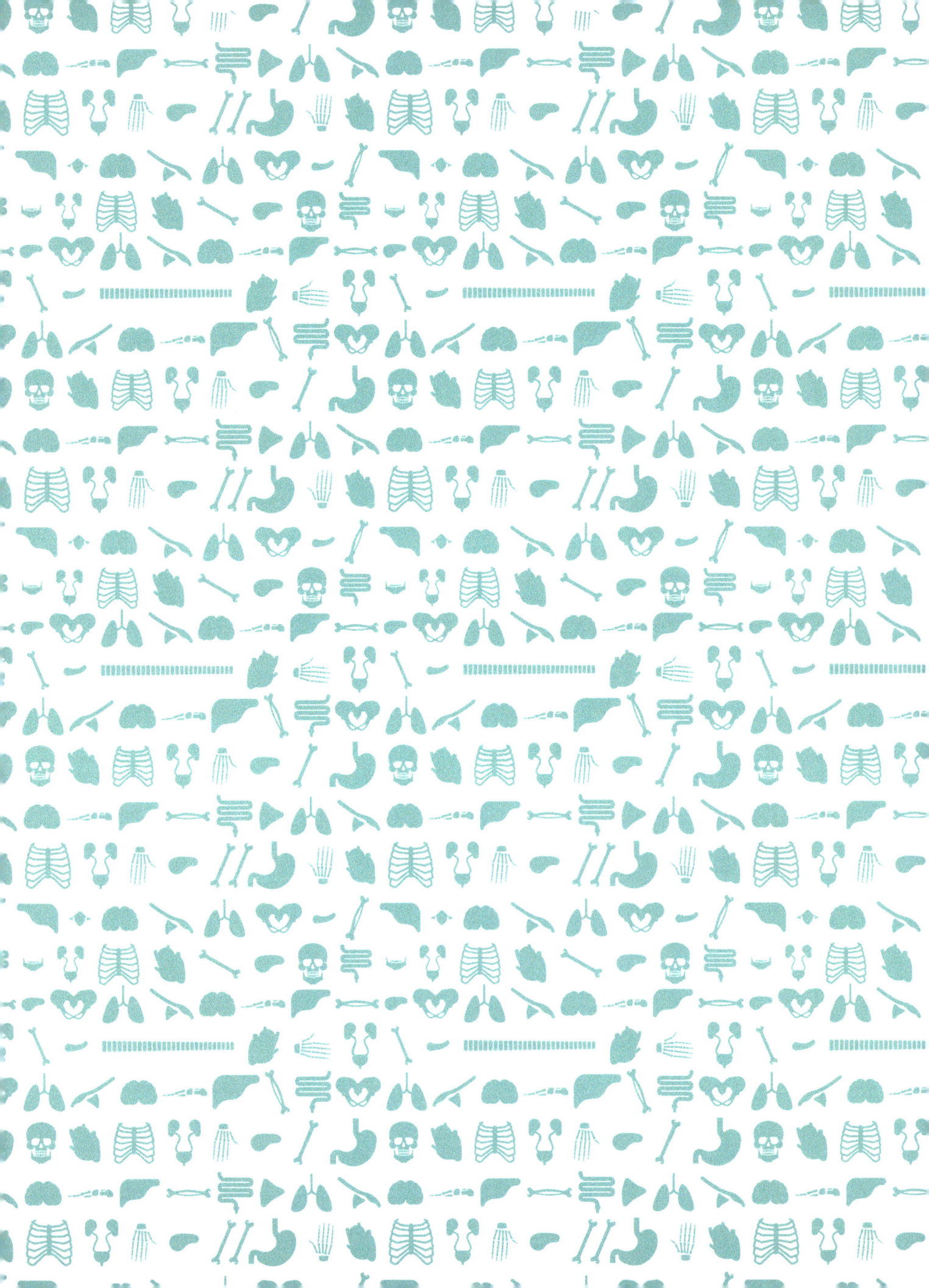

Anatomy Art Study

The
Vitruvian
Man

by Leonardo da Vinci
c. 1492

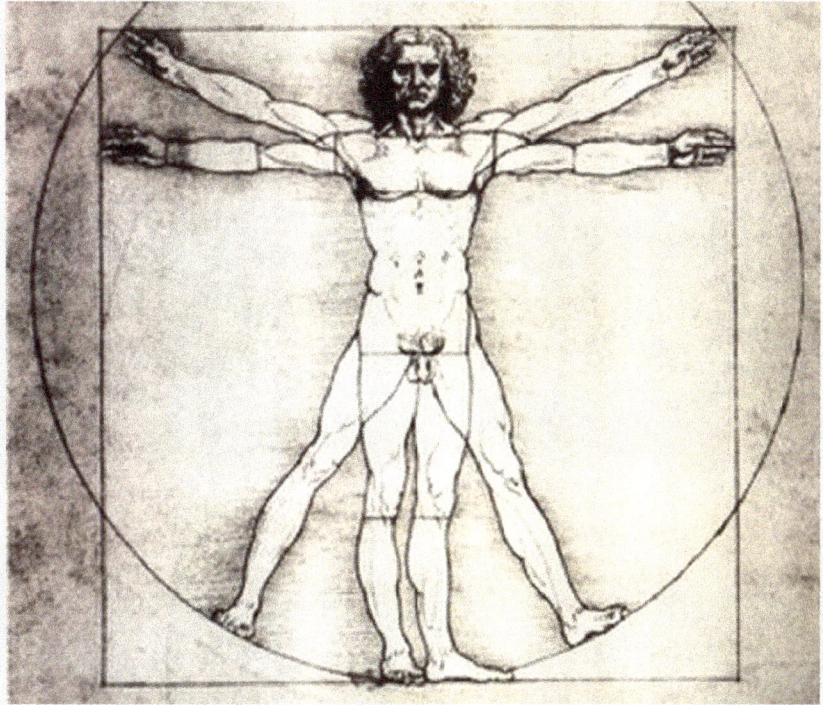

Libyan Sibyl

by Michelangelo di Lodovico Buonarroti Simoni
c. 1511

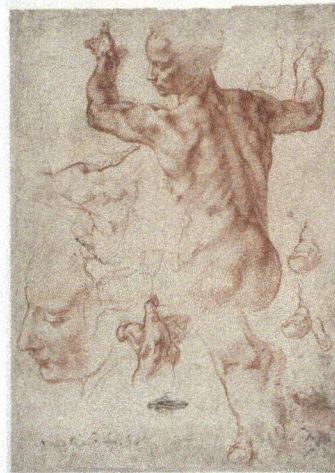

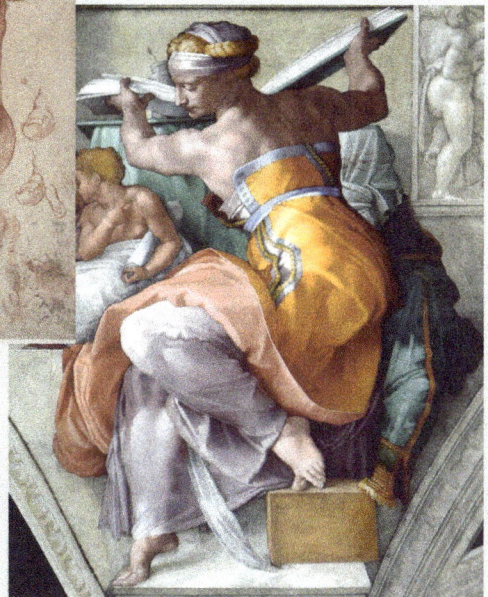

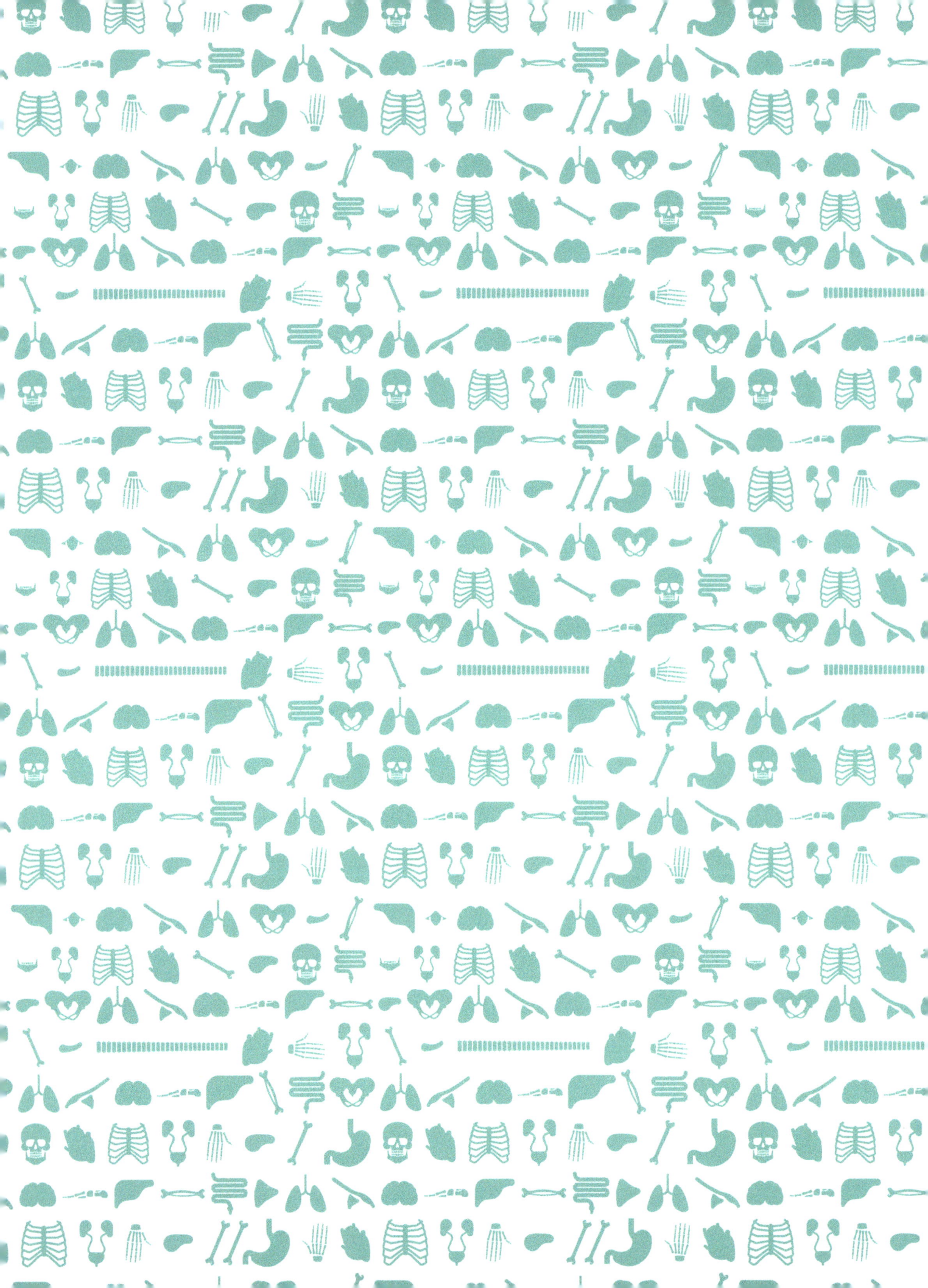

Anatomy Art Study

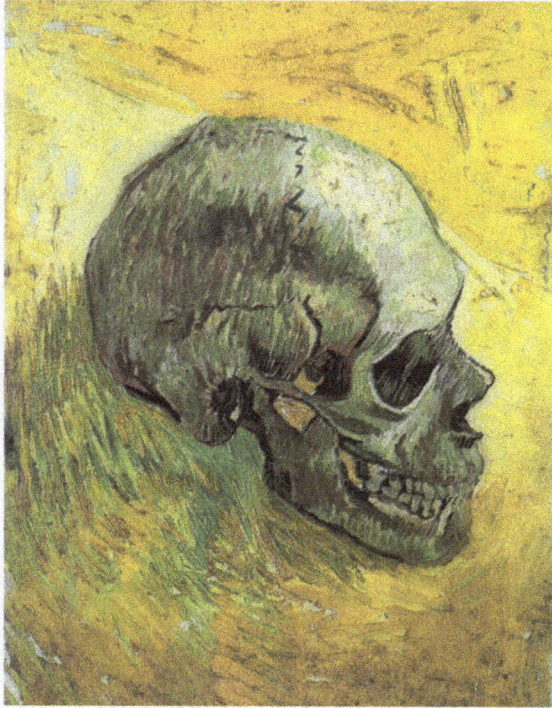

Skull

by Vincent Van Gogh
c. 1888

Las Dos Fridas

by Frida Kahlo
c. 1939

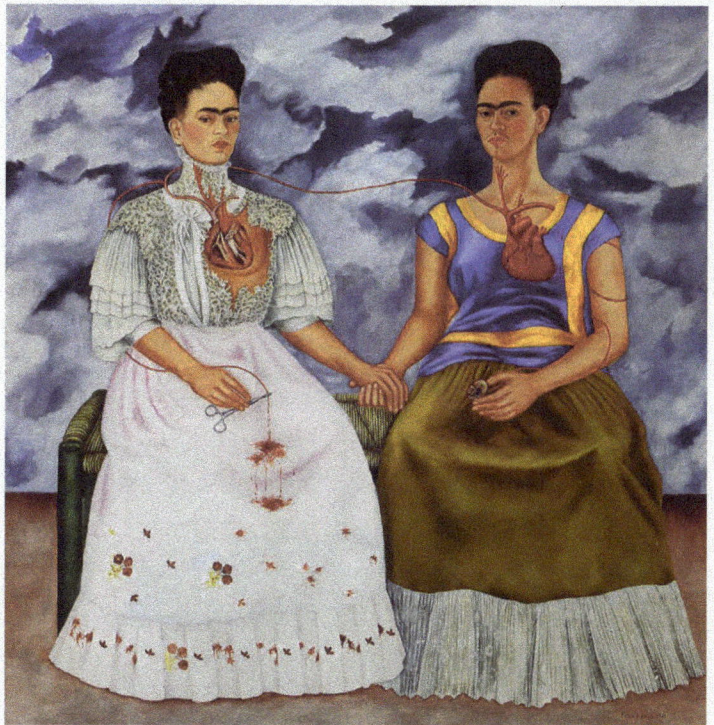

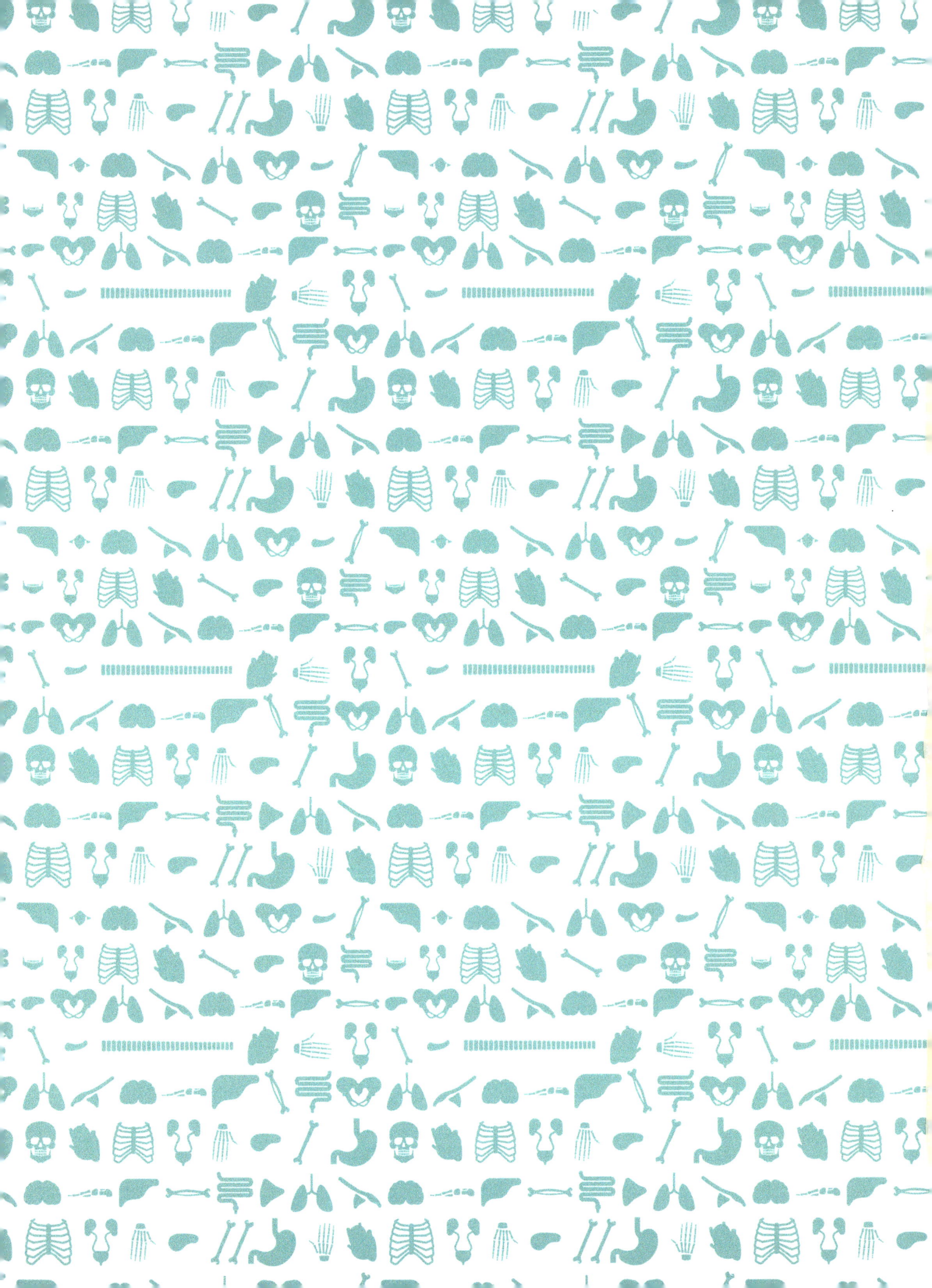

Savy Activities

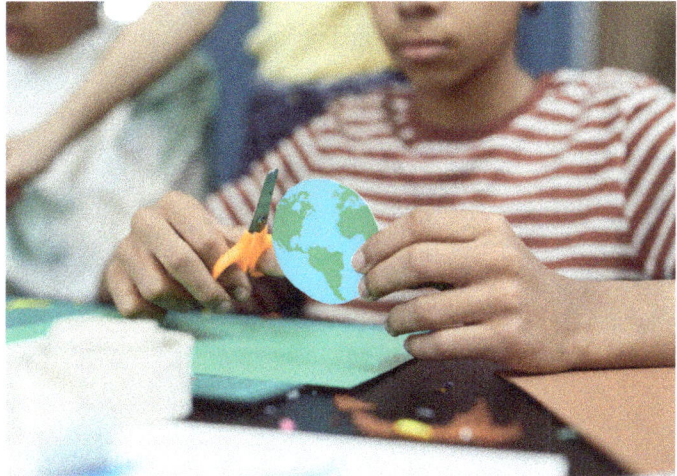

Travel the world through the interactive learning activities of **Savy Activities**; these hands-on resources provide parents, caregivers and educators practical ways to teach children about the world around them. Each book features a country, location or time period where subjects such as geography, history, vocabulary, reading, language, science, mathematics, music and art come alive by engaging auditory, visual and kinesthetic learning styles.

All activity books include geography with applicable maps, landmarks and locations. Historical events and time periods are visually represented with full color posters and flashcards, if applicable. Each book includes a set of fun-fact cards, poster and flag, if applicable. Paper models allow children to create 3D creations of major landmarks and structures. All books include a life cycle and anatomy of a plant, animal or organic compound, with flashcards and 3-part cards featuring important structures applicable to the theme.

Children learn scientific principles through active experiments and activities. Traditional customs, festivals, toys, clothing and art are also explored. Each book includes an exclusive themed mini-story featuring historical events or traditional mythology and folklore to promote vocabulary and reading. Where applicable, world languages are introduced through engaging flashcards, posters and tracing work. Each country has been meticulously researched by interviewing native persons and/or personal travel experiences to ensure the authentic culture is fully explored.

Savy Activities utilizes concepts from multiple educational methods to create unique resources allowing children a tangible and enjoyable way to explore their world. The **Savy Activities** series should not be viewed as a curriculum, but rather complimentary thematic resources to enhance traditional education. Because the individual needs and knowledge of children varies within standardized grade levels, **Savy Activities** resources have the flexibility to be used with preschool learners through early to mid-elementary years. For younger learners, adult supervision and/or assistance may be needed and activities presented in a simplified version. For older learners, resources may be paired with additional content from other materials to meet learning outcomes.

Check out our other products and resources at **www.SavyActivities.com**

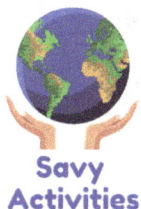

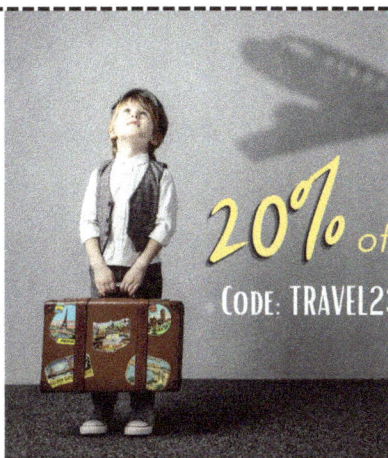

www.ingramcontent.com/pod-product-compliance
Lightning Source LLC
Chambersburg PA
CBHW061220270326
41926CB00032B/4787